Healing
and
History

Prefatory Note

This book has had a saddening history. It was planned early in 1977 as a festschrift, a volume to be written and published quietly, then presented to George Rosen at his retirement in the spring of 1978. With George's sudden death in the summer of 1977, the project became, unexpectedly and tragically, a memorial volume instead of the festive commemoration of a long and distinguished career.

I would particularly like to thank Dr. Beate Rosen who helped throughout the project and especially in the choice of authors; we had hoped to assemble a group of contributors who represented both the range of George's intellectual interests and his equally varied range of personal friends. I would also like to thank Neale Watson, the publisher of this volume, and Gerald Lombardi, its editor, for an extraordinary mixture of graciousness and professionalism. Their help was consistent and indispensable. The authors, of course, have all found time in busy schedules to contribute in memory of a friend and teacher.

Charles E. Rosenberg
June 3, 1978

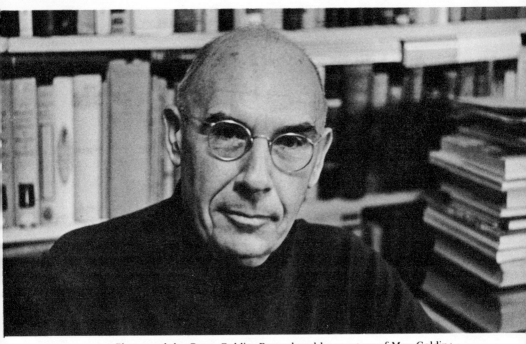

Photograph by Grace Goldin. Reproduced by courtesy of Mrs. Goldin.

Healing
and History

Essays for George Rosen

EDITED BY CHARLES E. ROSENBERG

Dawson

Science History Publications

1979

First published in the United States of America
by Science History Publications/USA *a division of*
Neale Watson Academic Publications, Inc.
156 Fifth Avenue, New York 10010

© 1979 Neale Watson Academic Publications, Inc.
(CIP DATA on final Page.)

Published in Great Britain
by Wm. Dawson & Sons, Ltd.
Cannon House Folkestone,
Kent, England
ISBN 0-7129-0927-3

Designed and manufactured in the USA.

Contents

George Rosen

and the

Social History of Medicine

CHARLES E. ROSENBERG

In some ways it is difficult to define George Rosen's place in the history of medicine; his work illuminated so many subjects, touched on so many countries and every century from the Renaissance to the present. One is continually amazed at his energy and fertility of imagination, at the nine books and more than 200 articles which he wrote in four decades of scholarship.[1] Yet, George Rosen's contribution to the history of medicine can be explained without difficulty, for a central theme unifies his extraordinarily diverse writings.

George Rosen was not simply an historian of public health or of social medicine—all medicine was social medicine to him. There was no aspect of the healing art from the definition of disease categories to the development of specialism that did not reflect social and economic, demographic and attitudinal factors. The labelling of witches, the nineteenth century's broadening conceptions of insanity were as much a product of intersecting social forces as the diseases which afflicted sixteenth-century miners or the rickets which crippled children in Europe's new industrial cities.[2] Not surprisingly, George Rosen's work has never seemed more relevant than it does in the 1970s as a growing number of social historians and critical laymen turn toward the history of medicine and health.

In some ways, indeed, this general shift of interest has made it easy to forget how original George Rosen was, how much he anticipated interests which seem timely and innovative in the 1970s. But in the three decades between the mid-1930s and the mid-1960s, his scholarly interests were still atypical among medical historians, while general historians were little concerned with the history of medicine. Through the 1950s the ultimate reality of medicine was to most of its chroniclers—for the most part, practicing physicians themselves—a logically integrated structure of ideas and techniques. It was a structure shaped by an inexorable and laudable accretion of scientific insight; it was a structure inevitably

1

beneficial to man in its accumulation of skill and understanding.

Needless to say, this was a political as well as a sociological posi-tion—though most of its advocates would hardly have understood it as being either. In the past century, the claims of medicine to auton-omy have increasingly rested on its claims to a scientific identity—and to the interest free and inevitably beneficial implications of that view of the profession. Certainly, no historian of medicine would deny that practice was often less than ideal in the past, or that many practitioners were unworthy of the status implied by their scientific identity. But the moral compromises and intellectual inadequacies of individual priests have never compromised the Church's view of its ultimate spiritual meaning; there was a similar awkward asymmetry between medicine as a body of knowledge and ethical truths and the day-to-day transactions of many of its practitioners. Had not modern medicine increased the length of man's life and made those surviving years increasingly free from pain and discomfort? The widespread scepticism of the 1970s toward the reality and moral impact of such putative achievments hardly existed when George Rosen began to study the history of medi-cine. And in many ways, indeed, Rosen shared the optimism implicit in this pervasive faith in medicine as inevitably progressive; but Rosen also assumed that medicine's humanitarian potential could only be reached through careful and intelligent analysis of medicine's place in society. Perhaps, indeed, that society itself would have to alter before medicine could assume a different aspect. For George Rosen and like-thinking critics realized how wide the gap was between knowledge and its applications, how sensitively medicine mirrored social values and the forms of economic power. He could not share the vision of a medicine unsullied by the realities of class interest, of social prejudice, of economic constraint.

In removing medicine from a largely intellectualistic and neces-sarily benevolent framework, Rosen helped bring it not only into the marketplace of social interactions, but into culture construed in its broadest terms. He consistently emphasized how both medicine's in-tellectual life and its institutional realities reflected extrinsic factors, intellectual, economic, and social. He suggested, for example, that mercantilist ideas shaped both medical theory and health policy in the eighteenth century—in some ways, indeed, they were inextricable.[3] He emphasized, in parallel fashion, the role of certain Enlightenment conceptions of epistemology in helping create the necessary precondi-tions for the achievements of French medicine in the early nineteenth century.[4] Rosen saw the line between social ideology and scientific inquiry as a subtle and shifting one as he examined the classical texts of medicine and social policy. Medicine was always a pervasive social function to George Rosen, not a neatly ordered structure of ideas and techniques; it was a reflection of society's total being, not a cool and distant intellectual activity.

But perhaps it should be no surprise that a poor Jewish boy who came of age in New York City in the late 1920s and early 1930s and was then denied admittance to an American medical school should have failed to appreciate such medical claims to transcendent legitimacy. And in a climate of bitter social criticism—both in New York and Berlin where Rosen studied medicine and began his work in medical history—it is only natural that he might have seen the development of medicine as a continuing interaction of the healing arts with the society which nurtured them. Of course, Rosen was not alone in adopting this broadly cultural—and necessarily relativist—view of medicine. In the United States, for example, Richard Shryock, a scholar from a backround very different from that of Rosen, pioneered at almost the same time in writing a history of medicine incorporating social and cultural factors. In Germany, even more influentially, such historians as Henry Sigerist, Owsei Temkin, Erwin Ackerknecht, and Walter Pagel all sought in their diverse ways to relate medical ideas to the culture in which they were elaborated. Even Pagel, of this group the most consistently oriented toward the internal texture of ideas, saw medical and biological ideas as parts of a more general world-view. In elucidating the influence of philosophical and religious ideas in the works of van Helmont, Paracelsus, and Harvey, Pagel emphasized the interpenetration of ideas between realms which previous generations of biomedical historians had preferred to maintain as separate; the landmarks of science were not to be confused with the crabbed theology and archaic cosmologies which encrusted them.[5] Let me cite another example: Owsei Temkin's first article, on the social context in which syphilis was perceived and treated, provides another illustration of how young scholars of Rosen's generation brought problems conventionally medical into the sphere of culture generally.[6] Nurtured in the intellectual atmosphere of Weimar Germany, Henry Sigerist's explicit political commitments are too well-known to demand comment. A sense of social concern and a view of medicine as cultural artifact were fundamental to the work undertaken at Sigerist's Leipzig Institute; it was entirely consistent with the social attitudes and intellectual predispositions of the young George Rosen who returned from Berlin to practice medicine during America's worst depression.

George Rosen also soon undertook another line of inquiry, one particularly significant in historiographical retrospect. This was his deployment of social science literature and perspectives in shaping an understanding of past medicine. As early as the 1940s, Rosen turned to academic sociology and wrote what is in some ways his most influential study—on the origins of specialism—as a doctoral dissertation in Columbia University's department of sociology.[7] Rosen had found a prestigious, putatively scientific, and unavoidably relativist point-of-view from which to interpret the role of medicine in society and of science in medicine.

Many of Rosen's themes have, as we have suggested, become the commonplaces of contemporary social criticism. When critics of psychiatry see its diagnostic categories as socially determined labels for deviance, not absolute and scientifically grounded truths; when the women's movement proclaims medical thought as one ideological prop for male dominance; when sceptics cite the data and authority of sociology and anthropology to demythologize medicine's claims to interest free benevolence; when economically oriented critics of the profession insist that medicine must be seen as at least in part a marketplace phenomenon they are all elaborating themes implicit or explicit in the work of those context conscious students of medical history who came of age in the 1920s and 1930s. As increasing numbers of younger historians turn to the social history of medicine, they will discover a long and sophisticated concern with medicine as a social institution. In this tradition, no name looms more prominently than that of George Rosen.

Notes

1. For a complete bibliography of Rosen's books, articles, and translations, see below, p. 252.

2. Most of Rosen's conclusions on the place of mental illness in society are to be found in his *Madness in Society. Chapters in the Historical Sociology of Mental Illness* (Chicago: University of Chicago, 1968). The mention of miners' ailments refers to Rosen's *The History of Miners' Diseases. A Medical and Social Interpretation* (New York: Schuman's, 1943).

3. "Cameralism and the Concept of Medical Police," *Bull. Hist. Med.*, 27 (1952), pp. 21–42.

4. "The Philosophy of Ideology and the Emergence of Modern Medicine in France,"

ibid, 20 (1946), pp. 328–339. Much, of course, has since been written on this subject. See, Erwin Ackerknecht, *Medicine at the Paris Hospital, 1794–1848* (Baltimore: The Johns Hopkins University, 1967).

5. In citing Pagel's work, I have deliberately chosen a historian who might seem, at first glance, to have little in common with Rosen's approach in the hope of emphasizing this area of overlap. See Walter Pagel, *The Religious and Philosophical Aspects of van Helmont's Science and Medicine.* Supplements to the Bulletin of the History of Medicine No. 2 (Baltimore: The Johns Hopkins University, 1944); *Paracelsus. An Introduction to Philosophical Medicine in the Era of the Renaissance* (Basel and New York: S. Karger, 1958); *William Harvey's Biological Ideas* (Basel and New York: S. Karger, 1967).

6. Temkin's important essay *"Zur Geschichte von Moral und Syphilis,"* which appeared originally in *Sudhoff's Archiv* (*19* (1927), pp. 331–348) has been translated by C. Lillian Temkin, and appears in Owsei Temkin's *The Double Face of Janus and other Essays in the History of Medicine* (Baltimore and London: The Johns Hopkins University, 1977), pp. 472–484. The title essay is autobiographical and pages 3–12 provide a number of significant recollections of Sigerist and the Leipzig years.

7. *The Specialization of Medicine with Special Reference to Opthamology* (New York: Froben Press, 1944, reprinted: New York: Arno Press, 1972). Erwin Ackerknecht's influential work in medicine and ethnology undertaken in the late 1930s and 1940s provides a significant parallel to Rosen's work in sociology; both, however, were atypical in their formal commitment to the social sciences.

Medical Ethics and Honoraria
in Late Antiquity

OWSEI TEMKIN

George Rosen's work on *Fees and Fee Bills* has shed much light on the economic reality of medical practice in the United States.[1] What he did for the nineteenth century can, unfortunately, not be done for all other periods and certainly not for late Antiquity, the span of Western history from about the end of the second century to the end of the sixth. Indeed, the little we know about the actual amounts paid as medical fees is mainly anecdotal and will not be our theme here.

Late Antiquity was a period of profound change in political and economic structure, as well as in religious and moral outlook. This change, which prepared the ground for feudal European society and marked the victory of Christianity over paganism, also affected medicine and the relationship between physician and patient expressed in the attitude toward the remuneration for medical services. We shall approach our exploration of this change in attitude by first analyzing a well-known law issued by Emperor Valentinian I in A.D. 368.[2] Then we shall consider some early medieval Latin testimonies dating from the sixth to the tenth centuries, yet in many cases reaching back to earlier compositions.

The imperial law reads:

> There should be appointed as many archiaters as there are regions in the city [i.e., Rome], except those of the portus Xysti and of the vestal virgins. Having in mind that salaries in the form of supplies are furnished them from the provisions for public services, they had better choose to dedicate themselves honestly to the poor than shamefully to serve the rich. Furthermore, we permit them to accept what the healthy present to them for their dedication, not what those in peril of death promise for being saved. If a fatal disease or some chance has removed one from the number of archiaters, another should be put in his place: not by patronage of the very powerful, not by the favor of one examiner, but by the faithful and circumspect choice of all of them. And he should be one who is deemed worthy of their fellowship, of the dignity of the archiatral rank, and of our approval. His name will have to be reported to us forthwith.

To avoid misunderstandings, "the poor" of the translation must not simply be identified with the indigent. The Latin term *(tenuiores)* used here, just as the Greek word for poor *(penēs)*, was broader. It included people of small means, such as craftsmen, who had to work for a living, not merely the dependent.[3] Many of the poor were, therefore, able to show their appreciation for what the archiater had done for them.

The law is a piece of social legislation, providing for an archiater in each of the regions of Rome, except two which probably had their own physicians. Together, these archiaters formed a college, as is evident from the rules of election of new members, as well as from a supplementary law in which Valentinian regulated the rank and salary of an archiater who was to be promoted when a member died or dropped out for some other reason.[4] We have no information about the duties the office involved, nor do we know whether the law founded or merely reorganized archiaters in Rome;[5] other cities had long had public physicians.

Election to the college of archiaters bestowed compensation (in natural products, as was usual at the time) and prestige, of which a new candidate had to be worthy. It may, therefore, be assumed that its members enjoyed the immunity from taxation, military service, billeting, and burdensome civic obligations which the Roman emperors since Vespasian had granted to physicians. The Emperor Antoninus Pius (138–161) had fixed the number of physicians on whom immunities were bestowed in accordance with the size of the city that granted them.[6]

Valentinian's law guarded the college against individual arbitrariness and the patronage of "the very powerful," which was in line with the character of an emperor said to have "hated the well dressed, the learned, the rich, and the high-born."[7] Also in line with it were his appeal for dutiful behavior by the archiaters and the stipulation that they might accept only what patients offered them for their *dedication* after they had been cured.[8] But, as I shall try to show, appeal and regulation are substantially part of an ethical tradition that had been formed long before.

The so-called Hippocratic collection, i.e., the medical writings attributed to Hippocrates, though the work of many authors between the fifth century B.C. and the first century A.D., contains a number of deontological texts, of which the famous *Oath, Decorum,* and *Precepts* are the most important in our context. Though not unmindful of the physician's reward,[9] the author of *Precepts* warns against discussing fees at the outset, for the sick will think that the physician may leave him or neglect the treatment if he does not agree. Such worries would affect the patient adversely, especially if the disease were acute. The good physician will think of his reputation rather than of what is due to him: "It is better to upbraid those who have been saved than to shorten [the life of] those in danger of death."[10]

On the principle that what is frowned upon must have existed, it can be inferred that some physicians did mention the fee when called. Indeed, probably not much later than *Precepts* was composed, the older Pliny (died A.D. 70) castigated the physicians of Rome in these words: "Let me not even bring charges against their avarice, *their greedy bargains made with those whose fate lies in the balance,* the prices charged for anodynes, the earnest-money paid for death. . . . The result is that the brightest side of the picture is the vast number of marauders; for it is not shame but the competition of rivals that brings down fees."[11] Pliny may have scorned the haggling rather than the mentioning of a fee. The late law of the Visigoths, in the portions designated as old *(antiqua),* speaks of agreements entered upon as soon as a wound has been seen by the physician or an illness diagnosed. The agreements legally guaranteed payment of the fee, which was forfeited if the patient died.[12]

Precepts opposed raising the question of a fee at the outset, but it expected the patient to pay; otherwise the physician would upbraid him after a successful cure. As a general rule, physicians all through Antiquity expected to be paid and usually were paid. Seneca, whom we shall discuss later, mentioned the physician's fee as a matter of course,[13] and legal documents discussed whether expenses for medical care could be charged to a partnership, and similar problems.[14] Whether remuneration under such conditions and expectations constituted a fee or an honorarium is a question I must leave to experts in Roman law to decide.[15] At any rate, the remuneration of the archiaters in Rome constituted a true honorarium, for as a gift in appreciation of such dedication as had been shown, it might be accepted but not demanded. Acceptance of an honorarium was a concession to these salaried physicians, limited further by the Hippocratic aversion to exacting fees from despairing patients.

Since the honorarium was voluntary, indigent patients presumably paid nothing, and if the others did not appreciate his services, the archiater might conceivably remain unremunerated.[16] Being salaried, he would not starve; but the idea of practicing without remuneration, though probably contrary to the common rule, was not completely unknown. Galen claimed never to have demanded a fee from a patient and often to have provided for their wants. As a man of independent means, living on the income from his patrimony, Galen could afford such generosity.[17] He did, moreover, accept gifts from grateful patients.[18] Galen himself would have cited philanthropy as a motive for his behavior. In his opinion,

> Some practice the medical art for the sake of making money, some because of the exemption from public services given to them by law, others for the sake of philanthropy, while others do so because of the glory or reputation accruing therefrom. In their quality of producers of health, they have the common appellation of physician. But in as far as their activities serve different purposes, one is called philanthropic, another ambitious of repute, another ambitious of glory, and still another a man of business. For physicians as such, the goal does not lie in honor or in profit, as Menodotus the Empiricist wrote; such was his, Menodotus's goal, but not that of Diocles, nor of Hippocrates and Empedocles, nor of quite a number of other ancients, who treated men for philanthropy's sake.[19]

Hippocrates was Galen's model of philanthropy, and his name meant not only the author of Hippocratic books, but also the hero of the legend that had begun to form around him in Hellenistic times.[20] By the end of the second century, this legend had found its documentation in fictitious correspondence and decrees, in biographies where truth is hard to separate from myth, and in various authors, notably Galen himself. The Hippocrates of the legend showed a deep contempt for money. In a letter to a famous rhizotome (a herbalist, literally a "roots cutter"), he exclaims: "Oh that you, Crateuas, could cut out the bitter root of the love of money, so that no remnant of it showed forth! Know that we would purge the sick souls of men together with their bodies!"[21] Galen himself stated that instead of taking up permanent residence at the court of the king of Macedon, Hippocrates "treated the poor in Cranon, Thasos, and the other small cities."[22]

Since "the poor" (the reference probably is to patients mentioned in the Hippocratic *Epidemics*) included all those who had to work for a living, the remark need not mean more than that Hippocrates was content with a small fee. This, as well as Galen's own provision for patients in need, indicates that medical philanthropy, as conceived in

the second century, was not indifferent to the patient's circumstances.
It could go beyond the advice given in *Precepts:*

> Sometimes give your services for nothing, calling to mind a previous
> benefaction or present good will. And if there be an opportunity of
> serving one who is a stranger in financial traits, give full assistance to all
> such. For where there is love of man [*philanthropiē*], there is also love of
> the art [i.e, the patient will love the medical art].[23]

The inclusion in philanthropy of consideration for the needy
may seem obvious to us. But for ancient philanthropy, this was not
true.[24] It has been said that "broadly speaking, pity for the poor had
little place in the normal Greek character, and consequently for the
poor, as such, no provision usually existed; the idea of democracy
and equality was so strong that anything done must be done for all
alike; there was nothing corresponding to our mass of privately or-
ganised charities and hospitals."[25] For medicine, as we have just
seen, this statement is perhaps too sweeping; nevertheless, it is true
to the extent that consideration for the needy, although included in
philanthropy, was not its primary aim. Galen claimed never to have
demanded a fee from *any* patient; *Precepts* did not teach consideration
for the poor as such. According to the Hippocratic *Decorum,* "a physician who is a philosopher is god-like;" greediness and avarice had no
place where medicine was cultivated in a philosophical spirit.[26] This
sentiment corresponded to Galen's efforts to cultivate medicine in a
philosophical-scientific spirit, for he thought of himself as both philosopher and physician.

Several inscriptions from Greek cities, from the second and first
centuries B.C., praise public physicians for their devotion and, especially in times of disaster, for having served all alike, sometimes gratis and at personal expense. Thus we read that one Damiadas showed
"unlimited energy and devotion . . . in serving fairly all alike,
whether poor or rich, slaves or free or foreigners," and that "he
maintained a blameless reputation in all respects, providing proper
attendance, which was open to all, as befits a man of culture and
moral sense."[27]

What the inscriptions tell us as having actually been done by some
public physicians was idealistically elaborated by some authors of the
first century. In the preface to his little book on medical prescriptions,
the Roman, Scribonius Largus, wrote: "The very profession of medicine demands that the physician's mind be imbued with compassion

[*misericordiae*] and humaneness [*humanitatis*]; otherwise he is bound to be hated by gods and men. . . . Medicine does not value human beings for their fortune or standing, rather, by means of its remedies, it promises succor equally to all who ask for it, and it professes never to harm anybody."[28] The prohibition of poison for murder, suicide, and abortion in the Hippocratic *Oath* allowed Scribonius Largus to refer to this document, the first mention of the *Oath* known to us. For Scribonius Largus, Hippocrates was an educator of physicians toward humaneness. The *Oath* had been silent on the social and economic circumstances of the patients,[29] a silence that could easily be interpreted as "equality of all human beings"[30] but did not allow inferences to fees or honoraria. Scribonius Largus mentions compassion and humaneness, and we are free to believe that this included consideration of the needy.

The same is true of a poem by Sarapion, probably a contemporary of Plutarch (died *ca.* 120), that extols the physician's ethical duties: "Let him cure not only with (professional) skill but also with blameless character . . . like a savior god, let him make himself the equal of slaves and of paupers, of the rich and of rulers of men, and to all let him minister like a brother; for we are all children of the same blood. Therefore let him not hate any one nor hide envy in his heart, nor be lifted up with price."[31] The "savior god," of course, makes us think of Asclepius, who cured rich and poor equally and, as the Emperor Julian the Apostate (361–363) was to say, without hope of remuneration.[32]

To a man like Galen, the notion of philanthropy may thus have appeared incompatible with demanding fees, and lust for money with the exercise of medicine in a philosophical spirit. Whether Galen was actually motivated by benevolence, or displayed it as becoming to a philosopher, need not be decided here. *Precepts* had not appealed to a feeling of compassion, and the great orator Libanius, a contemporary of the Emperor Valentinian, gave a sober reason for behaving in a manner somewhat similar to Galen's. In a fictitious speech accusing an imaginary physician turned poisoner, Libanius depicted the ideal physician in words even more glowing than Sarapion's. The physician must cultivate philanthropy, answer a summons immediately, suffer with his patient, and rejoice with him when relieved. Depending on the patient's age, the physician must be brother, son, or father to him; he must do all he can and never rest in the exercise of his profession.[33] After having set forth what the physician should do and feel, the prosecutor continues:

The physician must deem these [precepts] to come to him from the [medical] art. They have been heeded, gentlemen, to our advantage, by all those physicians who, rather than striving for money, strive for the fame [derived] from having conquered disease. Indeed, I know many physicians who, instead of receiving [money], have themselves spent [money] for poor people. Reasonably so! For the art also affords them respect in the cities. And we look upon the most outstanding of them as if they were gods, believing that in them, next to the gods, lies our hope for deliverance.[34]

Here, at last, free treatment of the poor is positively stated. But it is interpreted as the physician's due to the city where he gains respect beyond the reputation of being an experienced craftsman.[35]

A similar kind of reasoning may also have guided Galen, who valued the reputation of medicine as a liberal art.[36] Medicine, Seneca had said, conveyed the benefits of health and life, benefits not to be measured by remuneration.[37] It might be demeaned by the exaction of a fee. Moreover, to the many conceivable motives actuating Galen, who was on familiar terms with members of the court, that of emulating the Roman gentleman barrister must be added. The fame and glory a barrister obtained for a successful plea in court, and which smoothed his way to high political office, were originally deemed a sufficient reward. Only reluctantly was compensation permitted, which, however, must not exceed 10,000 sesterces (a relatively modest sum) and could be given only after the matter had been closed; no fee might be given or promised before the proceedings in court. In form at least, the award was an honorarium, not a contractual fee.[38] The younger Pliny (a rich barrister and the nephew of the author of the *Natural History*) boasted of having "always refrained from making any bargain, or accepting any fee, reward, or so much as a friendly present." To this he added as a maxim: "One ought, no doubt, to avoid whatever is dishonorable [*inhonesta*], not so much because it is illegal, as because it is shameful [*pudenda*]".[39] This old ideal of the Roman gentleman may have influenced Galen, and it may still have echoed in Valentinian's law.

Inscriptions and authors like Sarapion and Libanius have given us an idealized picture of honest dedication. From other authors we can obtain an idea of what "shameful" service to the rich must have meant. Seneca raised the question why we remained under obligation to our physician and our teacher of the liberal arts. "Because," he answered, "from being physician and teacher they pass into friends, and we are under obligation to them, not because of their art, which they sell, but because of their kindly and friendly goodwill."[40] The personal devotion Seneca expected of his physician included that "though a host of others called for him, I was always his chief concern; that he took time for others only when my illness had permitted him."[41]

As one patient's friend (or, figuratively speaking, father, brother, or son), the physician could easily appear neglectful of other patients. This is all the more important because ancient dietetic medicine demanded intimate acquaintance with the patient in order to judge his condition. The physician was believed to be better able to deal with patients who were his friends than with others.[42] Highly educated and philosophically trained physicians were more likely to be friends of men like Seneca than of poor, uneducated citizens or slaves. But one-sided devotion became overtly shameful if it turned into servility to the rich, as is evident in Galen's criticism. When ill, the rich "summon those with whom they have been most familiar and who are also the greatest sycophants, who will give something cold when asked and, if urged, will permit bathing and snow and wine to those yearning for these things, and who will servilely do everything that is commanded, like men sold into slavery."[43] His own friends urged Galen to pay his respects to the rich and mighty in the morning and sup with them at night.[44] It is not necessary to insist on Galen's influence to realize that shameful servility in Valentinian's law suggested more than mere preference for treating rich people who could afford a large honorarium. Not the treatment of the rich as such was condemned, but the manner in which they were served while others were neglected.

Valentinian's law did not transcend the tradition of pagan medical ethics. It insisted on decent treatment for all, emphatically including "the humbler classes," for whom Valentinian (himself a tolerant Christian) showed much concern,[45] and it aimed at protecting them. Our information on the duties of ancient town physicians, Greek as well as Roman, is too scanty to permit us to say whether the law *intended* to socialize medicine in Rome, i.e., to provide free medical care for all inhabitants by salaried physicians, with honoraria being optional.[46] Before making such a claim, we ought at least to know whether archiaters could be consulted by any inhabitant, at any time, for any medical complaint. At the time of Valentinian, Rome numbered around 500,-000 people.[47] If the law refers to the traditional 14 regions of Rome, as is usually assumed,[48] and if we also assume an equal distribution of the population over the fourteen regions, every region would have counted approximately 35,000 inhabitants. One to thirty-five thousand would thus have been the physician to population ratio for each of the regions expressly provided with an archiater. Even if we assume that the law did not intend, but merely implied the possibility of unrestricted free treatment,[49] the potential patient load could not easily be reconciled with the dignity of the office, of which the edict spoke.[50]

However this may be, our concern here is not with the role of the archiaters as such. The point to be made in our context is this: although the law contrasts the rich and those relatively poor, and although the physicians involved are salaried and thus independent of fees, the poor are not singled out as a class for free medical care to be denied to the rich.

The care of the sick imposed by St. Benedict (480–543) upon monks of his order was made a matter of monkish study by Cassiodorus after his retirement to Vivarium, the monastery he had founded about 550. His famous chapter, "On the care of the sick that the monks should have in mind," begins with these words:

> But you too, I exhort, illustrious brethren, who deal with the welfare of the human body with diligent inquisitiveness and devote the services of holy piety to those who take refuge in the abodes of the saints, [you] who are saddened by others' sufferings, who grieve over those in danger, are pierced by the pain of those you take into your care, and always stunned by grief over the misfortunes of others: Serve the sick with sincere dedication as knowledge of your art directs, expecting a fee from Him who can give eternal rewards instead of temporal ones. And therefore, study the nature of herbs and perform the mixing of the [various] species with solicitous attention; but do not put your hope in the herbs nor your trust in human counsel. For though it can be read that medicine is ordained by the Lord [Ecclesiasticus 38:1ff.], yet it is without doubt He who makes [men] healthy and who grants life. For it is written: whatever you do in word or deed, do all in the name of the Lord Jesus, giving thanks to God and the Father by him [Colossians 3:17].[51]

Clearly recognizable within the first part of Cassiodorus's appeal is the old Hippocratic saying: "The physician sees terrible things, touches what is loathesome, and from others' misfortunes harvests troubles of his own."[52] In its original context, this statement was to prove that medicine belonged to the arts beneficial for others and a public good, but troublesome and grievous for the practitioners.

It was taken up by the "physicians of the soul," the pagan philosophers and the Christian theologians, who saw in Jesus the great physi-

cian who had suffered for the sins of men.[53] In Cassiodorus, the saying
is elaborated, and the emphasis has shifted from a sigh over the burdensome lot of the good physician to praise of the compassion and zeal
of the monk who will find his reward in heaven.

It does not seem surprising that ancient medical deontology survived into the Middle Ages. At some as yet undetermined time, probably not later than the sixth century, Latin translations of Greek texts
were made, copies of which, in various forms with or without changes
and elaborations, are found in medical manuscripts from as early as the
ninth century.[54] Some of these early medieval texts show no clear
Christian influence at all, as for instance an alleged letter by Soranus,
who practised in Rome in the early second century and whose name
was famous in the early Middle Ages. In this letter we read:[55]

> [The physician] should be kind in manner and modest, with due probity.
> He should not lack chastity,[56] nor should he be proud but should give
> equal treatment to poor and rich, slaves and free men, for medicine is one
> for [all of] them. If indeed remuneration is offered, let him accept and not
> refuse. If, however, it is not offered, he should not demand it, because
> however much anyone may offer, the remuneration cannot equal the
> benefits of medicine.

In what follows, the Hippocratic *Oath* is cited and the physician's
desirable appearance and bedside manner are discussed. Even in details, dependence on ancient sources is traceable,[57] including the remark on the inestimable value of medicine that we already met in
Seneca.

The passage on remuneration is somewhat sweeping, especially in
view of the advice not to refuse it if offered! The text does not mention
any salary. Conceivably, the Christian writer thought of monks, who
should not humiliate the patient by a refusal of what was freely given,
the only point where the text possibly went beyond what we found in
pagan Antiquity. The idea of Christian charity, however, found expression in another text: "What is given should not be refused and should
not be demanded if not given; but all, poor and rich, should be loved
one and the same; before the Lord, [the physician] cannot consider his
pay."[58]

We may, therefore, say that in Christianity the pagan Hippocratic
ideals persisted,[59] though accommodated to a world of different values. Philanthropy for all became love and charity for all; pagan virtue
became a religious command whose fulfillment entailed a reward that

was not of this world. But philanthropy also acquired another, more specific, meaning: loving care for the needy, especially the indigent, the beggars.[60] With Christianity dominant in society and state, religious duty acquired institutional forms. The main beneficiaries were the poor, the sick, and the homeless, who found care, support, and protection in hospitals and other charitable foundations.

All this is too well known to need elaboration. Yet another feature of the transition is easily overlooked. In living up to the demands of ancient medical ethics, the pagan physician found a reward in social prestige and fame, values that were even dearer to the Ancients than to us, and which were also promised to the physician faithful to the Hippocratic *Oath*. Ancient medical ethics were not quite as idealistic as they appear, if by idealistic we understand unselfish and spiritual. However, although aware of its material promises, moral philosophers treated them as a by-product. According to the dominating philosophy of educated pagans of late Antiquity, virtue carried its own reward. Christianity, however, though it removed the reward from this world, definitely promised it for the other and also threatened damnation for disobedience to its teachings. Agnostics and disbelievers of the nineteenth century, who broke away from Christianity while remaining faithful to Judeo-Christian ethics, have accustomed many of us to overlook, or to underestimate, the pervasive eschatology of Christianity (and of late Judaism and of Islam). The eschatological expectations of the gospel together with its radical devotion to the needy must be kept in mind, if we wish to understand a significant feature of Christian medical ethics.

A few of the early medieval texts, although unmistakably colored by Christian doctrines, inject quite different advice:[61] "Accept at least half of the remuneration without hesitation, for he who wishes to buy [your services] is disposed to pay and to beg [for treatment]. Get it while he is suffering, for when the pain ceases, your services also cease."[62] A pronouncedly Christian text belonging to a different category but to an equally early period (early ninth century) will be discussed presently.[63] It strikes the same note.

The question has been raised, whether this "brutally practical factor" may have been "Salerno's first contribution to the despiritualization" of medicine.[64] In Salerno, or at least in a medical poem ascribed to Salerno under such titles as *Schola Salernitana* or *Regimen sanitatis*, a cynical materialism was voiced that hardly finds its equal in later medical literature:

I did not study gratis, neither will the clever muse of Hippocrates serve the sick on the streets without gifts. When disease is present, the physician is promised the world, but when the disease recedes, the physician soon escapes the mind. He should press right away for money or for a pledge, for a secure pledge keeps an old friend unchanged. If you make your demand later, you will be taken for an enemy. While the sick man is in pain, the physician should be firm about the pledge; [once the patient] is relieved, he is sorry for the pledge he gave. Therefore, ask for the reward while the pain harasses the patient, for when the disease is gone, the giving stops and quarreling remains. Medicine bought dearly is wont to help; if given gratis, it is of little benefit.[65]

The repetitiousness of the sentiment expressed in the above lines, as well as in subsequent lines of the poem, can be explained by accretions from different years or from different places, or both.[66]

This Salernitan poem, originating not before 1100, obviously takes up the idea we found in texts of about 300 years earlier. In late medieval Italian cities a mundane spirit, pushing for trade, can well be cited in explanation of the poem.[67] It is the wisdom of the trader, unmitigated by pagan or Christian ethics. The early medieval texts, on the other hand, can hardly be explained by an urban, mercantile spirit for which there is little evidence around 800.

Before venturing on an explanation, we must remember that the reality of medical life in late Antiquity did not always correspond to the ethical postulates. Pliny's complaint about haggling over fees with severely ill patients and the provisions for an early contract in the Visigothic laws suggest that early payment or a binding contract were common practice in late Antiquity. We may also think that the texts containing the mundane outlook on fees were intended for freely practicing lay physicians who could not be satisfied with the promise of a heavenly reward, as could monks sheltered by their monasteries and mainly having sick monks for their patients. In view of the fragmentary survival of ancient literature, the possibility cannot even be excluded that there existed older deontological texts containing the harsh note about fees and that a peculiar fate played just these versions into the hands of those copyists who left clear traces of their Christianity.

Nevertheless, even if all this were true, it does not contain the whole truth, since it does not account for a different aspect such as is discernible in a treatise of the early ninth century written in defense of Christian occupation with worldly medicine:[68] "I am compelled to answer those who say that I wrote this book in vain because it contains little that is true. But I, as if deaf, have not heard their words, because I considered the requirements of those in need, rather than the censure of those who rage against me. Therefore, I shall answer them not in my words, but in the words of Holy Writ, that human medicine is not to be totally rejected, since it is certainly not unknown to the divine books."[69]

Human medicine, in contrast to divine medicine, was rejected by Christians who set their trust in faith and prayer alone (James 5:14–15). Distrust of physicians manifested itself in the story of Jesus's cure of the woman with a bloody flux, who suffered much from many physicians, on whom she had spent her substance without being helped (Mark 5:26). It is against such enemies of secular medicine that the theologically trained author argues at length, with quotations from the Bible and from Christian authorities. He includes the exhortation that Cassiodorus had addressed to the monks of Vivarium, and having paraphrased the latter's reference to Colossians 3:17, he himself reminds his readers that, in visiting the poor, they visit Christ.[70] "Indeed," he writes, "the abundance of the rich assures for them the visits of the physicians."[71] Then he continues:

> Remember the deeds of the Lord, who did not disdain to help the centurion's servant when he was crushed by disease, yet disdained to attend the princeling's son with his bodily presence.[72] Here, indeed, our pride is blunted, who revere in men not [their] nature, whereby they are made in the likeness of the Lord, but honors and riches. Behold, He who comes from heaven is not above helping a servant; should we, who are dust and ashes, disdain to go to the sick who are poor? Therefore, do not set your sight upon the reward you may receive in this world, but in that which is to come. For you will be blessed if you apply your care to *those of whom you know that they cannot repay us.* You must not demand anything from them, if you wish to find reward in eternal rest, because it is more blessed to give than to receive [Acts 20:35][73] . . . Therefore learn to have compassion with the poor, that the Lord may sometime have compassion on you. For blessed are the merciful, for they shall obtain mercy [Matthew 5:7].[74]

In addition to the free treatment of paupers, they have a preferred status over the rich, who can easily obtain medical services. Jesus showed his preference: although he cured the princeling's son, he did not deign to enter this man's house, in contrast to his behavior toward the centurion's servant.

This note is struck even more distinctly in a Latin poem that immediately follows the above text.[75] It begins:

> Cosmas, Damianus, Hippocrates, Galen, whom medicine celebrates as illustrious teachers of the world, are the men to whom this page refers. Gifts are due the physician while one is ill; once the patient gets up, there comes no [recompense?[76]]. You who are sick: Give the physician what you owe him, lest the evil recur and nobody comes back again to you. Physician: Attend the poor as well as the mighty with his wealth; their unequal condition has to be taken into account differently. If the patient is wealthy, let this be a proper occasion for profit; if a pauper, any reward is sufficient for you.[77]

The different handling of fees for rich and poor is here made a matter of deliberate policy. We are on our way to the advice given by Geiler of Keisersberg, a popular preacher around 1500: "A physician should have compassion with everyone, especially with the poor man who has not much to give him. He should help him not only out of compassion and for God's sake, but he should also be on hand for him every day and should afterwards take all the more from the rich, who can afford to pay."[78]

I believe that the two texts of this manuscript of the early ninth century reflect the Christian discrimination between rich and poor. Love goes to all men; but the unfortunate of this world are in a privileged position. This holds true of the sick,[79] all of whom have to be attended, and also of the poor. "Blessed be ye poor [*ptōchoi*, literally, beggars]: for yours is the kingdom of God [Luke 6:-20]." Merely being very poor opens the doors of God's kingdom. The rich, in turn, are condemned, unless they distribute all they have to the poor (and then are no longer rich), as the rich young man was told. "It is easier for a camel to go through the eye of a needle, than for a rich man to enter into the kingdom of God" [Matthew 19:24 and Luke 18:25]. After their deaths, Lazarus the beggar "was carried by the angels into Abraham's bosom," whereas the rich man went to hell and was told: "Remember that thou in thy lifetime receivedst thy good things, and likewise Lazarus evil things: but now he is comforted, and thou art tormented" [Luke 16:22–25].[80]

With such a bias in favor of the very poor, and against all the rich, the way was open for a double standard in medical pay. Pagan Graeco-Roman medical ethics had praised the physician who treated poor and rich alike. As late as Valentinian's law of 368, this meant that the poor were to receive the same attention as the rich; it also meant that the rich were not to receive treatment tailored to their whims. It was left to the individual physician to consider the patient's economic status. For this we have corroboration from the time of Valentinian from John Chrysostom (died A.D. 407). In one of his sermons, abounding in comparisons of physicians with Jesus as a healer, John Chrysostom draws a parallel between the fee of the physician and the faith of those whom Jesus cured:

> As physicians, healing the same disease, take a hundred pieces of gold from some patients, half [of it] from others, less [still] from others, and from some nothing at all, so Christ accepted much and marvelous faith from the centurion, less from this one [*i.e.* the paralytic of Matthew 9:2 ff.], and from the other [*i.e.* the invalid of John 5:5 ff.] not even a modicum —and, nevertheless, healed them all.[81]

We are not told the physicians' motivation, whether they took what the patients happened to give them (as Valentinian expected from the Roman archiaters) or what the patients could give them, or whether they considerately adapted their demands to the patients' circumstances—much from the rich to nothing from the indigent. The comparison tells us that physicians were expected to heal regardless of their fee. By his comparison John Chrysostom sanctioned what he depicted as medical practice. From here it was but a step to turn practice into religious duty, insistent on equal treatment for all, yet putting the indigent under special protection through institutions and by claims upon the conscience of all physicians, who were free to compensate themselves by high demands on those patients able to pay. Christianity neither introduced nor favored bargaining over fees or exploiting the rich. But its victory in late Antiquity removed some of the moral restraint upon doing so or, at least, doing it openly.

Notes

1. George Rosen, *Fees and Fee Bills: Some Economic Aspects of Medical Practice in Nineteenth Century America,* (Baltimore: Johns Hopkins Press, 1946) (Supplement to the Bulletin of the History of Medicine, no. 6).

2. *Codex Theodosianus* 13. 3. 8; *Theodosiani libri XVI cum constitutionibus Sirmondianis et leges Novellae and Theodosianum pertinentes,* ed. by Theodor Mommsen and Paul M. Meyer (Berlin: Weidmann, 1905) vol. 1, pt. 2, p. 742.

3. See Hendrik Bolkestein, *Wohltätigkeit und Armenpflege im vorchristlichen Altertum*

(Utrecht: Oosthoek, 1939), pp. 181–99 and 327–29, and Hands (below n. 23), pp. 62–76. Bolkestein has little to say about medicine and physicians, a neglect which, at times, accounts for an undue radicalism in his comparison of all-embracing Graeco-Roman philanthropy and oriental (i.e., in Egypt and Israel) charity for the poor. Nevertheless, his contraposition is fundamental and, together with the wealth of material contained in the book, offers a general background for much of what the present article attempts to show for medicine in a later period.

4. *Codex Theodosianus* 13. 3. 9; p. 742. The Latin text of both laws can also be found in A. H. M. Jones, *The Later Roman Empire 284–602*, 2 vols. (Norman: University of Oklahoma Press, 1964), II, p. 1293, and is discussed *ibid.*, II, p. 1012. For French translations see Briau (below n. 6), pp. 84–85, 89.

5. Darrel W. Amundsen, "Visigothic medical legislation," *Bull. Hist. Med.*, 45 (1971), pp. 553–569; see pp. 556–557, ftn. 15.

6. On public physicians see Louis Cohn-Haft, *The Public Physicians of Ancient Greece* (Northampton, Mass.: 1956) (Smith College Studies in History, vol. 42), and Karl-Heinz Below, *Der Arzt im römischen Recht* (Munich: C. H. Beck, 1953)(Münchener Beiträge zur Papyrusforschung und antiken Rechtsgeschichte, fasc. 37), who also discusses in detail the immunities granted. There also existed imperial archiaters who enjoyed a very high rank (see Below, pp. 44–48). René Briau, *L'archiatrie romaine* (Paris: Manon, 1877), is somewhat antiquated.

7. Ammianus Marcellinus 30. 8. 10; Loeb edition vol. 3, pp. 366–367 (Rolfe's translation).

8. See A. H. M. Jones (above n. 4) vol. 2, p. 1012. If my memory serves me right, the existence of the antitheses: honestly—shamefully, and dedication—servility was emphasized by Dr. Donald W. Peterson in a seminar several years ago.

9. *Precepts* 5; W. H. S. Jones' edition of *Hippocrates*, Loeb, vol. 1, pp. 318–319, but the Greek text is very uncertain; cf. Jones's notes p. 318. On the dates of *Precepts* and *Decorum* see Ludwig Edelstein, "The professional ethics of the Greek physician," reprinted in *Ancient Medicine: Selected Papers of Ludwig Edelstein*, ed. by Owsei and C. Lilian Temkin (Baltimore: Johns Hopkins Press, 1967), pp. 319–348; see pp. 329–331. This volume will be cited as *Ancient Medicine* for this and other publications of Edelstein's reprinted therein. This article of Edelstein's, together with his essay on the Hippocratic *Oath* (*Ancient Medicine*, pp. 3–63), is fundamental for the history of Greek medical ethics. With it should be consulted Fridolf Kudlien, "Medical ethics and popular ethics in Greece and Rome," *Clio medica*, 5 (1970), pp. 91–121.

10. *Precepts* 4; p. 316. I have translated *promussein* in analogy to Plutarch, *Moral Essays* 798 b, where it means "to snuff a lamp," the only certain meaning we have for this verb.

11. Pliny, *Natural History* 29. 8. 21. I have quoted the translation by W. H. S. Jones, vol. 8, p. 197 of the Loeb edition. The italics are mine.

12. For text and translation see Darrel W. Amundsen (above n. 5) pp. 559ff.

13. Seneca, *Moral Essays* 6. 15. 1; vol. 3, p. 392 of the Loeb edition (John W. Basore's translation).

14. Below (above n. 6), pp. 61–81.

15. Below, *ibid.* and p. 108, discusses these questions.

16. Amundsen (above n. 5), pp. 556–557.

17. Owsei Temkin, *Galenism: Rise and Decline of a Medical Philosophy* (Ithaca, N.Y.: Cornell University Press, 1973), pp. 37 and 47.

18. Galen, *De praenotione ad Posthumum* 8; ed. Kühn, vol 14, p. 647.

19. Galen, *De placitis Hippocratis et Platonis* 9.5. My translation is from the edition of this passage in Karl Deichgräber, *Die griechische Empirikerschule* (Berlin: Weidmann, 1930), pp. 213–214.

20. See Temkin (above n. 17), pp. 35 and 48.

21. *Letters* 16; Littré ed. of the Hippocratic works, vol. 9, p. 344, lines 5–8.

22. Galen, *Quod optimus medicus sit quoque philosophus* 3; *Claudii Galeni Scripta minora*, ed. J. Marquardt et al., 3 vols (Leipzig: Teubner, 1884–1893), 2:5.

23. *Precepts* 6; p. 319 (W. H. S. Jones's translation where, however, I have substituted "present good will" for "present satisfaction.") For the interpretation see Edelstein, *Ancient Medicine*, p. 321, and, differently, Huldrych M. Koelbing, *Arzt und Patient in der Antiken Welt* (Zurich: Artemis, 1977), p. 130. The passage is an example of the reciprocity of philanthropy, on which cf. A.R. Hands, *Charities and Social Aid in Greece and Rome* (Ithaca, N. Y.: Cornell University Press, 1968), pp. 35–36. For remuneration according to circumstances, see Hermann G. Frings, *Medizin und Arzt bei dem griechischen Kirchenvätern bis Chrysostomos* (Bonn: Dissertation, 1959), p. 91.

24. Bolkestein (above n. 3), p. 110: philanthropy was *"volks*freundlich . . . nicht *armen* freundlich." On the general development of the Greek concept of philanthropy and its reception by the Romans and the Church Fathers, see John Ferguson, *Moral Values in the Ancient World* (London: Methuen, 1958), pp. 102–117. On its development in medicine, see Edelstein, *Ancient Medicine*, pp. 320–324 and 329–331.

25. W. W. Tarn and G. T. Griffith, *Hellenistic Civilization*, 3rd ed. (1952), reprinted by The World Publishing Company, Meridian Books (1963), p. 118. To this, however, cf. Hands (above n. 23), p. 11 and ch. 6.

26. *Decorum* 2 and 5; Loeb ed., vol. 2, pp. 278–280 and 286.

27. Quoted from Hands (above n. 23), p. 205. For a discussion of this and similar inscriptions, see A. G. Woodhead, "The state health service in ancient Greece," *Cambridge Historical Journal* 10, 3 (1952), 235–253; Cohn-Haft (above n. 6), pp. 32–45; Hands, pp. 131–141; Fridolf Kudlien, *Die Sklaven in der griechischen Medizin der klassischen und hellenistischen Zeit* (Wiesbaden: Steiner, 1968), pp. 39–40 (Forschungen zur antiken Sklaverei, vol. 2). James H. Oliver, "The empress Plotina and the sacred Thymelic synod," *Historia* 24 (1975), pp. 125–128, on pp. 125–126, gives an inscription for one Heraclitus, who had been "honored with exemption from liturgy" and had "served without charge as physician," presumably as town physician to Rhodiapolis.

28. Scribonius Largus, *Conpositiones*, ed. by Georg Helmreich (Leipzig: Teubner, 1887), p. 2, lines 17–26. On his broader concept of philanthropy compared with that of *Precepts*, see Edelstein, *Ancient Medicine*, pp. 337–44, and Kudlien (above n. 9), pp. 95–96 and 101.

29. The only reference to such conditions in the *Oath* is to the household to which the physician is admitted and refers to all its inmates, not only to the patient, as Joseph Vogt,

Sklaverei und Humanität (Wiesbaden: Steiner, 1965), p. 11, and Kudlien (above n. 27), pp. 5–6, seem to think.

30. See Edelstein, *Ancient Medicine*, p. 35, ftn. 115, and Kudlien (above n. 27), p. 25.

31. Quoted from James H. Oliver, "Two Athenian poets," *Hesperia*, Supplement 8, American School of Classical Studies at Athens, 1949, pp. 243–258 (see p. 246). The original (incomplete) reconstruction of the poem was published in an article by Oliver and Paul Maas, "An Ancient Poem on the Duties of a Physician," *Bull. Hist. Med.* 7 (1939), pp. 315–323. The poem is discussed by Edelstein, *Ancient Medicine*, pp. 344 and 347, and by Kudlien (above n. 9), p. 96.

32. For text and translation of the passage in Julian's *Letters*, see Emma J. and Ludwig Edelstein, *Asclepius*, 2 vols. (Baltimore: Johns Hopkins Press, 1945), 1:164. At most, Asclepius demanded a nominal fee for his miraculous cures, with which alone we are concerned here; see *ibid.*, 2: 173–178.

33. Libanius, *Kata iatrou pharmakeōs* 7; ed. of his works by Richard Foerster, vol. 8 (Leipzig: Teubner, 1915), pp. 184–185. This passage has been translated by Edelstein, *Ancient Medicine*, p. 345.

34. Libanius, *ibid.* 8; p. 185, lines 8–17. Not every word in this fictitious speech should be taken at face value. But even a literary exercise in traditional style could hardly make claims at obvious variance with reality.

35. Hands (above n. 23), p. 137, discusses prudence as a motive for waiving fees (though possibly accepting an honorarium) rather than "any deep emotional feeling" see also his chapters 3 and 4.

36. For material on medicine as a liberal art see Below (above n. 6), pp. 57–60. The matter has now been discussed in detail and with regard to fees by Fridolf Kudlien, "Medicine as a 'Liberal Art' and the Question of the Physician's Income," *Journal of the History of Medicine and Allied Sciences*, 31 (1976), pp. 448–459. To my regret this essay has come to my attention (through the courtesy of Dr. Jerome Bylebyl) only after completion of the present article.

37. Seneca, *Moral Essays* 6. 15. 1–2.

38. Pliny, *Letters* 5. 9; Loeb. ed., vol. 1, pp. 404–407; see John Crook, *Law and Life of Rome* (Ithaca, N.Y.: Cornell University Press, 1967), pp. 90–91 for the remuneration of barristers.

39. Pliny, *ibid.* 5. 13; p. 417 (translation by W. Melmoth and W. M. L. Hutchinson).

40. Seneca, *Moral Essays* 6. 16. 1; vol. 3, p. 397 of the Loeb ed. (John W. Basore' translation, modified).

41. *Ibid.* 6. 16. 5; p. 397 (Basore's translation, modified). Seneca speaks of "my" physician in a generalizing sense. Nevertheless, these references to the physician and the teacher of the liberal arts (especially the philosopher) make us think of the upper strata of Roman society.

42. See Owsei Temkin, "The scientific approach to disease: specific entity and individual sickness," reprinted in *The Double Face of Janus and Other Essays in the History of Medicine* (Baltimore: Johns Hopkins University Press, 1977), pp. 441–455 (see pp. 445–446).

43. Galen, *Methodus medendi* 1. 1; Kühn ed., vol. 10, p. 4. For the role of the layman

and of money in choosing the physician, see Jutta Kollesch, "Arztwahl und ärztliche Ethik in der römischen Kaiserzeit," *Das Altertum,* 18 (1972), pp. 27–30.

44.   Galen, *ibid.,* p. 1; *cf.* Temkin (above n. 17). p. 36. For additional references on shameful behavior, see Deichgräber, *Medicus gratiosus* (below n. 57), p. 17.

45.   A. H. M. Jones (above n. 4), vol. 1, pp. 144–145: "Valentinian's care for the humbler classes is most notably exemplified in his treatment of the office of *defensor civitatis,"* whose function it was "to be patron of the *plebs* against the injuries of the powerful." Even if Christian influences were credited with Valentinian's concern for the poor (so Briau, above n. 6, pp. 85–86), they would only account for the motivation for issuing the law, without imposing a distinctly Christian character upon it. The law does not appeal to the archiaters' charity but to their being paid from public funds!

46.   A strong plea for the existence of a medical care system in Greece has been made by Woodhead (above . 27), to which, however, *cf.* Cohn-Haft (above n. 6), pp. 32–45 and Hands (above n. 23), ch. 9.

47.   A. H. M. Jones (above n. 4), vol. 2, p. 1040 mentions between "half and three-quarters of a million in the early fourth century." Considering the steady decline in population, I have taken the lower figure for the time of the law.

48.   *E.g.,* A. H. M. Jones (above n. 4), vol. 1, p. 708. I have, however, not been able to identify the portus Xysti and the district of the vestal virgins with any of the traditional fourteen regions, for which see article, "Rom," Pauly-Wissowa, *Real-Encyclopadie der classischen Altertumswissenschaft,* 2. Reihe, 1. Halbband, col.1038. Briau (above n. 6), p. 86, and Below (above n. 6), p. 50, speak of fourteen archiaters, and so does Rudolf Pohl, *De Graecorum medicis publicis,* Diss. Berlin, 1905, pp. 54 and 65–66, who explains that the two exempted regions each had its own archiater. This seems an arbitrary assumption, and the total number of archiaters may have been twelve or more than fourteen.

49.   See Amundsen, above n. 5.

50.   Symmachus, *Relationes* 27, suggests that high ranking Romans also desired the position of archiater. The case is sketched by A. H. M. Jones (above n. 4), vol. 1, p. 690.

51.   Cassiodorus, *Institutiones* 31. 1; ed. by R. A. B. Mynors, Oxford: Clarendon Press, 1937, pp. 78–79. On Cassiodorus see Loren MacKinney, *Early Medieval Medicine* (Baltimore: Johns Hopkins Press, 1937), pp. 49–52.

52.   Hippocrates, *Breaths* 1; Loeb ed., vol. 2, p. 226.

53.   Eusebius, *Historia ecclesiastica* 10. 4. 11. There exists quite a large literature on the afterlife of this Hippocratic saying.

54.   They have been translated into English by Loren MacKinney, "Medical Ethics and Etiquette in the Early Middle Ages: the Persistence of Hippocratic Ideals," *Bull. Hist. Med.,* 26 (1952), pp. 1–31.

55.   For the Latin text, see Valentin Rose, *Anecdota graeca et graecolatina,* reprinted (2 vols. in one) (Amsterdam: Hakkert, 1963), 2, p. 245, lines 10–15, and the reproduction from the Chartes ms. 62 in MacKinney (above n. 54), p. 13. In part I have utilized MacKinney's translation, p. 12.

56.   Rose: *sanctitas.* MacKinney, who translates "he should be neither lacking in knowledge," seems to have read *scientias.* The word is not legible in the reproduction.

57. See Karl Deichgräber, *Medicus gloriosus: Untersuchungen zu einem griechischen Arztbild* (Wiesbaden: Akademie der Wissenschaften und der Literatur Mainz)(Abhandlungen der geistes-und sozialwissenschaftlichen Klasse, 1970, no. 3), pp. 79–84 and appendix 1 (pp. 88–107).

58. Translated from cod. Sangallensis 751, saec. ix-x, p. 368, as edited by Ernst Hirschfeld, "Deontologische Texte des frühen Mittelalters," *Archiv für Geschichte der Medizin* (now *Sudhoffs Archiv*), 20 (1928), pp. 353–371; see p. 363.

59. See the title of MacKinney's essay, above n. 54.

60. See Bolkestein (above n. 3), on comparisons of ancient philanthropy and Christian charity, see also Hands (above n. 23) especially ch. 9, on "Health and Hygiene," and Demetrios J. Constantelos, *Byzantine Philanthropy and Social Welfare* (New Brunswick, N. J.: Rutgers University Press, 1968), pp. 10–11.

61. See MacKinney (above n. 54), pp. 8 and 23–24 for the translation from Glasgow ms. Hunter v. 3. 2, which he believes of southern Italian provenance and assigns to the early tenth century, and Hirschfeld (above n. 58), pp. 370–371, for the texts from cod. Turicensis C 128/32 and cod. Vat. Angel. N 1502 (V.3.9) that he assigns to the eleventh and twelfth centuries respectively. For the Glasgow ms. *cf.* Augusto Beccaria, *I codici di medicina del periodo presalernitano* (Rome: Edizioni di Storia e Letteratura, 1956), p. 243; the Zurich ms. is not listed here, and the Rome ms. is outside the chronological scope of the book.

62. Quoted from MacKinney (above n. 54), pp. 23–24.

63. See below n. 68.

64. MacKinney (above n. 54), p. 23, ftn. 37.

65. For the Latin text see Salvatore De Renzi, *Collectio Salernitana*, 5 vols., (Naples: Filiatre-Sebezio, 1852–1859), 5, pp. 102–103, lines 3450–3462.

66. The exact wording and date of the original version are uncertain.

67. See MacKinney (above n. 54), pp. 22–26. Moreover, the lighthearted tone of the poem, reminiscent of medieval student poetry, should not be overlooked.

68. The treatise contained in the Bamberg cod. med. 1 (L. III. 8), for which see Beccaria (above n. 61), pp. 193–197, was published by Karl Sudhoff, "Eine Verteidigung der Heilkunde aus den Zeiten der 'Mönchsmedizin,' " *Archiv für Geschichte der Medizin* (now *Sudhoffs Archiv*), 7 (1913), pp. 223–237. It is also discussed by MacKinney (above n. 54), pp. 5–6.

69. Sudhoff, *ibid.*, p. 224, lines 1–8. We are not told which book by the author had been attacked.

70. *Cf.* Matthew 25: 36 ("I was sick and ye visited me") and 40 ("In as much as ye have done it unto one of the least of these my brethren, ye have done it unto me").

71. Sudhoff, *ibid.*, p. 232, lines 334–435.

72. The reference is to John 4: 46–53, which tells the story of the officer in the royal service whose son Jesus cures without going to his house as requested. Our author, following the Vulgate, refers to the man as *regulus* which bestows an exalted status upon him. In contrast, Jesus was willing to go to the centurion's house to heal his servant (Matthew 8: 7–8), and Luke 7:1–7).

73. Sudhoff (above n. 68), p. 232, lines 336–348. Italics are mine.

74. *Ibid.*, lines 351–354.

75. Published by Sudhoff, *ibid.*, p. 237.

76. *Ibid.*, p. 237, line 5: "nulla laguna venit." The meaning of *laguna* escapes me.

77. Line 11: "si pauper, merces sufficit una tibi." MacKinney's (above n. 54), p. 6, ftn 7, translation: "if poor, let one reward [spiritual] suffice," makes the contrast even stronger.

78. From the original German as quoted by L. Kotelmann, *Gesundheitspflege im Mittelalter*, Hamburg-Leipzig: Voss, 1890, p. 203.

79. See Henry E. Sigerist, "The Special Position of the Sick," in *Henry E. Sigerist On the Sociology of Medicine*, ed. by M. I. Roemer and J. M. Mackintosh, New York: MD Publications, 1960, pp. 9–22, especially pp. 16–18.

80. Bolkestein (above n. 3), pp. 383–84, 407–409, and 424–425, traces the idea of the different fate after death awaiting the poor and the rich back to ancient Egypt. In Judaism, and even more so in Christianity, there was, moreover, a tendency to identify the poor with the pious. In the story of Lazarus and the rich man, Bolkestein, p. 409, sees the idea of retaliation in a form which "could only originate and find followers among the poor as satisfying a sublimated need for vengeance."

81. *Homilia in paralyticum per tectum demissum* 4; Migne, *Patrologia Graeca.* vol. 51, columns 55–56; see also Frings (above, n. 23). According to Chrysostom the faith of the centurion was immense, because he believed that Jesus only had to say the word. "This one" refers to the paralytic of Matthew 9:2 ff., who was brought to Jesus in the hope of a cure; "the other" is the invalid of John 5: 5 ff., who did not know Jesus and expected nothing. Him too Chrysostom calls a paralytic.

The Impact of Hugo van der Goes's Mental Illness and Late-Medieval Religious Attitudes on the *Death of the Virgin**

SUSAN KOSLOW

In the fifteenth century, the southern Netherlands was the leading artistic region in northern Europe. This densely populated, urbanized area was the center of trade and finance in northern Europe and the seat of the resplendent Burgundian court. The happy confluence of bourgeois prosperity and courtly grandeur favored the emergence of a distinctive "modern" style that rivalled the contemporaneous artistic innovations of Italy. As in Italy, the principal artistic concern was the "imitation of nature," but whereas in the south this notion was informed by the classical heritage and scientific objectives (crystallized in the theory and practice of single focus perspective), Netherlandish artists preferred a photographic naturalism that recorded the appearance of all natural phenomena, be they as commonplace as the grain of weathered wood or as brilliant as the lustre of gold and sparkling gems.[1]

The emphasis on textural specificity in Netherlandish art arose from two sources, one secular, the other religious. Appreciation of material richness and variety was undoubtedly fostered by the daily encounter by merchants with their goods.[2] Given the artistic objectives and representational innovations of the fifteenth century, materiality could be satisfied by pictorial means. This interest did not originate solely with the urban bourgeoisie; the Burgundian court, famous for its ostentation and lavish display of wealth, also contributed to the preference for a detailed reproduction of the natural world. The second stimulus originated in a theological belief current in this period, namely that all aspects of nature and artifacts of man could be imbued with a symbolic meaning.[3] Before the advent of naturalistic art, symbolism was overt and ordered in a non-realistic fashion.

The rise of representational realism, however, necessitated a new mode of symbolic language. In Netherlandish art, panel painters intro-

27

duced their symbols into a naturalistic setting thereby hiding or "disguising" their meaning. The untutored observer would thus see mere reality, whereas the initiated would perceive beneath the objective data of nature a divinely ordered world invested with sacred truths. This approach to religious symbolism justified and probably intensified the realism of fifteenth-century Netherlandish art. Two painters are credited with the invention of this new style, or *"ars nova,"* as Erwin Panofsky coined it, Robert Campin (1375?–1444) and Jan van Eyck (fl. 1422–1441).[4] Drawing upon certain realist tendencies of the fourteenth century, they formulated a comprehensive naturalism that directed the course of painting for the remainder of the century.

In the second half of the fifteenth century, after the death of Rogier van der Weyden (1400–1464), a young artist rose to preeminence in the Netherlands, Hugo van der Goes.[5] His activity can be documented from 1467 until his death in 1482.[6] Although his birth date has not yet been discovered, his birthplace was Ghent, where he established his workshop and became one of the leading citizens. At least twice, he was elected dean of the painter's guild. Soon after winning these responsibilities and honors, van der Goes apparently experienced a *crise de conscience* and retired to the monastery of the Red Cloister in the forest of Soignies outside of Brussels.[7] This monastery was affiliated with the Windesheim Congregation, a late medieval reform movement associated with the Canons Regular of St. Augustine.[8] As a converse brother, he was allowed to continue his artistic pursuits.[9] Probably in 1480–1481 while returning from Cologne with a group of Windesheim monks, including his half-brother who also resided at the Red Cloister, van der Goes experienced a psychotic episode during which he tried to commit suicide and raved repeatedly that he was a lost soul doomed to perdition. The severity of the attack required forcible restraint. When the group arrived in Brussels, the prior of the Red Cloister who had been informed of van der Goes's illness and had gone to meet the travellers, ordered musical therapy and spectacles to be performed for him. This treatment proved to be ineffective, and van der Goes returned to the Red Cloister incapacitated. He remained severely depressed for some time but eventually recovered sufficiently to participate in the life of the community.

Hugo van der Goes's illness is recorded in a chronicle detailing the history of the Red Cloister and its most noteworthy members.[10] Such chronicles were not uncommon in the Windesheim Congregation.[11] The author, Gaspar Ofhuys, who had been personally ac-

quainted with van der Goes, presents a detailed account of van der
Goes's illness, its symptoms, diagnoses, treatment, and causes.[12] Ofhuys only refers to van der Goes's artistic activity in order to identify
him and when it relates to the description of the painter's illness. Since
Ofhuys was not writing a humanist biography intended to exalt the
individual and his accomplishments and perpetuate his fame, none of
van der Goes's paintings are described. Ofhuys does stress the moral
and spiritual dangers attendant upon those who have achieved worldly
renown.

The chief danger of fame is that it may deter the individual from
following the path of humility, the virtue most highly esteemed by the
Windesheimers because it fosters contempt for the world.[13] Hugo's
biography therefore has a moralizing and didactic purpose. It illustrates how God chose to punish and thereby save one sinner, Hugo,
and also teaches, by example, the perils of pride. Ofhuys's account of
Hugo has been characterized as manifesting sanctimonious malice and
betraying self-righteousness and even jealousy.[14] This evaluation of
Ofhuys is, I believe, mistaken. The criticisms levelled against Hugo by
Ofhuys are not personal expressions of disapproval but judgments
founded on the beliefs of the Windesheim Congregation. In a sense
Ofhuys can be considered as a spokesman for the monks of the Windesheim Congregation.

It was not Hugo's excellence in his craft or the craft itself that
Ofhuys considered dangerous. The most widely practiced form of
manual labor among members of the Windesheim Congregation was
manuscript and book production.[15] Writing and illuminating these
texts were the responsibility of the houses in which they originated.
Panel painting was not as ubiquitous, nor were there any masters even
approaching Hugo's eminence within the Order, but Hugo's craft was
certainly not frowned upon by his fellow monks. In fact, the continua-
tion of his work within the cloister was probably welcomed because
payments made to him would have been given to the monastery. Ofhuys attributes Hugo's spiritual difficulties to the artist's worldly in-
volvements resulting from his craft. Although he retired to the Red
Cloister ostensibly to sever his ties with the world, Hugo continued to
be sought after by persons of high station.[16] During these visits the
rules of the Order were set aside, so that Hugo would participate in
the dinners held in honor of the guests. The special privileges granted
Hugo and his continued contact with persons of rank were, according
to Ofhuys, largely responsible for van der Goes's excessive pride. To

save Hugo from eternal damnation, God visited on the painter a debili-
tating and humiliating disease that showed him the true path to salvation—humility.[17] Quite possibly, Hugo himself believed that he was
not sufficiently humble.

Whatever Hugo's psychological dysfunctions may have been, their
form and their expression were rooted in the social conventions of his
time. As a monk, one of the afflictions which might have beset him was
scrupulosity.[18] Religious who are affected by this condition are tormented by a sense of sinfulness which they fear to be mortal and which
no devotions can assuage. An obsessive, terrifying fantasy of damnation and eternal suffering haunts them. The Wittkowers have plausibly
suggested that Hugo's illness, as described by Ofhuys, is typical of the
scrupulous.[19]

One might also suggest that since the Windesheimers stressed
humility, Hugo's failure to embrace this aspect of his new life entirely
to his satisfaction as well as to meet the expectations of his brothers,
might have precipitated a breakdown. The roots of his illness undoubtedly originated before his monastic retirement and probably
prompted him to seek solace within the confines of the Red Cloister
in the first place.[20] However, rather than discovering the hoped for
consolation and relief from guilt, van der Goes's withdrawal seems to
have exacerbated his mental anguish and resulted finally in psychosis.
Hugo's mental state after the disappearance of the most distressing
symptoms was apparently subdued. Ofhuys mentions approvingly that
Hugo now dined with the lay brethren rather than with the religious
as he had done formerly.[21] Not only was he thus following the Cloister's rules, but it also showed that he was sincerely desirous of being
humble. The conclusion of Ofhuys's biography of Hugo affirms the
positive value of humility, how it saved van der Goes, who upon the
remission of his illness, at last understood the power of this virtue.[22]

The work almost universally accepted as Hugo van der Goes's
earliest painting is the Monforte Altarpiece.[23] Only the central panel
is extant, and that unfortunately is severely trimmed. It depicts the
adoration of the Magi, a theme frequently represented in Netherlandish art. The painting exhibits total mastery of the concerns of Netherlandish painting: convincing portrayal of varied textures, magnificent
fabrics, sensuous, rich color, and natural light diffused by atmosphere.
What is instantly striking about the painting is its insistence on monumental, volumetric figures capable of articulate movement and placed
in ample space that seems designed in accordance with the rules of

single focus perspective. The astonishingly mobile monumentality of the figures contrasts dramatically with the slender gothicism that had, by the 1460's, become the prevailing fashion in Netherlandish art as exemplified by Rogier van der Weyden's last major work, the Columba altarpiece.[24] Hugo continued to pursue the problems set forth in the Monforte altarpiece in his subsequent development modifying his manner as he matured.

Three works are associated with the last years of his life executed presumably after he had entered the Red Cloister: the Edinburgh wings, the Berlin *Nativity* and the Bruges *Death of the Virgin.* [25] Although these works reveal certain stylistic affinities, particularly the Berlin *Nativity* and the *Death of the Virgin,* [26] the latter manifests the most profound break with the intentions of Hugo's previous paintings. No longer do we find the harmonious color schemes, breathtaking displays of richly embroidered materials, active, plastic figures, and rationally ordered space. Instead, Hugo has created an image austere in content and formal realization. Dissonant, sharply contrasting colors, a total lack of textural specificity, a congested composition betraying no interest in the conventional Netherlandish interior setting, and figures sharply articulated by angular linearity separate the *Death of the Virgin* from all of Hugo's other paintings.

Was the motivation personal for this dramatic reformation of artistic aims? Was it prompted by religious and social factors or by a combination of both? Most historians accept the former reason, basing their explanation on the data recorded in Ofhuys' biography of Hugo in the chronicle of the Red Cloister. The historians who subscribe to this explanation believe that the progression of his psychosis can be traced in his art.[27] Accordingly, the works assigned to his earliest phase do not manifest signs of distress, whereas traces of the incipient stages of the breakdown are noted in works produced during his middle period, and those paintings placed at the conclusion of his activity reveal either the imminent onset of psychosis or the after effects of illness. The correlation of style and personality is predicated on the widely held belief rooted in classical culture that art reveals the character of the creator or conversely that the creator imprints his character on his work.[28] Although there can be no doubt that every work is a constellation of distinctive features deriving from the uniqueness of the individual, it does not follow that either mental health or pyschological dysfunction will be projected directly in the form and content of the artist's production. Only under special circumstances will this occur, that is, when influential segments of society encourage creative independence and place a positive value on subjectivity and even irrationality. Rarely has this occurred in the visual arts because art generally was produced for specific cultural functions (propaganda, decoration, instruction, etc.) necessitating legibility and communication in commonly understood symbols. In the fifteenth century individual manners were encouraged, but manifest deviations from a prevailing style based on irrational distortions of reality would not have been accepted. An artist would have isolated himself and lost the patronage necessary for his activity and very existence. According to Ofhuys, Hugo's fame increased rather than decreased during his monastic life, and it was said that he could not have completed his commissions in nine years.[29] To explain, therefore, the evident stylistic peculiarities of his late work, and in particular the qualities manifested in the *Death of the Virgin,* recourse to other than psychological explanations must be considered. The most promising approach is to investigate the iconography of the altarpiece, its destination and function and to situate it in the context of the spiritual concerns of the religious community to which Hugo van der Goes belonged.

Although neither the contract for the altarpiece of the *Death of the Virgin* nor any other documentation regarding its date and creator has been discovered, it is nevertheless possible to establish its provenance and deduce with a fair degree of certainty the donor and its location.[30] In an inventory published in 1848 of the paintings owned by the Abbey of the Dunes, a major Cistercian monastery that had once been located on the seacoast outside of Bruges, one of the items listed was "La Mort de la Vierge, tableau ancien, bien dessiné, 5 pieds × 4 pieds."[31] This is the earliest record of the altarpiece. Although recognized as the work of a Netherlandish primitive, it was not attributed to Hugo van der Goes until 1902. Since then its authorship has never been questioned.

The Abbey of the Dunes was one of the largest and most famous Cistercian foundations in the Netherlands.[32] By the second half of the thirteenth century, a little more than a century after its establishment, grandiose structures had been erected providing quarters for 400 monks and a spacious church consecrated in 1262. In the fourteenth century its growth was checked by several factors. The mendicant orders attracted large numbers of recruits who formerly would have inclined to the Cistercians, and warfare between the Netherlands, England, and France interferred with the Abbey's commercial affairs. In

1338 rebellion broke out in the monastery, and the Abbey fell into
serious decline.

However, in the following century, the Abbey of the Dunes experienced a revival under the leadership of learned and politically
astute abbots. The abbot who held office when the altarpiece of the
Death of the Virgin was painted was Jean Crabbe.[33] His term lasted from
1457 to 1488. Like so many religious of his day, his services were
enlisted by the Burgundian court. He became councillor to Mary of
Burgundy and Maximilian and presided as president of their council.
His abilities were also recognized by his Order which appointed him
Vicar General. Although these duties required his frequent absence
from the monastery, he nevertheless maintained an abiding interest in
its affairs. According to a biography written by a sixteenth-century
chronicler of the Abbey, he commissioned manuscripts for the Abbey's
library and enriched the building itself with decorations. Unfortunately, Adrien de But, the chronicler, does not describe the decorations, but one may assume that van der Goes's painting was among
them. Even though its location within the church is not documented,
there was one chapel, the Maes chapel, which, because of its use and
dedication, may well have sheltered the altarpiece. Constructed in
1400 by Abbot Jean Maes, the chapel, dedicated to the Blessed Virgin,
functioned as a memorial foundation for defunct and living abbots,
daily masses being celebrated on their behalf at its altar.[34] As the
altarpiece's subject is mariological, it would have been appropriate for
a chapel dedicated to the Virgin and particularly one established to
commemorate the deceased leaders of the monastic community.

That Abbot Jean Crabbe commissioned the altarpiece from
Hugo van der Goes rather than from the leading Bruges painter of
the day, Hans Memling, not only underscores the popularity of the
Goesian style in the ambience of the Burgundian court, but also indicates a possible prediliction for van der Goes's art by a fellow monk,
albeit of a different Order. In many respects the Cistercian Order
presages the Windesheim Congregation, and it has been claimed that
aspects of the Modern Devotion, the spiritual basis of the Windesheim Congregation,[35] originated in the practices of the Cistercians.[36] Both were reform movements that insisted upon austerity
and simplicity in all facets of life and removal from worldly affairs. In
their respective periods, each order was quickly constituted and
spread rapidly because they appealed to individuals who perceived
the ills of contemporary institutions and desired an alternative that

would assist them in obtaining salvation through spiritual enlightenment.

In Hugo's day the Cistercians were no longer as exacting as in the twelfth and thirteenth centuries, the heyday of the movement, but the ideal of strictness was still upheld.[37] Their daily life was devoted to three activities: the celebration of the liturgy, reading of sacred texts, and manual labor. They built their monasteries in uncultivated regions in order to avoid the privileges and obligations attendant upon foundations in more densely populated areas. Cistercian architecture was chaste and unadorned, functional without superfluous embellishments as were their liturgical appurtenances and church ornaments. Only painted wooden crosses were permitted; gold and silver were prohibited. Vestments were fashioned either from wool or linen, and none was decorated with precious threads of gold, silver, or silk. Simplicity was also the hallmark of the Cistercian rite. Since the impetus for founding the Cistercian movement originated in the desire to return to the strict observance of the Rule of St Benedict occasioned by a reaction against the Cluniac Order, especially its material splendor, temporal power, and its overwhelming emphasis on the celebration of the Divine Office to the exclusion of all other occupations prescribed in St Benedict's Rule, it is not surprising that the Cistercians embarked on a campaign to excise all accretions and superfluities from the Cluniac rite.

In certain respects the Windesheim Congregation professed aims comparable to those of the Cistercians. They also embraced a simple, austere existence removed from worldly concerns, and their days were occupied by similar activities: celebration of the liturgy, manual labor, and spiritual exercises. The Windesheim Congregation which belonged to the Canons Regular of St Augustine and its lay counterpart, the Brethren of the Common Life, constituted "the strictest form of late medieval monastic piety and reform,"[38] based on the ideals and practices of the Modern Devotion formulated by Gerard Groote (1340–1384). The Modern Devotion is characterized by its Christocentrism, asceticism, anti-speculative bias, and rejection of learning, both secular and religious.[39] In pursuit of salvation, the Devotionalists emphasized imitation of Christ's human nature, self-abnegation, contempt of the world, and the practice of spiritual exercises, specifically meditation and introspection.[40] The latter are the quintessence of the Modern Devotion as they indicate that deliverance can only be achieved, if God is to grant it at all, through personal purification and not by rote performance of prescribed acts. Introspection required the individual to examine his conscience to discover whether any vices or destructive passions existed that could sway him from the path of virtue. The practitioner of introspection constantly reminded himself of his shortcomings through continual self-examination, self-criticism, and self-correction. Meditation, the second spiritual exercise, was conducted continuously throughout the day. A subject was chosen from Christ's life and Passion and the Four Last Things (Death, the Last Judgment, Heaven, and Hell) for each day's meditation, alternating between those that inspired fear and those that gave comfort. Each monk was expected to ruminate on the given topic throughout his waking hours. The purpose of this spiritual exercise was to impress upon the Devotionalist the model of Christ's human nature and man's redemption through His sacrifice.

The Cistercian order and the Windesheim Congregation agreed in yet another respect: Both groups were under the patronage of Mary, the former dedicating their churches to Mary, Mother of God,[41] the latter to Our Lady of the Assumption.[42] The patronal feast of the Cistercian Order was the Assumption of the Virgin,[43] which helps to explain why the theme of the death of the Virgin was chosen by Jean Crabbe for an altarpiece in the church of the Abbey of the Dunes. This feast originated in the East where its official title was the Falling Asleep of the Mother of God.[44] Its purpose was to commemorate the death of Mary and her reception into Glory. The feast did not appear in the West until the seventh century. Shortly after its introduction in Rome under the title of the Dormition, its designation was changed to the Assumption. This shift signaled a change in the object of the feast: It became a celebration of Mary's triumphal entrance into heaven rather than a commemoration of her death. Despite the changes, the feast continued to recall Mary's demise.

To understand Hugo's representation of the death of the Virgin, it is necessary to review the iconographic tradition of this theme and the textual sources on which it is based.[45] Neither the Gospels nor the Acts of the Apostles mention the death and assumption of the Virgin. The primary textual sources regarding Mary's life are found in the Apocryphal Gospels of Greco-Syrian and Coptic origin written in the fifth and sixth centuries. Later authors embellished and varied these narratives according to their predilictions. From the late thirteenth century on, the principal textual source was the *Golden Legend* of Jacopo de Voragine written before 1264.[46] This book recounts three versions of the Virgin's death that were based upon the Greco-Syrian textual tradition. According to the principal narrative, an angel appeared to Mary and informed her that she would die shortly. She requested that the apostles be present at her death. Miraculously transported from distant places to her bedside, they comforted her during her last hours and were present when Christ took Mary's soul with Him to Heaven. After Mary's death, the Apostles transported her body to her grave. For three days they stood guard at her tomb, until Christ reappeared to wake his mother and transport her bodily to Heaven where, after her body and soul were reunited, she was crowned Queen of Heaven.

The representation of the death of the Virgin first appeared in Byzantine art, which established a compositional pattern that remained constant. The West continued this Byzantine pattern until the late fourteenth century when important modifications were introduced, specifically in Germany and the Netherlands. Elsewhere the Byzantine-type persisted, although updated in certain respects in keeping with current artistic and religious movements.

The classic Byzantine formula depicts the Virgin enveloped in a mantle recumbent on her death bed which is situated parallel to the picture plane. At the head and foot of the bed is an apostle inclining towards Mary's body. Behind the bowing apostles the others congregate in two groups betraying signs of restrained grief. Christ appears in the center of this group holding Mary's soul portrayed as a doll-like figure in his arms. In some examples Christ appears above the bed either holding the soul in his arms or receiving it from angels who transport it to Him.

Some of the major transformations that occurred in the representation of the theme of the death of the Virgin in the fourteenth and fifteenth centuries were sparked by the pictorial revolution of the Renaissance. A new spatial design occurred as a consequence of a shift in the position of Mary's bed. An oblique orientation rather than one parallel to the picture plane fostered by a desire to show depth encouraged the representation of perspectively coherent interiors and allowed for greater variety in the arrangement and actions of the apostles. The apostles are portrayed in diverse poses. Some stand, others kneel or sit beside the Virgin's bed. Almost invariably the Last Rites are being celebrated. Usually these are conducted by St. Peter who is assisted by several other apostles.

Although Hugo van der Goes's painting is indebted to the iconographic traditions of the fourteenth and fifteenth centuries, there are significant changes that represent a shift in the interpretation of the theme and its presentation. Hugo portrayed Christ in an unprecedented manner, hovering above Mary, gazing downwards at her, genuflecting and raising his hands so that the wounds in His palms are visible.[47] A brilliant aureole of light surrounds His figure and the choir of attending angels.[48] Christ's gesture is characteristic of the Saviour in gothic representations of the Last Judgment and signifies intercession, redemption, and triumph over death.[49] These meanings are retained in the new context. Before taking up Mary's soul, Christ reveals Himself to his mother and indicates by means of His gesture the fulfilment of His promise of eternal life.[50]

Mary is the only person in the scene who is aware of Christ's presence as evidenced by her upturned eyes fixed on the miraculous apparition.[51] She is clearly still alive when she beholds Christ. Her animate state is shown not only by the fact that her eyes are open and that she gazes above her, but also by the ceremony enacted by St. Peter. He is taking a lighted candle from St. Paul to place in Mary's hands.[52] This candle, known as the "candle of death,"[53] symbolized the soul's "expectation of Christ" and "Eternal Light" and was given to the dying person during the rite of the *commendatio animae* which was celebrated after the sacrament of extreme unction.[54] Its purpose was to commend the soul to God's mercy by invoking the intercession of Christ, Mary, and the saints. To this end prayers were recited by the dying person and by his companions as he expired.

The iconographic reform of the theme of the death of the Virgin was introduced to stress Mary's experience of dying and Christ's assurance of salvation to her and originates ultimately in the late medieval preoccupation with death.[55] Coping with the fear of death in the fourteenth and fifteenth centuries profoundly affected religious and social life. Chantries and obits proliferated; memorials, tomb monuments, and altarpieces were commissioned at an unprecedented rate; the Dance of Death and the Meeting of the Three Living and Three Dead Kings became especially popular themes in art and literature. The transcience of earthly happiness, beauty, love, and worldly pleasures was frequently expressed in poetry and prose. It is not surprising, then, that in this period a handbook on dying was written. Popularly known as the *Ars moriendi,* this treatise instructed the Christian in the "business of dying."[56] The treatise teaches Moriens, the dying person, how to endure his physical, emotional, and spiritual anguish and advises Moriens's comforters on their role in the universal drama which they witness and will also experience one day.

In this context the Virgin's death acquired a special significance. It became a model of "good dying," preparing the faithful, as the *Ars moriendi* did, for dying well.[57] Mary, by virtue of her spiritual purity experienced a painless death untroubled by the devil, willingly relinquishing her soul, without fear, to her son. All Christians aspired to a comparable death, desiring release from this world without suffering, protection against the final temptations of the devil, and ultimately eternal life. Van der Goes's portrayal of the *Death of the Virgin* expresses these hopes. Mary is shown calmly accepting death as she perceives her son in her last conscious moments appearing to her as the Saviour. By His gesture Christ demonstrates His sacrifice and triumph over death and his promise of redemption to all who commit themselves to Him.

By the second half of the fifteenth century, the prevailing trend depicted the scene of the Virgin's death within a room localized by secular furnishings to indicate that the event was taking place within the Virgin's home. The most important fixture was Mary's bed. In van der Goes's painting, only the most minimal references to a room are introduced. On the left side of the composition, the corner of the chamber appears behind an open curtain. Except for this feature and a shallow floor area, no other architectural elements—walls, windows, ceiling—are incorporated in the design. The orientation of the bed is based on the oblique arrangement of earlier works but is radically different in effect. It is viewed in emphatically foreshortened perspective, so that the Virgin appears to be lying diagonally across it. Other artists had represented beds in a similar manner but with the intention of producing the effect of spatial depth. Hugo did not. Although depth is implied, van der Goes contradicts it by the arrangement of the apostles. Clustered closely on the sides and front of the bed, they do not diminish in size the farther they are from the picture plane. Also they extend laterally to the edges of the panel and are cut arbitrarily. The apostles' bodies, though designed with consummate perfection, are not modeled to suggest weighty, solid forms. There is a pervasive sense of *horror vacui* that even extends to the area above Mary's bed which is filled with Christ and angels and the encompassing radiance. In keeping with the anti-naturalistic treatment of depth, light too is not logically explicable. A uniform brightness with no apparent source either natural or supernatural illuminates the scene. Atmosphere does not soften the light so that a linear definition of form predominates. Eschewing the "modern" devices of pictorial structure and linear and aerial perspective, van der Goes reasserts the potential of overlapping forms and contrasting colors to indicate sequences in depth.

Only a small range of colors is used.[58] The principal one, blue, appears in varying shades for the Virgin's mantle, the bed cover, curtain, the robes of Christ, the angels, and two apostles.[59] Green, pale red, and white comprise the other basic hues. They are disposed in a balanced fashion to achieve an abstract surface harmony, if not a naturalistic spatial order.

Artistic concerns that one would expect to discover in a Netherlandish painting—textural passages and embroidered fabrics, or at least decorated forms—are not encountered in this painting. The austerity and negation of the Netherlandish artistic heritage has been remarked upon by several historians, but no satisfactory explanation accounts for it. Two hypotheses, however, can be entertained. Both depend upon the notion that Hugo consciously opted for certain stylistic objectives and rejected others. To stress the solemnity of the event and its miraculous nature, van der Goes may have decided that material richness would be distracting and indecorous, particularly for an altarpiece depicting the death of the Virgin commissioned by Cistercians whose professed ideals were at variance with material splendor. The second hypothesis, though similar to the first, does not correlate style with specific religious precepts but rather with secular aesthetic objectives: style should correspond to or be approriate to the content. This aim was formulated within the matrix of Italian humanist culture.

One of the disciplines most widely studied by humanists was classical rhetoric.[60] Its application was not restricted solely to oration and literary pursuits but was extended to other realms as well.[61] In the visual arts rhetorical distinctions provided a critical language that affected the analyses and appreciation of art. A basic rule of rhetoric insisted that the form of expression be suited to the content. If Hugo observed this rule, the austere aspect of his painting could be explained by a desire to express, in formal terms, the highly serious nature of the event. All embellishments in this case would be viewed as detracting from the gravity of the scene. Instead of exercising his skill on decorative passages, the artist focused his craft on the essential elements of the narrative—Christ, Mary and the apostles—emphasizing the cognitive and emotional responses of the latter. In this sense the *Death of the Virgin* could be considered the most classical work of the artist. Although the figures are not derived from classical prototypes nor reveal the qualities associated with classical beauty, Hugo's overriding interest in the expression of feeling and thought through the attitudes, gestures, and expressions of the personae of the drama corresponds theoretically with classical objectives.

Although knowledge was considered a vain pursuit by the followers of the Modern Devotion, it is nevertheless possible that van der Goes might have been familiar with humanistic treatises on art and in particular with Leon Battista Alberti's *On Painting*. [62] In this treatise, the first modern European book on painting, Alberti considers the elements that constitute a painting. In his discussion of variety, one of the elements of a good painting, Alberti uses the term in reference to color and figural attitude. In both cases according to Alberti, there should be diversity and contrast. As an example of variety properly applied, he cites and describes the *Navicella* "in which our Tuscan painter Giotto put eleven disciples, all moved by fear seeing one of their companions walk on the waters, because he represented each figure with its face and action indicating a disturbed mind, so that each had its own diverse movements and attitudes."[63] The latter part of the description could just as well describe Hugo van der Goes's *Death of the Virgin* as the Trecento mosaic. Twelve male mourners, at least half of whom are elderly, are individuated. Physiognomies, expressions, postures, and gestures differ and are wonderfully expressive of deeply experienced emotion and thought. The resemblance between Hugo's and Giotto's results (as described by Alberti) may be simply fortuitous, caused by the resolution of comparable problems, or one might speculate that van der Goes, after either reading or hearing about Alberti's text, might have been challenged to emulate or surpass the paradigm quoted by the Italian author.

According to the *Golden Legend,* when the angel informed Mary of her impending death, she requested that all the apostles be assembled at her bedside during her final hours. This wish was granted. Little is said in the *Golden Legend* of the apostles' actions. Once having miraculously arrived, they awaited Mary's death, keeping watch and discoursing in her honor. The sketchiness of their role allowed artists freedom in their representation. The Byzantine artists as noted above, showed the apostles standing and grieving quietly in two groups at the head and foot of the bed. In Western representations the apostles are frequently shown celebrating the Last Rites.[64] St. Peter presides while the other apostles hold the requisite liturgical objects—censer, candles, holy water vessel, and cross. By the end of the fourteenth century, further changes were introduced. The apostles assume new poses and are engaged in more varied actions. Rather than portraying all of them standing, artists now placed some apostles on the floor frequently showing two in front of the bed as if they were guarding the Virgin.[65] Grief is expressed by restrained gestures and mournful expressions in keeping with the pictorial tradition that appears to have been inspired by the injunction in the apocryphal Gospels, where St. John the Evangelist bids his brothers not to evidence grief because the Jews will then cast doubt on their belief in the resurrection and claim that they fear death. One of the most significant qualities that characterizes the apostles in all representations is the sorrowful mood and expression of common grief even when the chorus-like unity of the Byzantine tradition gives way to naturalistic individuation and the physical separation of the apostles.

Van der Goes has maintained the grave mood associated with this group but has not followed the iconographic tradition of showing the apostles grieving in unison. Rather, his apostles, though in close physical proximity to one another are emotionally isolated and do not exhibit attitudes or expressions specific to mourning. Except for Peter and Paul, who celebrate the Last Rites, none of the other apostles interact, sharing thoughts and feelings.[66] They pray and meditate in isolation. Even the two apostles seated at the foot of the bed, who in other interpretations of this subject are represented attentively reading or telling their beads, have, in van der Goes's painting, set aside their devotional aides and stare off into space.

The unusual, if not unique, portrayal of the apostles has been explained by reference to van der Goes's mental illness; the introspective attitudes of the figures are viewed as projections of the artist's morbid fancies. This romantic yet modern, "scientific" explanation has been so ubiquitous that other approaches have not even been considered. Throughout this paper the beliefs and practices of van der Goes's religious community and the community for which the altarpiece was painted have been cited to explain and understand aspects of the work. Again, it is the conventions of these groups that provide the key to understanding Hugo's intentions. The peculiarities of the apostles were introduced by van der Goes to communicate one of the most important aspects of the life of the Modern Devotionalists—the pivotal role of medication and prayer in the attainment of enlightenment and spiritual purification. Interestingly, van der Goes did not design the apostles in traditional poses of meditation and reflection; these attitudes may have been associated too closely with the attain-

ment of worldly knowledge to convey the particular qualities that the
Devotionalists believed incited devout effective meditation—sinless-
ness, fervor, humility, silence, withdrawal. Indeed, these qualities
could be said to characterize the apostles in Hugo's painting.[67] Van der
Goes invented new, expressive conventions. The apostles' faces are
grave and solemn. Their brows are contracted and furrowed; their lips
compressed; and the corners of their mouths are ever so slightly drawn
downwards. Some gaze downwards, others above, and yet others
straight ahead. None focus on the same object or place. This is one
significant way that van der Goes uses to express solitary experience
and cognition. Not only are faces expressive vehicles, but hands can
also indicate mental and psychological states.

Delineated with exquisite subtlety, the slender hands seem to
move of their own accord communicating the apostles' intense emotions. These gestures recall the *chiropsalterium* devised by the Winde-
sheimer Jean Mombaer, a native of Brussels who joined the monastery
of St. Agnietenberg near Zwolle in 1477–1478.[68] To assist himself and
other monks in their spiritual life, Mombaer wrote the *Rosetum.* This
book encourages the Devotionalist to tend his three important rose
gardens—the Hours, communion, and meditation—and supplies him
with systems for each devotional activity. "Ladders" were devised for
communion and meditation while a hand zither or *chiropsalterium* was
invented for the Hours. Twenty-eight brief, pious thoughts were sys-
tematically distributed on the palms and inner digits of the left hand.
As the psalms were recited for the Hours, the Devotionalist ran his
right hand thumb over the places on the left hand where the notations
corresponding to the ideas and feelings expressed in the psalms were
situated.

Although the eloquent, articulate gestures in Hugo's painting do
not accord precisely with Mombaer's hand zither, van der Goes may,
nevertheless, have been alluding to this devotional aid in the design
of the apostles. Mombaer's *chiropsalterium,* first published in 1486, was
probably composed several years earlier, allowing for the possibility
that van der Goes was acquainted with it. Even if he was not, comparable systems not recorded in print may well have been employed by the
monks of the Red Cloister and other monasteries of the Windesheim
Congregation.

The distinctive aspects of the apostles' appearance have been
interpreted in this study in conjunction with the devotional ideals
and practices of the Windesheim Congregation, yet the altarpiece

commissioned for this religious group but for the Cistercians. Could these ideals and practices have been transferable from one group to the other? As there is no specific documentation for the devotions of the Cistercians at the Abbey of the Dunes, we can only speculate on their nature. But considering the ideological congruity and generative association between the Cistercians and the Windesheim Congregation, it does not seem farfetched to hypothesize that the attitudes of the Windesheimers at the Red Cloister were congenial to the brothers at the nearby Abbey of the Dunes and to its abbot, Jean Crabbe. Austerity, simplicity, and meditation were esteemed and fostered by both groups. We may conclude, therefore, that the iconographic novelties in this altarpiece, though inspired or affected by the Modern Devotion, suited the spiritual sensibilities of the patron and of his religious order.[69]

In this extraordinary painting, Hugo van der Goes has created an unforgettable image, voicing the doubts, fears, and hopes of his contemporaries in the face of life's inevitable conclusion, death. Rejecting the constraints of his Netherlandish artistic heritage and the theme's traditional iconography, the artist has forged a work that expresses the specific concerns of his religious community and those that embraced all sectors of society. Its spirit at once presages the tormented mood of the work of the archmannerist Pontormo and recalls an earlier, more primitive manner.

The Janus-like character of this painting suggests a parallel with the creator's own life. Van der Goes is both the quintessence of the late-medieval man suffering from an overwhelming sense of sin, and the modern genius whose psychological anguish is released through the agency of his art.

Hugo van der Goes, may, in his last moments have received comfort from the very image that he had created. Perhaps like Mary in the *Death of the Virgin,* he heard celestial music and saw in a radiant circle of light the Saviour, who appeared to redeem, Hugo, the sinner and painter, of whom it was said "that on our side of the Alps there was no one his equal. . . ."[70]

This paper has questioned the widely accepted belief that a simple connection exists between Hugo van der Goes's mental illness and the stylistic and iconographic novelties apparent in his painting, the *Death of the Virgin.* Examination of the painting in its historical context indicates that explanations based upon the artist's psychopathology are not required in order to understand the unique features of this work and by extension, other late paintings associated with it. This approach does not deny the importance of the individual sensibility which governs the creative processes and imprints its character on the completed work. But this sensibility or personal vision is structured by specific cultural elements. For Hugo van der Goes, certain artistic traditions of the renaissance were informed by the religious beliefs and devotional practices of his ambience. The Modern Devotion particularly influenced his perceptions and attitudes. In turn, van der Goes's pyschopathology prior to the onset of his psychosis undoubtedly helped to create a new pictorial vision in which the ideals of the Modern Devotion could be communicated.

Notes

*For my father, my first teacher.

The research for this paper was supported by a grant from the City University of New York PSC-BHE Research Award Program.

1.   See Erwin Panofsky, *Renaissance and Renascences in Western Art* (New York: Harper Torchbook ed., 1969), chaps. 3, 4.

2.   For a stimulating and persuasive discussion of the interrelationship between pictorial and social conventions, see Michael Baxandall, *Painting and Experience in Fifteenth Century Italy* (Oxford: Clarendon, 1972), chap. 2.

3.   See Erwin Panofsky, *Early Netherlandish Painting. Its Origin and Character* (Cambridge: Harvard, 1953), chap. 4.

4.   Panofsky, *Early Netherlandish Painting,* p. 150 ff.

5.   The most significant monographs on Hugo van der Goes are (in chronological order): Hjalmar G. Sander, "Beiträge zur Biographie Hugo van der Goes und zur Chronologie seiner Werke," *Repertorium fur Kunstwissenschaft* 35 (1912): 519–545; Joseph Destrée, *Hugo van der Goes* (Brussels, Paris: G. van Oest & Cie, 1914); Panofsky, *Early Netherlandish Painting,* pp. 330–345; Friedrich Winkler, *Das Werk des Hugo van der Goes* (Berlin: Walter de Gruyter, 1964); Max J. Friedländer, *Early Netherlandish Painting, IV, Hugo van der Goes,* trans. H. Norden (Leyden, Brussels: A.W. Sÿthoff 1969); Colin Thompson and Lorne Campbell, *Hugo van der Goes and the Trinity Panels in Edinburgh* (National Gallery of Scotland: 1974).

6.   For documents concerning van der Goes, see E. de Busscher, "Recherches sur les anciens peintres gantois," *Messager des sciences historiques* (1859): 105–271; Antoine de Schryver, "Hugo van der Goes' laatste jaren te Gent," *Gentse Bijdragen tot de Kunstgeschiedenis* 16 (1955–1956): 193–211. De Schryver discovered documents in the Ghent archives that show that Hugo van der Goes rented a house from the Van der Zickele family in Ghent from May, 1473 until May, 1477. This data indicates that van der Goes remained in Ghent longer than had been previously supposed before entering the Red Cloister.

This event is generally dated 1475–1476; if De Schryver's arguments are accepted the painter's retirement to the Cloister must be situated 1477–1478.

7. For the Red Cloister see Alphonse Wauters, *Histoire des Environs de Bruxelles* (Brussels: Editions Libro-Science, 1969, reprint of 1851 edition) p. 352 ff.; Johannes G.R. Acquoy, *Het Klooster te Windesheim en Zijn Invloed* (Utrecht: Van der Post, 1875–1880) 3:16.

8. For the Windesheim Congregation see Acquoy, *Windesheim;* Karl Egger, "Windesheim," *Lexikon für Theologie und Kirche* (Freiburg i. Br.: Lexikon fur Theologie und Kirche, Verlag Herder, 1965), 10: 1177–1178; Regnerus R. Post, *The Modern Devotion. Confrontation with Reformation and Humanism* (Leiden: E.J. Brill, 1968); G. Spahr, "Monastery of Windesheim," *New Catholic Encyclopedia* (New York: McGraw-Hill, 1967) 14:956.

9. See S. Hilpisch, "Conversi," *New Catholic Encyclopedia,* 4: 285; Acquoy, *Windesheim,* 1:111.

10. The original Latin manuscript written by Gaspar Ofhuys was acquired from the collection of Camberlyn d'Amougie by the Royal Library, Brussels: Brussels, B.R., ms. II, 48 017. The section on van der Goes, f.115v–118r, was first published in translation (French) by Alphonse Wauters, "Originale Cenobi Rubevallis in Zonia propre Bruxellam in Brabantia," *Bulletin de l'Académie royale de Belgique,* 2(1863): 723–743. English translations appear in Wolfgang Stechow, *Northern Renaissance Art 1400–1600, Sources and Documents* (Englewood Cliffs, N.J.: Prentice-Hall, 1966) pp. 16–18 and William A. McCloy, *The Ofhuys Chronicle and Hugo van der Goes,* unpublished doctoral dissertation. State University of Iowa, 1958, pp. 16–26 (Latin text, pp. 10–15). McCloy's translation will be cited in this study.

11. Post, *Modern Devotion,* pp. 382–383.

12. The most recent and thorough account of the medical aspects of Ofhuys's biography of van der Goes is found in McCloy, *Ofhuys Chronicle.* McCloy was the first scholar to recognize Ofhuys's dependence on Bartholomeus Anglicus's *De proprietatibus rerum.* In this thirteenth-century encyclopedia there is a discussion of the causes of madness. Under the entry for *amentia,* Bartholomeus observes that there are three natural causes for mental illness: certain foods and alcoholic beverages, worry and too much study, and "aggravation of a predisposition." This passage quoted verbatim from Bartholomeus as McCloy demonstrated (pp. 30–32), was used by Ofhuys as a diagnostic schema when discussing the natural causes of van der Goes's malady. Ofhuys pointed to instances of these habits and conditions in the artist's behavior. When dining with guests he drank wine, hence the belief that Hugo was a chronic alcoholic: "He was exceedingly worried about how he was to carry out the paintings he had undertaken. . . . He spent a great deal of his time studying in a Flemish book." (McCloy, *Ofhuys Chronicle,* p. 22). In addition to McCloy, Sander, *Beiträge* should also be consulted for an informed discussion of Hugo's illness in relationship to medical knowledge in the fifteenth century.

13. Acquoy, *Windesheim,* 2: 284. Thomas à Kempis expressed the ideal of humility in his classic work, *The Imitation of Christ:* "If a humble man is humiliated his peace is not disturbed because he does not live by the world—his life depends on God. Only when you think yourself of less importance than everybody else may you consider that you have made some progress." Quoted from Thomas à Kempis, *The Imitation of Christ,* trans.

B.I. Knott (London, Glasgow: Wm. Collins Sons & Co. Ltd, Fontana Books, 1963), pp. 86–87. To teach humility and contempt for the world, the Brethren at Deventer and Zwolle—and probably in other houses as well—were humiliated by being slapped on the cheek by the rector and by wearing old, torn clothing in public. The Canons Regular of the Windesheim Chapter experienced the same humiliations. See Post, *Modern Devotion*, pp. 309–375.

14.   See Panofsky, *Early Netherlandish Painting*, p. 331; Friedlander, *Hugo van der Goes*, p. 14; McCloy, *Ofhuys Chronicle*, p. 52.

15.   The monks of the Windesheim Congregation were expected to spend four to five hours a day copying manuscripts. Acquoy, *Windesheim*, 2: 194, 229 ff.

16.   "And since he was so very eminent as a painter he was visited by high standing persons and many others notably by the most illustrious Archduke Maximilian." McCloy, *Ofhuys Chronicle*, pp. 52–53.

17.   "For this convert brother was exalted highly in our order on account of his special gifts, was made more famous than if he had remained a layman, and since he was only human like the rest of us, by the honors shown him and the various visits and salutations his heart was elevated, wherefore the Lord, not wishing him to perish, out of compassion sent him this humiliating infirmity, by which justly he was reduced to great humility." McCloy, *Ofhuys Chronicle*, p. 23.

18.   See Richard P. Vaughan, *Mental Illness and the Religious Life* (Milwaukee: Bruce, 1962), pp. 59–68.

19.   Rudolf and Margot Wittkower, *Born Under Saturn* (New York: Random House, 1963), p. 112.

20.   For a review of the diagnostic literature pertaining to van der Goes's illness see McCloy, *Ofhuys Chronicle*, pp. 93–99.

21.   McCloy, *Ofhuys Chronicle*, p. 23.

22.   McCloy, *Ofhuys Chronicle*, pp. 23–24.

23.   Friedländer, *Hugo van der Goes*, plate 28.

24.   Max J. Friedländer, *Early Netherlandish Painting, II, Rogier van der Weyden and the Master of Flemalle*, trans. H. Norden (Leyden: A.W. Sÿthoff, 1967), plate 70.

25.   See Thompson and Campbell, *Hugo van der Goes*, for recent literature on the dating of these paintings.

26.   Spatial ambiguities, similar physiognomic types, and linear definition of form are some of the features shared by these works. Yet there are still significant differences. In the Berlin *Nativity* textured surfaces, mobile, plastic figures, harmoniously ordered hues, and palpable atmosphere indicate that the *Nativity*, despite its late dating, still betrays a strong allegiance to some of the primary concerns of van der Goes's early and mature paintings. The same observations hold true for the Edinburgh panels. In this supremely austere work van der Goes evidences his continuing fascination with the specific appearance of substances—witness his superb painting of Edward Bonkil's diaphonous surplice and the fur amice folded over his arm.

27.   For the most eloquent statement of this position see Panofsky, *Early Netherlandish Painting*, p. 332 f.

28. Wittkower, *Born under Saturn*, p. 281 f.

29. McCloy, *Ofhuys Chronicle*, p. 22.

30. For complete documentation see Alin Janssens de Bisthoven and Remi A. Parmentier, *Le Musée Communal de Bruges (Les Primitifs Flamands, Corpus de la Peinture des Anciens Pays-Bas Meridionaux au Quinzième Siècle*, Vol. I) (Antwerp: De Sikkel, 1951), pp. 50–54.

31. Ferdinand van de Putte, "Cabinet de tableaux de l'abbaye des Dunes," *Annales de la Société d'Emulation pour l'étude de l'histoire et des antiquités de Flandre*, 6, 2nd ser. (1848): 182.

32. For the Abbey of the Dunes see Joseph M. Canivez, *L'Ordre de Citeaux en Belgique des origines (1132) au XX siècle* (Forges les-Chimay, Belgium: Abbaye cistercienne de N.-D. de Scourmont, 1926); M.-A. Dimier, "Les Dunes," *Dictionnaire d'histoire et de géographie ecclesiastiques* (Paris: Letouzey it Ané 1960) 4: 1039–1042.

33. For Jean Crabbe de Hulst see Adrianus de But, *Cronica abbatum monasterii de Dunis, per fratrem Adrianum But. Recueil de Chroniques, chartes et autres documents l'histoire et les antiquites de la Flandre—Occidentale. Publiee par La Societe d'emulation de Bruges. ser. l. Chroniques des monasteres de Flandre* (Bruges: Vandecastule-Werbrouck, 1839), pp. 35, 48, 177; Frederick Hartt, G. Corti and C. Kennedy, *The Chapel of the Cardinal of Portugal* (Philadelphia: University of Pennsylvania, 1964), pp. 36–37, 42.

34. A. Dimier, "L'Eglise de l'Abbaye des Dunes," *Bulletin Monumental* 112 (1954): 246.

35. For the Modern Devotion see Post, *Modern Devotion;* R. Garcia Villoslada, "Devotio Moderna," *New Catholic Encyclopedia*, 4: 831–832.

36. Kolumban Spahr, "Zisterzienser," *Lexikon für Theologie und Kirche* (Freiburg i. Br.: 1965) 10: 1384.

37. For the history, art, and liturgy of the Cistercians, see Archdale A. King, *Liturgies of the Religious Orders* (London: Longmans, Green, 1955), pp. 62–156.

38. Steven E. Ozment, *The Reformation in Medieval Perspective* (Chicago: Quadrangle, 1971), p. 157.

39. The characterization of the Modern Devotion presented here is based on Garcia Villoslada, "Devotio Moderna," pp. 831–832.

40. Post, *Modern Devotion*, pp. 323 ff.

41. Acquoy, *Windesheim*, I: 193.

42. King, *Liturgies*, p. 108.

43. King, *Liturgies*, p. 109.

44. Martin Jugie, *La Mort et l'Assomption de la Sainte Vierge, Studi et Testi* (Vatican City: Biblioteca Vaticana, 1944)

45. For the iconography of the death of the Virgin see Louis Réau, *Iconographie de l'art chrétien, 2, Iconographie de la Bible, pt. 2 Nouveau Testament* (Paris: Presses Universitaires de France, 1967), pp. 601–604; Gertrud Holzherr, *Die Darstellung des Marientodes im Spätmittelalters* (Tübingen: 1971); Josef Myslivec, "Tod Mariens," *Allgemeine Lexikon der Christlichen Ikonographie* (Freiburg i. Br.: Verlag Herder, 1972), 4: 333–338. These articles and the dissertation cite earlier literature and describe numerous examples which serve as the basis for the following discussion.

46. Jacques de Voragine, *La Legende Dorée*, trans. J.-B. M. Roze (Paris: Garmier Flammarion, 1967), 2: 82–111.

47. Holzherr, *Die Darstellung des Marientodes*, p. 107 states that only other depiction of the death of the Virgin, a painting in Donnersmark, shows Christ exhibiting his wounds. In that work Christ is enthroned and holds a crown in readiness for the Virgin.

48. Holzherr, *Die Darstellung des Marientodes*, p. 106 claims that "the phenomenon of light" is an innovation. It is derived from the mandorla frequently found in Italian depictions of the death of the Virgin. Holzherr observes that the radiance in van der Goes's painting closely resembles those painted by Grunewald in the *Resurrection* and *Annunciation to the Shepherds* in the Isenheim altarpiece. Although no direct connection can be established between the Isenheim altarpiece and the *Death of the Virgin*, the aureoles portrayed in these paintings have a similar appearance which seems to depend upon a common belief: Light possesses medicinal powers. This belief, based upon astrological theory, attributed to "glowing light, the color of the sun and gold itself" protective qualities against disease (see Andrée Hayum, "The Meaning and Function of the Isenheim Altarpiece: The Hospital Context Revisited," *The Art Bulletin*, 59 (1977): 515). Hayum has linked this theory with the dazzling radiances that appear in the Isenheim polyptych, an altarpiece originally located in a hospital complex. The glowing radiance in Hugo's painting could conceivably have been introduced for the same reason: to allude to the spiritual protection and ameliorative power of Christ. In addition to medicinal associations, light is a metaphor for, or symbol of God. In Scripture God is described as light and as the source of light. Christ, "the light of the world," has a vivifying effect on man just as natural light has on organisms. See below, fn. 52.

49. Panofsky, *Early Netherlandish Painting*, p. 337 observed that Christ is depicted as he appears in His Second Coming. Holzherr, *Die Darstellung des Marientodes*, p. 107 disagrees with Panofsky's interpretation. She does not accept his view that the wounds allude to the Last Judgment and that Christ is the Just Judge.

50. By excluding all references to Mary's coronation as Queen of Heaven, a theme frequently associated with depictions of the death of the Virgin, van der Goes has stressed Mary's mortal nature.

51. Holzherr, *Die Darstellung des Marientodes*, p. 105 asserts that Mary's pale complexion and half-shut eyes signify that she has died. I cannot agree with this conclusion. I believe that van der Goes, had he wanted to represent Mary as moribund, would have shown her with closed eyes in accordance with the traditional depiction of the dead. Ritual also indicates that Mary is still alive: She is not holding the candle of death; St. Peter is taking it from a fellow apostle in preparation for placing it in Mary's hands. By showing Mary dying rather than dead, van der Goes has emphasized Mary's human nature and likeness to Christ; like the rest of mankind and even Christ, the Virgin must depart from this world. But because Mary's death was the perfect death, painless, and protected by Christ (as van der Goes makes apparent by depicting Christ hovering above Mary), it gives all men solace and hope.

52. For the symbolism of light see Editor, "Licht, Lichterscheinungen," *Lexikon der christlichen Ikonographie*, 3: 95–99. For candles see Ferdinand Cabrol, "Cierges," *Dictionnaire d'Archéologie et de Liturgie* (Paris: Letouzey et Ané, 1914) 3: 1613–1622.

53. Theodor Schnitzler, "Sterbekerze," *Lexikon für Theologie und Kirche* (Freiburg i. Br.: 1968) 9: 1054.

54. For the *commendatio animae* see B. Lowenberg, "Commendatio animae," *Lexikon für Theologie und Kirche*, 3: 19; P. van Dijk, "Commendatio animae," *New Catholic Encyclopedia* 4: 8–9.

55. See Johan Huizinga, *The Waning of the Middle Ages*, trans. F. Hopman (New York: Doubleday, 1954), pp. 138–151; *Europe in Torment*, exhibition catalogue, Brown University (1974), pp. 71–118; *Image of Love and Death in Late Medieval and Renaissance Art*, exhibition catalogue, The University of Michigan Museum of Art (1975–1976).

56. See Sister Mary C. O'Connor, *The Art of Dying Well. The Development of the Ars Moriendi* (New York: Columbia University, 1966); Nancy L. Beaty, *The Craft of Dying. A Study in the Literary Tradition of the 'Ars Moriendi' in England* (New Haven, London: Yale University, 1970).

57. Paul Guérin, *Les Petits Bollandistes, Vie des Saints* (Paris: Bloud et Barral 1888) 9: 548 sets forth several reasons for the necessity of Mary's death; the third, fourth, and fifth are summarized here. By dying, Mary eased the suffering all mankind experiences in death. Whereas Christ's death is heroic, violent, Mary's is a tranquil, natural death. Just as she has taught us to live better, so her death teaches man to die better. Finally, Mary's death makes her the advocate and patroness of all who die, allowing the dying to invoke her aid in their last hour. The late medieval association between the Virgin's death and dying well is attested by tomb monuments and funereal tablets decorated with depictions of this theme. Holzherr, *Die Darstellung des Marientodes*, p. 52 ff.

58. W.H. James Weale, "Mélanges et nouvelles vandalisme à Bruges," *Le Beffroi*, 2 (1864–1865): 237–238 asserted that the painting had been damaged by poor cleaning. As a result, the old glazes were removed, the bed and curtains were transformed from violet to blue, and the apostles' garments were changed. Recent examination of the altarpiece has established that the condition of the painting is good and that the original paint has been preserved except in those areas which are restored. See Janssens de Bisthoven and Parmentier, *Le Musée communal de Bruges*, p. 53.

Color of course had a symbolic aspect based upon liturgical color canons. Blue signified hope, green, regeneration, red, love and white, purity. The pervasive use of blue in the *Death of the Virgin* underscores one of the altarpiece's principal themes, hope in eternal life.

59. As a rule the appropriate color for Mary's feasts was white but blue was apparently also used.

60. Michael Baxandall, *Giotto and the Orators. Humanist Observers of Painting in Italy and the Discovery of Pictorial Composition* (Oxford: Clarendon Press, 1971), p. 1 ff.

61. Baxandall, *Giotto and the Orators, passim*.

62. Leon Battista Alberti, *On Painting*, trans. J.R. Spencer, rev. ed. (New Haven, London: Yale University, 1966); Michael Baxandall, *Painting and Experience in Fifteenth Century Italy* (Oxford, 1972) pp. 114 ff.

63. Baxandall, *Painting and Experience*, pp. 134–135.

64. The Last Rites are divisible into two ceremonies, extreme unction and the *commendatio animae*. The former, a sacrament, cleanses the dying person of venial sin whereas

the latter is a ceremony of prayer commending the soul to God. Performed after extreme unction, the *commendatio animae* is carried out as the person actually dies.

65. Holzherr, *Die Darstellung des Marientodes*, p. 21 ff. discusses the deliberate paralleling in late medieval art between Mary's death and Christ's. To suggest the similarity, the motif of the crouching soldiers guarding Christ's tomb were transformed into the seated and kneeling apostles at the foot of Mary's bed.

66. For the prominence accorded St. Peter in the celebration of the Last Rites, see Holzherr, *Die Darstellung des Marientodes*, pp. 39–46.

67. Post, *Modern Devotion*, p. 545.

68. For the *chiropsalterium* see Pierre Debongnie, *Jean Mombaer de Bruxelles, Abbé de Livry. Ses Ecrits et ses Reformes* (Louvain, Toulouse: 1927), pp. 172–184.

69. Wittkower, *Born under Saturn*, p. 111 are the only scholars who have attempted to discover connections between van der Goes's art and the beliefs of the Windesheim Congregation. The Wittkowers observed that ". . . strangely enough, modern students have not noticed that in his interpretations of the Holy Stories he was profoundly indebted to the teaching of Thomas à Kempis."

70. McCloy, *Ofhuys Chronicle*, p.16.

The "Epidemia Rheumatica" Described by Lancisi (1711)

SAUL JARCHO, M.D.*

As numerous bibliographies and indices tell us, the history of public health is one of the many areas which Dr. George Rosen illuminated by his industrious investigations. This subject was never far from the center of his thoughts. Accordingly, I hope that he would have been interested in this essay, which I have written as a complement and compliment to his researches.

The fame of Giovanni Maria Lancisi (1654–1720) exempts the essayist from the need to burden the editor, the publisher, and the reader with Lancisi's complete *curriculum vitae*. It is sufficient to recall that Lancisi was an excellent student of the classics; that he was diverted from theology to the sciences; that he was graduated from the *Sapienza* at Rome at age eighteen; and that he professed anatomy there for thirteen years.

In 1688 he began a long period of service or servitude as papal physician. Just as his work as professor of anatomy included not only teaching and research in normal anatomy but extended also to pathologic anatomy and probably to physiology—such being the scope of anatomical study at that time—his services to the popes required him to act not only as personal physician to the pontiffs, but also as advisor to the Vatican on problems of public health, research, and publication.

These complex and onerous responsibilities, of which he complained to his friend Morgagni, are reflected in Lancisi's writings. In 1705 and 1706 an apparent increase in the incidence of sudden death at Rome impelled Pope Clement XI to order an investigation by Lancisi. The research, as is well known, was partly epidemiological but chiefly anatomical and was embodied in Lancisi's famous treatise on sudden death, the *De Subitaneis Mortibus* (1707). Much later, in 1728, it was to find full development in the posthumous volume *De Motu Cordis et Aneurysmatibus*.

Between 1711 and 1717 Lancisi published three epidemiological works: his treatise on the Roman climate (*Dissertatio de Nativis, deque Adventitiis Romani Coeli Qualitatibus*, Rome, 1711); his book on bovine plague (*Dissertatio Historica de Bovilla Peste ex Campaniae Finibus Anno MDCCXIII Latio Importata,* Rome, 1715); and the treatise on noxious emanations from swamps (*De Noxiis Paludum Effluviis,* Rome, 1717). These three works can be regarded as a crescendo, in that the first—which forms the subject of the present analysis—is scarcely known, whereas the second is mentioned occasionally, and the third is accepted as a classic contribution.

Let us now return to the first of the three treatises. In true eighteenth-century style, its ample title comes close to being a table of contents:

> *JO. MARIAE LANCISII*
> *Intimi Cubicularii, & Archiatri Pontificii*
> *DISSERTATIO*
> *De Nativis, deque Adventitiis*
> *Romani Coeli Qualitatibus,*
> *Cui Accedit*
> *HISTORIA*
> *Epidemiae Rheumaticae, quae per hyemem*
> *Anni MDCCIX. vagata est.*
> *Romae,*
> *Apud Franciscum Gonzagum MDCCXI.*
> *Superiorum Permissu.*

The English translation is less stately but no less informative:

> *By Johannes Maria Lancisi/Domestic Councillor and Chief Papal Physician/a Treatise/on the Natural and Adventitious/Qualities of the Roman Climate,/to which is added/a History/of the Rheumatic Epidemic, which during the winter/of the year 1709 was disseminated. . . .*

As its title shows, the volume contains two essays. The first, on the natural and adventitious qualities of the Roman climate, runs to 190 pages, divided into 31 chapters. Its text opens with a discussion of the individual winds, e.g., the *sirocco* and the *auster,* and the general healthfulness of Roman waters. Next comes a systematic, quantitative analysis of individual waters, such as those in the baths of Diocletian, those in the Tiber, and those on the Janiculum. The analyses attempt gravimetric determination of the waters and qualitative analysis of the sediments. Then, in two intercalated chapters, Lancisi discusses the prevalence of aged persons as evidence of general salubrity.

In the remainder of the essay, Lancisi discusses what he calls the "adventitious" factors in the Roman climate, by which he means the features that have been added or modified by man. Accordingly, he summarizes the ancient, medieval, and modern history of public health in Rome, with emphasis on official civil or ecclesiastical actions. Then he discusses the baths, the mines of sulphur and vitriol, and the drainage of swamps and ponds, especially after flooding.

The remaining 65 pages of the text form a separate treatise, amply titled (in English translation) "The rheumatic epidemic which, with acute fevers, raged at Rome especially in the winter of the year 1709; together with a history of the actions that were taken through the foresight and vigilance of the Most Holy Father Clement XI to investigate, correct, and forestall the causes of the disease. Described by the same Johannes Maria Lancisi. . . ."

What was the "rheumatic epidemic," announced on Lancisi's title-page with this fanfare of phrases and clauses?

The text, Coan in its major inspiration, opens (p. 193) with a thoroughly Hippocratic comment to the effect that changes of weather should be given special attention in connection with epidemics. With this sound advice Ballonius, Sylvius, Sydenham, Ramazzini, and various obscure fuglemen had agreed. In accordance with Hippocratic admonition, Lancisi points out that the summer of 1708 was followed by a warm autumn. His statement is *calidumque experti sumus, ut producta velut aestas,* an elegant Latin description of what Americans call an Indian summer. Soon the pleasant weeks gave way to the inordinately severe winter of 1708–1709. Then epidemic diseases of the chest— *epidemici pectoris morbi*—appeared. At the beginning these consisted of coryzas and rheums *(rheumata)* with slight cough. In the sixteenth and seventeenth centuries, such diseases were apt to be dubbed *morbus castronis.*

A few comments on nomenclature must now be made. Lancisi's reference to coryzas and rheums as diseases of the *chest* suggests abandonment of the long-lived Greek opinion that such diseases came from the head and caused humors to drip down into the thorax. Second, the term *castronis* (p. 196)—condemned by Lancisi and others—is easily mistaken for typhus *(morbus castrensis,* camp fever), or the *febris castrensis* —mainly malaria—later discussed by Lancisi in his book on swamp fevers, or the so-called camp fevers that were described by J. J. Woodward during the American Civil War.[1] Lancisi demonstrates the great age of the term *castronis* by citing authors of the two preceding centuries. The great Italian etymological dictionary of Battisti and Alessio[2] does not record an Italian cognate of this word. It presents *castrense* as a seventeenth-century word used for a disease that is propagated by encampments.

By the end of January 1709, the outbreak had increased in severity. The manifestations now included pain in the chest, angina—pharyngitis, not angina pectoris—pleurisy, and true pneumonia. Other features were initial lassitude followed by fever and chills, cough, reddish or turbid urine, dyspnea, and a yellow color resembling that of jaundice.

Inmates of the prison of the Holy Inquisition escaped the disease, allegedly because the building was protected from the north wind and was near a furnace. In the populace at large, women were less often attacked than men. Many patients recovered after having had nosebleeds, sweats, diarrhea, or diuresis.

The vaguely described postmortem findings (p. 198) are not devoid of significance. The precordia—perhaps this means the epicardium, the pericardium, or the substernal tissues—as far as the diaphragm were red and were blackened by coagulated blood, and there were "polyps" (coagula) in the great vessels. It was inferred from these observations that the patients suffered especially from fluids stagnating in the lungs. This interpretation probably is derived from ancient humoral doctrine, but it may also reflect Lancisi's interest in the stagnation of swamps, ponds, and other terrestrial waters. There is no mention of pleural effusion or of anything resembling pulmonary edema.

The long introductory explanations prepare the reader for a nineteen-page statement (pp. 204–222) in which Lancisi gives his opinion about the nature, causes, and remedies of the rheumatic epidemic. Whereas the introductory remarks, already summarized, make us suspect that the "rheumatic" disease of 1708–1709 was an epidemic—and presumably viral—infection of the respiratory tract, Lancisi in his statement of opinion offers a fact (p. 206) that is additionally significant to the modern reader, *viz.*, that the outbreak affected not only Rome and Italy, but nearly all of [Western] Europe. The "epidemia rheumatica," therefore, was almost certainly *pandemic influenza.* Hence, it is no surprise to find the outbreak listed in the tabulations of the faithful August Hirsch in his chapter on influenza.[3] Indeed Hirsch,[4] following Corradi and others, mentions "general diffusion" in Italy, France, Belgium, Germany, and Denmark. Corradi uses the term "influenza catarrale".[5]

After mentioning the wide dissemination in Europe, Lancisi reiterates that the epidemic disease was of rheumatic character. In individual cases the illness started with simple pain in the chest unaccompanied by fever or with coryza accompanied by cough, but in those who harbored a hidden collection of noxious humors *in quibus noxii humores collecti latent*—this refers to a preexisting latent reservoir of harmful humors—the disease soon became an acute fever, to which were added inflammations of the throat or larynx or pleura of all the precordial organs. Hence, says Lancisi (p. 207), it is very clear that in the outbreak under discussion the principal disease is fever and its symptoms are inflammations *(constat . . . febrem morbum esse praecipuum, cujus symptomata sunt ejusmodi inflammationes)*. Moreover, the diversity of anatomical findings in different autopsies (p. 207) does not imply diversity of cause but merely evidences diversity of habitus.

In analyzing this explanation of pathogenesis, it is necessary to consider several subtleties in the meanings of words. In the passages just cited, the term *febris* should not be interpreted as fever in the sense of a simple elevation of body temperature. Instead, it should be taken to mean a febrile affection, just as malaria and typhoid are designated as fevers. Hence, Lancisi's dictum should be translated into the statement that the principal disease is a febrile disease and its symptoms are inflammations. In this version it seems less startling.

Lancisi's use of the word *symptoma* presents greater difficulties. Liddell and Scott's *Greek-English Lexicon* defines this word as *"anything that happens, a chance occurrence . . . mishap, mischance . . . property, attribute . . . in diseases, symptom. . . ."* In the present context we are justified in disregarding the attribution to chance and are obliged to retain the last-mentioned meaning, *viz.,* symptom. In modern practise we are not in the habit of saying that pleurisy is a symptom of influenza. We are more likely to designate it as a complication, a sequel, or perhaps a manifestation. Whatever the term chosen, the pleurisy is regarded as subordinate to the influenza. To this extent Lancisi's concept agrees with ours.

Lancisi's use of the term *symptoma* agrees with that of Boerhaave and Blancardus. The former[6] states, somewhat less than clearly, that a symptom is something abnormal which in the sick body arises from disease and is caused by it, yet can be distinguished from the disease itself and from its proximate cause. Blancardus the lexicographer[7] says that a symptom is an abnormal thing *(res contra naturam)* that arises from a disease in the body. It is, he adds, either a disease that has arisen from a disease or a cause that has arisen from a disease.

Lancisi's use of the term *rheumatica* obviously derives from the old concept of *rheuma,* a flux. In the present instance the flux was a nasal and faucial discharge, whereas, as is well known, our use of the term 'rheumatic fever' commemorates the old idea of a flux into joints.

It is interesting that the Spanish language retains the cognate forms *romadizarse* and *romadizo.* In the current, nineteenth edition of the *Diccionario de la Lengua Española* issued by the Royal Spanish Academy (Madrid, 1970, p. 1154), these words are presented as follows:

> romadizarse. (Del Lat. *rheumatizare,* y este del gr. *rheumatizo, de rheuma, -atos,* flujo) . . . Contraer romadizo.
>
> romadizo. (De *romadizarse.*) m. Catarrho de la membrana pituitaria.

These forms are akin to the French *rhume* and *enrhumer.*

When he explains the etiology (pp. 208 ff.) of the rheumatic epidemic, Lancisi involves himself in intricacies of hypothesis, and his sentences become long and tortuous. This stylistic shift is often to be observed in Latin medical authors when they turn from clinical fact to medical theory, the thread of Ariadne being long and anfractuous.

During the mild autumn of 1708, Lancisi says, the volatile and igneous salts of the atmosphere became diluted and tempered, and became mixed with the fluids of the human body, especially the bile, a substance which becomes excessively incandescent under the influence of heat. Hence, a collection of harmful humors was formed in persons who were naturally weak or careless, or did not know how to correct the "exalted" (sublimated, strengthened) juices by a suitable regimen. Hence, the internal cause of the disease began to be accumulated and prepared.

Such was the harm that the autumn of 1708 had inflicted. The sudden severe winter of 1708–1709 added two pathogenic components. The cold interrupted all transpiration, both external transpiration from the skin and internal transpiration, especially that from the nose, throat, and lungs. In addition the force of the cold and the wind drove exogenous salts, mixed with air, into the body. "Experimental philosophers" (unnamed) had considered these salts to be nitrous and subacid. The admixture of volatile igneous salts with nitrous subacid salts (p. 209) readily produced fevers, which differed according to the constitutions of individual patients. At the same time the simple salt of the atmosphere caused stagnation of lymph in parts of the body that were in contact with the air or were infirm because of previous disease. Hence, the diversity of local morbid effects.

Those who have even a moderate knowledge of chemistry and anatomy, says Lancisi (p. 210), know that one and the same nitrous principle can produce widely differing effects in different parts of the body, e.g., puncture of nerves, disturbances of circulation, and stagnation of lymph.

While a complete analysis of Lancisi's proposed etiology is beyond the scope of the present study, several characteristics require mention. First, the alleged cause of the epidemic is chemical. Second, the allegations as to chemical causes are not supported by any definite evidence; Lancisi merely refers in a vague way to "experimental philosophers." Third, Lancisi's reasoning includes elements of observed fact, such as clinical observations, observations of incidence and distribution, anatomical observations, and simple observations of weather. Fourth, his hypothesis attempts to embrace all these kinds of fact. Fifth, his hypothesis is presented *as a fact.* As is so often the case in literature of the eighteenth and earlier centuries, fact and hypothesis are not distinguished as sharply as twentieth-century science requires. Sixth, there is no mention or consideration of facts that refute the hypothesis or in any way oppose it, and there is no mention of any observation that the hypothesis fails to explain. Seventh, Lancisi's reasoning, as might be expected, contains elements derived from ancient humoralism. Eighth, the influence of Hippocrates and Galen is all-pervasive.

It should be added that Lancisi's opinions are approximately the same as those to be found in the writings of his contemporaries. His doctrine is not to be construed as original.

Lancisi's conclusions, which I have attempted to summarize as briefly as possible,[8] contain nothing that can be considered an addition to knowledge. Their value lies in the clarity with which they exemplify the condition of epidemiology in 1711 and in the distinctness with which they reveal the thoughts and actions of an energetic, mature eighteenth-century investigator supported by a humanitarian and liberal pontiff. All of these components were soon to reappear—heightened and accentuated—in the great *De Noxiis Paludum Effluviis.*

Notes

*Investigation assisted by National Institutes of Health (LM-02561).

1. J.J. Woodward, *Outlines of the Chief Camp Diseases of the United States Armies* (Philadel-

phia: Lippincott, 1863; New York: Hafner, 1964). For an introduction to contemporary epidemiological thought, see W.G. Smillie, *Public Health Its Promise for the Future* (New York: Macmillan, 1955).

2. C. Battisti and G. Alessio, *Dizionario Etimologico Italiano* (Florence: Barbera, n.d. (1968?)), p. 800.

3. A. Hirsch, *Handbook of Geographical and Historical Pathology*, translated by Charles Creighton (London: New Sydenham Society, 1883–1886), I, p. 9, s.v. 1709.

4. Hirsch, *l. c.*, pp. 9, 43.

5. A. Corradi, *Annali delle Epidemie Occorse in Italia* (reprinted, Bologna: Forni, n. d. (1972–1973)), II, 307.

6. H. Boerhaave, *Institutiones Medicae*, S. 801, in his *Opera Omnia Medica* (Venice: Basilius, 1757), p. 112.

7. S. Blancardus, *Lexicon Medicum* (Jena: 1683; Hildesheim: Olms, 1973), pp. 462–463.

8. I omit from consideration Lancisi's suggestions as to therapeutics (pp. 217–221), based mainly on Hippocrates, Sydenham, and Willis, his simple recommendations as to prevention (pp. 221–222), and the official edicts (pp. 248–258) that were issued.

Health and Mental Health in the Thought of Philippe Pinel: The Emergence of Psychiatry during the French Revolution*

. . .il ne faut qu'un homme de génie pour donner
une nouvelle impulsion à l'esprit humain . . .
Philippe Pinel, 1793

. . . during the first half of the nineteenth century
. . . ideas of public service, public interest, and
social utility provided the seed-bed in which ger-
minated new views on the relations between
health, medicine, and society.
George Rosen, 1956

DORA B. WEINER*

As Western Europe entered the nineteenth century, preoccupation with health moved from the periphery to the center of private and
public concern. Advances in the basic and the medical sciences raised
hopes for reform of sanitation, nutrition, nursing, hospital and medical
care, therapy and disease prevention. A sense of urgency pervaded the
Enlightenment, particularly in France, where many feared violent social conflict. And indeed the French Revolution was fundamentally and
permanently to affect the development of medicine and health care.[1]

In a recent book, Michel Foucault has argued that the pursuit of
adequate health care for the people deepened the chasm between
"noso-politicians," who considered disease as a social and national
problem, and the physicians of the "medical market-place" intent on
a "clinical medicine strongly concentrated on individual examination,
diagnosis and therapy, with its explicit moral and scientific (but se-

The author wishes to record her gratitude to the following colleagues who have kindly given this
manuscript a critical reading: John Burnham, William Coleman, Nancy Frieden, Gerald N. Grob,
Y. Violé O'Neill and particularly the editor, Charles E. Rosenberg.

59

cretly economic) exaltation of the 'doctor-patient relationship' [*le 'colloque singulier'*]."[2] The socio-medical reformers wished to turn hospitals into "curing machines," the title of Foucault's book. The reader is startled to find that "curing machines" is an expression taken from Jacques Tenon, the great humanitarian revered by all historians of late eighteenth-century hospital reform, the very same Tenon who called the *Hôtel-Dieu de Paris* the "sanctuary of humanity."[3]

Foucault's thesis confronts the historian with two questions: first, whether late eighteenth-century French physicians can indeed be divided into those who pursued private practice and high fees, and another group of medical men preoccupied with the public health, including hospitalization for the poor. And secondly and more interestingly, whether medicine practiced on large numbers of people can be divorced from the pattern of individual examination, diagnosis, and therapy that Foucault stigmatizes as self-seeking—whether there are two ways of practicing medicine or not.

In an attempt to clarify our understanding of eighteenth-century medical views of sickness and health, it seemed promising to analyze the early writings of the greatest French clinician of that era, written before he reached prominence in Paris in 1793, at the height of the Terror. This paper tries to assess the concepts of health and mental health held by Philippe Pinel (1745–1826) at a unique historic moment when he found himself catapulted, at age 48, into the post of physician-in-chief of the Bicêtre Hospital. He had never before held a full-time job. He had published only brief and seemingly unconnected papers. During fifteen years residence in Paris, he had made some friends but joined only one major scientific society. He was unsuccessful and virtually unknown. And yet, within the next decade, Pinel helped revolutionize clinical teaching and laid the foundation of modern psychiatry.

Without the French Revolution Philippe Pinel would have died unknown. Without the reorganization of Parisian hospitals, he would have remained a theorist. Without the creation of the new revolutionary medical schools, he would have lacked students. Conversely, had his medical philosophy not been mature by 1789, the turmoil, confusion, violence, and emotional tone of the times would have precluded its rational elaboration. Pinel perfected his philosophy of medicine, a philosophy fundamental to modern psychiatry, during his long years of clerical, scientific, medical, and post-doctoral education in Toulouse, Montpellier, and Paris, at the high tide of the Enlightenment. After his appointment as hospital director in 1793, and particularly after he began teaching as Professor of Medical Physics and Hygiene at the Paris Health School in 1794, he published his three major books in rapid succession: *Philosophic Nosography* in 1798, *Treatise on Insanity* in 1801, *Clinical Medicine* in 1802.[4] His insistence on detailed and continuing case histories, the segregation of major syndromes for careful observation and treatment, the proscription of chains in favor of the straitjacket, the extensive use of the "moral method" (psychological therapy), the utilization of the asylum itself as a "therapeutic instrument"—these are models for modern psychiatry.

Pinel's career from 1793 till his death in 1826 is public knowledge, but his first 48 years are difficult to document. One is surprised to find that his biography remains unwritten.[5] Educated Frenchmen of the Revolutionary and Napoleonic era would have been dissatisfied with our modern, much publicized, image of Pinel the liberator, who struck the chains off the insane at the Salpêtrière. They knew Pinel primarily as a clinician, admired and loved by medical students for a quarter of a century; they knew him as a classifier, the author of the *Philosophic Nosography* of 1798. To the highly educated French public of his time, Pinel was a philosopher, an Ideologue.[6] His *Nosography,* a classification of disease according to a logical, orderly, comprehensive scheme, was a typical eighteenth-century attempt to subdivide a whole field of learning into neatly delimited areas, to group similar instances so as to facilitate generalization, in a word, to apply Francis Bacon's inductive method to medical diagnosis. Like Linnaeus in botany, Lavoisier and Priestley in chemistry, or Thomas Syndenham in medicine, Philippe Pinel in his *Philosophic Nosography* ordered, labelled, and categorized. A whole generation of medical students gratefully memorized his textbook.

Although steeped in the classical tradition—Hippocratic, Aristotelian, Stoic, and Patristic—Pinel cast his lot with modern medical science. He practiced the therapeutic skepticism and emphasis on observation so important to the Ideologues. This placed him in the broad stream of sensationalist philosophers descended from John Locke, represented in late eighteenth-century France by the disciples of the Abbé de Condillac. At Montpellier Pinel came to see medicine as a science distinct from the other sciences. Influenced by his teacher Barthez, a vitalist, Pinel eventually moved from iatromechanism towards the anthropologic dimensions of medicine. He was entirely in sympathy with the projects for reform then being passionately debated by physicians and wished to help transform medicine into a respected modern science, the "science of man."[7]

A biographer may scan the official life and the books published by this great physician for the facts about a career that began in 1793. But about the first 50 years of Pinel's life he would learn little; nor would official eulogies and centenary celebrations be of much help. The two official "éloges," at the Academy of Sciences by Georges Cuvier,[8] and at the Academy of Medicine by Etienne Pariset,[9] skim over Pinel's early years. And the plethora of brief, general articles, particularly those occasioned by the centenary of his death in 1926, predictably lack new information.[10] And yet, since Pinel reorganized the two major Parisian mental hospitals with speed and a sure touch, helped create modern clinical teaching, and wrote his three major books within four years, his medical thought must have been fully formed by 1793.

Four studies have been devoted to the mental, intellectual, and emotional growth of this great man before he reached Paris in 1778: Two of these focus on Pinel's psychiatric ideas;[11] the other two analyze his early education in great depth.[12] Nevertheless, there remains a conspicuous gap in our knowledge of Pinel before 1793. Except for a brief paper on his life in Paris between 1778 and 1793 by Pierre Chabbert, a French internist and the ranking Pinel scholar at this moment,[13] we lack information on the fifteen years during which Pinel acquired a post-doctoral education in Paris.

He was then a mature man, between the ages of 33 and 48, living at a unique and brilliant moment in human thought and culture; a rare concentration of talent, originality, daring, scientific progress, passionate dedication to human betterment, elegance, and refinement had created an intellectual milieu of unsurpassed stimulation. Whoever had not known Paris before the French Revolution, said Talleyrand, would never taste the pleasure of being alive.

In 1778, when Pinel walked to the capital from Montpellier in the company of a British student, his most precious baggage was his encyclopedic education.[14] Because of his precocious intelligence and his family's modest means, the teen-aged Pinel had begun his studies in 1762 with the Pères de la Doctrine Chrétienne at Lavaur, some 20 miles from Toulouse. Besides teaching Greek, Latin, and the traditional trivium and quadrivium, the Pères de la Doctrine enriched the curriculum with contemporary subject matter: Their teaching of grammar and rhetoric included modern literature, and their logic blended into philosophy. Arithmetic and geometry led them into physics, as did astronomy. Although the school did not yet have a laboratory, a microscope may have been available, and the botanical garden no doubt opened Pinel's eyes to natural history. He had always loved nature and, twice a week, walked the ten miles from school to his home. He even went hunting with his father, though not without a favorite book— Virgil, Horace, Cicero, or Tactitus—in his pocket. As a bachelor of arts, at 21, he moved on to Toulouse.

College meant the study of theology and mathematics; college also meant expenses for tuition, board, and lodging. Pinel always earned his own living: in Toulouse as a tutor in mathematics and philosophy. Three of his four younger brothers joined him to study surgery, the profession of their father and grandfather; in April, 1770 Pinel enrolled in his first medical school course. This was soon followed by the study of pharmacy, chemistry, biology, and botany, and the license and finally the doctorate of medicine, on December 21, 1773.

We do not know whether abandoning a clerical career meant an emotional wrench for the young man: he had taken no vows, although he had worn the clerical frock and bonnet for seven or eight years. Most likely he experienced an evolution common in those days when bright boys were sent to the schools of the Catholic teaching orders to receive a fine education. Few of the youngsters felt a real religious vocation. In any case, Pinel's change from theology to medical science did not signify a break with the past. Rather, it added Hippocrates, Galen, and Pliny to his beloved classical authors. It widened his concern from education and the care of souls, to man's physical existence and well-being within the natural environment. The transition was possibly initiated by the study of mathematics, especially geometry, for Pinel developed a life-long interest in structure. His first two papers were entitled: "On the Talent Needed to Apply Mathematics to the Human Body," and "On the Curves our Extremities Describe in their Various Movements."[15]

Both were read to the Royal Society of Sciences in Montpellier where Pinel moved in 1774, after he had learned all that Toulouse could teach him. His object in Montpellier was not to earn another medical degree but to broaden his knowledge: He attended lectures, studied in the excellent library, and followed medical rounds at the local hospital as he had done at Toulouse. To obtain a clear clinical picture for each patient, he began writing case histories. He trained himself in careful regular observation and meticulously recorded changed symptoms in each patient. Again, he earned a living as a tutor;

and in Montpellier he made friends who would be crucial to his career. He taught the brother of Pierre Bénézech (1775–1802), the future Minister of Internal Affairs under the Directory,[16] and became fast friends with another of his students, Jean-Antoine Chaptal (1756–1832), who would be Napoleon's Minister of Internal Affairs from 1801 to 1804. The help of these powerful supporters would be vital to Pinel's success as a hospital administrator in Paris.

It is not surprising that his quest for knowledge drove Pinel to Paris, the unique center of intellectual life in the French Enlightenment. In 1778 Rousseau, Voltaire, and Linnaeus died; Louis XVI and Marie Antoinette had been reigning for four years; Anton Mesmer came to Paris; Lavoisier and Guyton-Morveau were reforming chemistry; Condorcet and d'Alembert broke new ground in mathematics; Buffon was publishing his 44-volume *Natural History;* the *Encyclopédie* had recently been completed; Vicq d'Azyr headed the reform-oriented Royal Society of Medicine; Benjamin Franklin was gaining support for the new United States of America; Beaumarchais was preparing the *Marriage of Figaro.* In the Parisian salons, coffeehouses, theaters, academies, and learned societies, a unique intellectual stimulation awaited an eager provincial scholar.

Pinel did not go to Paris to seek success or fame, but to continue his education. He studied botany with his friend Desfontaines, chemistry with d'Arcet and Fourcroy at the Royal Gardens, attended lectures on Virgil at the Collège de France and meetings at the Academy of Sciences, followed the medical rounds of Desault at the Hôtel-Dieu, and socialized at the salon of Helvétius' widow at Auteuil where he met Franklin, Condorcet, Lavoisier, and Thouret—Michel-Augustin Thouret (1748–1810) who would become the first dean of the revolutionary medical school in 1794 and who would serve, with Pinel's friends P.-J.-G. Cabanis (1757–1808) and J.-A.-J. Cousin (1738–1800), on the three-man commission for Parisian hospitals during the Revolution. The groundwork for Pinel's career was being laid.

Meanwhile, Pinel, of course, continued to educate himself in obscurity and virtual isolation. Among all the learned societies that flourished in Paris, he joined only that for Natural History. It is instructive to find that Pinel's name does not appear among the members of the Agricultural or the Philomatic Society, and the Royal Society of Medicine (the group from which the reform of modern medical education originated), or the French Academy. These societies were quite large; their purposes coincided with Pinel's interests; he knew some of their members; and he was surely learned enough to be eligible. But he lacked powerful connections and political backing. He tried twice for the Diest prize—which would have permitted him to pursue the Paris medical doctorate gratis; he failed in 1782 and 1784. The jury's report for the 1784 examination reads in part:

> We judge that M. Pinel has scant learning and cannot easily be awarded the prize. In anatomy he carries little weight; in physiology he is better but far from remarkable; in surgery he does not stand out, either for theory or manual skill. He knows little chemistry, scarcely more medicine and pharmacy, and his deficiencies are numerous. . . . He has adequate notions in general pathology, but whenever related issues are raised, he seems to us to turn in endless circles. . . .
>
> . . . in the midst of all these difficulties one last hope remained: to analyze and develop the written questions . . . prove his wealth of medical knowledge, the skill and insight he had lacked in the oral test. Alas, this hope was dashed. . . .[17]

It is difficult, at a distance of 200 years, to pass judgment on the fairness of a jury. The running battle waged by the Paris Medical Faculty against the innovative ideas and practices of the Royal Society of Medicine in the 1770s and '80s suggests that Pinel may have been the victim of guilt by association. It is also true, however, that many biographers mention Pinel's awkward manner, his poor verbal delivery, his extreme reserve in social situations, his unprepossessing looks. Cuvier reports that Desfontaines once tried to secure for his impecunious colleague a post as physician to members of the royal family. The visit with the king's first physician, Louis-Guillaume Lemonnier, was quite lengthy: Pinel never said a word: ". . . his cursed timidity made him dumb . . . he gave the wrong impression and did not get the job. . . ."[18] He felt acutely ill at ease in the brilliant Parisian world of the Enlightenment, just as Jean-Jacques Rousseau had 30 years earlier. Also like Rousseau, he put pen to paper.

Pinel continued his life as a student, supporting himself as a tutor, as a ghost writer of medical theses, as an occasional medical practitioner, as a translator from the Latin and the English (Cullen, Baglivi, and four volumes of the *Transactions* of the Royal Society),[19] and as a medical journalist. In 1785 he presented to the Academy of Sciences a paper entitled "On the Application of Mathematics to the Human Body and on the Mechanism of Dislocations," later elaborated in detailed studies.[20]

At the beginning of this paper, Pinel emphasized the importance of knowing the *normal* structure when a physician wished to reduce a dislocated joint: "In order to remedy any kind of derangement, is not the natural approach first to form an accurate and precise idea concerning the disordered part?" This thought would guide Pinel's later work in psychiatry. He clearly identified himself as a "Modern" (in their controversy with the "Ancients") and argued for experience and dexterity in a surgeon against complex, antiquated machinery: ". . . no levers, pulleys or winches";[21] and he added that the physicians of antiquity were often brilliant but restricted to "the knowledge of their own times."[22]

From geometric structure, Pinel progressed to comparative anatomy, and he contributed studies on the shape of the elephant's head,[23] and on a new method for classifying quadrupeds based on the build and articulation of the jaw.[24] His methodology heralds that of a paper he published in 1800, entitled "Observations on the Insane and Their Division into Distinct Species."[25]

Pinel's interest in probability and statistics motivated some of his therapeutic strategies, as for example when, in 1803, as a member of the Vaccination Committee, he helped devise plans for preventing the spread of smallpox,[26] or when, in 1807, he submitted to the National Institute his "Observations and Tables to Determine the Degree of Probability for the Cure of Mental Patients."[27] Cuvier referred to Pinel in his eulogy before the Academy of Sciences—rather unkindly, I think —as a "geometer turned physician."[28]

While mathematics remained one of Pinel's lifelong sources of inspiration, he considered himself, in the early 1790s, a zoologist. In a paper on the preservation of quadrupeds and birds for natural history collections, he spoke of zoology as the science "with which I am more specially concerned."[29] And it was the Section for Zoology that eventually elected him to the National Institute in 1803—perhaps because this was the first available seat after Pinel had unsuccessfully competed against Georges Cuvier for the chair in comparative anatomy at the Museum of Natural History.

Thus, a passion to observe precisely and at length, an inclination to compare, and the ability to apply mathematical skills to science underlay Pinel's activities as a naturalist and physician during the years of his post-doctoral education. Yet, however involved he was in mathematics and the natural sciences, he agreed with the reformers at the Royal Society of Medicine in regarding medicine as a science in its own right: In his view, studies in the natural sciences and mathematics retained their importance for the physician, but as "accessory" to expertise in medicine. Significantly, he was to apply this point of view to mental as well as somatic illness. Raymond de Saussure has pointed out that Pinel was the first to make a systematic study of the "characteristic variations common to all mental diseases, namely variations of attention, memory, imagination and judgment," that he broke new ground when he described a case of mania in its daily manifestations, and that his insistence on observation and his rejection of every metaphysical hypothesis identified him as a scientist in medicine, and therefore as an innovator.[30]

Mathematics, natural history, clinical medicine, and Stoic philosophy have so far been identified as foci of Pinel's interests in the '70s and '80s. One should add a first glimmer of what one might justifiably call a concern for psychiatry—even though neither the term nor the field then existed. Pinel was shaken when a seriously depressed friend for whom he had been caring committed suicide in 1785. He also supervised the treatment of some mental patients in a private clinic.[31] Not until 1792, however, did he win a prize—not a first prize—for an essay submitted to the Royal Society of Medicine in answer to this question: "Indicate the Most Effective Means for Treating Patients Who Have Become Insane before Reaching Old Age."[32]

The diversity and disparity of topics treated by Pinel sometimes even verged on the trivial—as in the discourse on stuffing birds previously cited, or in a disquisition on improving laundry procedures that he described in *La médecine éclairée par les sciences physiques*.[33] One is puzzled by the spectacle of a mature and brilliant man living in a stimulating intellectual environment who is seemingly unable to commit himself to any major theme or labor. Perhaps it was precisely his many interests and what we would call a "psychosomatic" concept of human ailments, that prevented him for years from choosing any one approach. Others, it is true, published papers and even books of medical philosophy based on as thin a clinical experience as his. For Pinel, only wide exposure to clinical reality would eventually trigger the writer's creative impulse.

The apparent lack of a major theme in the thought of this outstanding physician before he reached age 50 seemed puzzling enough to warrant a close reading of all of Pinel's minor writings of the '70s, '80s, and '90s—of what has been called his "medical journalism."[34] During those years he wrote for the *Journal de Paris,* the *Journal de physique,* and the *Encyclopédie méthodique,* contributed to Fourcroy's *Médecine éclairée par les sciences physiques* and edited the *Gazette de santé* from 1784 to 1790. I hoped that Pinel's scattered minor writings might reveal a theme that connects his encyclopedic knowledge, so congenial to Enlightenment learning, to his medical philosophy that integrated psychiatry into the spectrum of clinical specialties. And, indeed, the disconnected articles in the *Gazette,* taken together, form a short treatise on hygiene, the discipline in which Pinel would be chosen as professor at the new Paris Health School in 1794. The fragments in the *Gazette* have never been reprinted or translated, though Pedro Marset has analyzed them in Spanish. He considers them the root of Pinel's psychiatric thought. A close look at this incomplete "treatise," indeed, reveals Pinel's view of hygiene or, to give this eighteenth-century term its modern meaning, health, including public and mental health.

This quest for health as the normal condition of man was a familiar theme for the educated French public of the 1780s. Rousseau's widely-read *Emile,* for example, advocated fresh air and exercise and encouraged mothers to breastfeed their babies. Nature was fashionable in this early phase of Romanticism. In medical thought—not impervious to cultural fashion—Romanticism emphasized the healthy development of mind and body: Attention to normal growth of healthy bones and structure had given rise to the specialty of orthopedics; attention to children as individuals, their growth and education, both mental and physical, encouraged the specialty of pediatrics; the normal needs of healthy man in his natural environment made hygiene—and soon public health and preventive medicine—timely subjects. Pinel's originality, of course, rests on his having added the dimension of mental health.

A close analysis of Pinel's articles on "hygiene" confirms that the theme preoccupying him was indeed health—health seen as balance and equilibrium between human physiology and the natural environment, in the classical Hippocratic tradition; health as the expression of a life well-lived *"mens sana in corpore sano;"* health, the result of care for the six Galenic non-naturals (air, food, bodily functions, exercise, sleep, and the passions),[35] where the physician only aids the *vis medicatrix naturae;* health—and this is the most creative aspect of Pinel's work —where disturbed mental functions are seen as imbalance, just as disturbed physiologic functions are seen as imbalance. Pinel considered insanity an illness and not an aberration or a crime. He urged that the patient's active collaboration be elicited, and that the healthy part of what we might call the the ego be put to work; Pinel's ultimate aim was to allow the patient to dispense with the physician's services and manage his own health: "I am working actively on my Hygiene," Pinel had written to Desfontaines on November 27, 1784, "and, to try it out on the public, I include occasional articles in the *Health Gazette*. I even have the impression that my approach is appreciated and that it is novel. . . ."[36]

By the fall of 1784, Pinel had tried out his new theme on his readers and found the response encouraging. During the subsequent six years, he elaborated his thought in brief signed essays captioned *"Hygiene"* in the *Gazette de santé*. This unfinished *Traité d'hygiène* abounds in Hippocratic notions and, as one would expect, Roman examples are stressed throughout: Pinel often quoted Celsus, Seneca, Galen, Suetonius, Plutarch, and especially Pliny. The central theme is *moderation*.

A fundamental consideration for the maintenance of good health is diet; Pinel reports that the Romans thought oysters excellent to start a meal and served them on snow. He advocates cool food as more digestible than hot, denounces hard liquor, and warns that tea causes tooth decay.[37] Diet is a personal matter: Regular habits are not an absolute *must;* rather, "a well thought-out plan based on the immutable laws of human structure and function" should be followed.[38] "By experimenting, each person can know what diet is best for his physical well-being. Quantities will vary with individual strength and daily activity but the general precept remains valid."[39]

Pliny cites the example of a "venerable" senior citizen who, at age 77 "enjoyed the full use of his senses." He would walk and study in the morning and talk with his friends; then swim and sunbathe in the nude, after which he played tennis, took a shower, and had a sparing lunch at his "frugal table."[40]

Food led Pinel to discuss fresh air, a subject of acute interest to Enlightenment philosophers because of the recent discovery of oxygen and of Lavoisier's experiments on respiration. Current debates about hospital reform usually included a discussion concerning the quantity of "respirable air" required for each patient. Pinel considered fresh air as man's natural environment to which he should be freely exposed:

"One should never frighten anyone of an element natural to man: air is the fluid in which we live from birth to death, it is an essential source of life. . . . One can see how babies, when they are undressed, respond to this pleasure: they stretch and flex their members and an innocent joy lights up their faces. This is why loose clothing is very favorable to health."[41]

Cold air "is a powerful stimulant and tonic, if not used excessively or for too long. Nothing is more important than to get accustomed to it young." Pinel contended that "children raised in a hardy manner resist colds and catarrhs, the sad lot of those brought up too delicately."[42] Pinel urged as well that "many nervous diseases could easily be cured if patients had the energy periodically to go jogging in the fresh air."[43]

Pinel spoke with empathy about a healthy upbringing for children, although he was not to marry until 1792:[44] "There are children who are so well that it is absurd to wish to make them healthier. All one needs to do is to toughen them to withstand the variations of air and light which are their natural elements."[45] The vogue for cold baths left Pinel unimpressed; these should be "continued if the child likes them and stopped if he dislikes them."[46]

> Under present social conditions, the general rule regarding cold baths must be applied with care. . . . M. de Fourcroy [J.L. de Fourcroy, *Les enfants élevés dans l'ordre de la nature, ou abrégé de l'histoire naturelle des enfants du premier âge* (Paris: Nyon, 1775).], while congratulating himself for having applied this method to his own children, confesses however that when his first-born was fourteen-months old, he so hated cold baths that these had to be discontinued for six months. Fourcroy attributes the child's irritation and discomfort to dentition. He also admits that the same boy, born very delicate and weak, continues to have a thin and frail body, is excessively nervous, cries easily and is often depressed. . . . It is hard to detect the admirable effect of cold baths in this case," concluded Pinel. "They may have preserved the child from colds, inflammations and whooping cough, but regular exposure to fresh air might have served as well.[47]

The passage also criticizes the indiscriminate use of cold baths for therapeutic purposes in mental illness, which was routine procedure at the Hôtel-Dieu. Pinel would soon minimize this practice, though he did not abandon it.

But Pinel did not always respond innovatively. For example, in his answer to a subscriber who wrote: "You will not expect, Sir, to be asked about a topic as frivolous as dreams, and yet that is the purpose of my letter. . . . I should like to know whether medicine can prescribe a regimen that will free nervous and overly imaginative persons from the torment of exhausting and stressful dreaming." Pinel's reply was utterly conventional: Hippocrates believed that sound sleep indicates good health. Disturbed sleep requires reducing food intake by one third, gradually returning to the usual quantities. "Walking, exercise, singing and declamation will be helpful."[48]

He was serious about singing and declamation, and, of course, cited Demosthenes: "Vocal exercise has the advantage that it can be done standing, lying or sitting, indoors or outdoors, but not on a full stomach. To combine it with walking is even better."[49] The great outdoors led him to speak of the seasons, of melancholy states brought on by the winter and manic phases by the spring. Persons subject to cold and fevers in the spring should be careful to avoid the customary bleeding and purging; they should instead eat simply and little, fish and vegetables rather than meat and rich sauces: "Nothing conforms more to the laws of Hygiene than the Church's prescription for Lent in the spring, if observed with regularity it can prevent certain sicknesses."[50]

Contagious disease, Pinel suggested, was not transmitted through the air. Unlike most of his contemporaries, he believed, that "these diseases are communicated by direct or indirect contact." His practical conclusions seem eminently reasonable. "During epidemics," he urged, "one cannot insist enough on cleanliness for all persons who deal with patients, encourage them to change their clothing as completely as possible and to wash and air it after use, to wash their hands and face frequently and meticulously after having touched infected clothes and linen." Only such precautions could arrest the contagion. "Unfortunately," Pinel noted, "they were everywhere neglected."[51]

In conclusion, he defines a good doctor as "an enlightened physician with firm principles who prescribes mild remedies sparingly, who is especially sensitive to psychological indicators [*"les circonstances de l'état moral"*] and whose therapy relies heavily on diet and daily habits . . . which is what all physicians do who observe their patients with care."[52]

Pinel's views on hygiene, as recorded in the *Gazette de santé* between 1784 and 1790, thus consist mainly of conventional eighteenth-century wisdom but reveal some surprising innovations. Most progressive physicians were skeptical about frequent bleeding, purging, and strong medication. They advocated a sensible diet and exercise and believed that the seasons and the weather influenced morbidity. They emphasized careful observation of signs and symptoms.

But it is remarkable that Pinel's reflections on *hygiène* give serious attention to the psychological aspects of ill health, to mental illness as illness suitable for diagnosis and therapy. He insists on precise and continuing observation and note-taking and encourages physicians to enlist the patient himself in the pursuit of his recovery. Furthermore, Pinel is interested in children, their education and maturation, and, while completely neutral in matters of religion, firmly insists on the benefits of sobriety and morality. There is no dogmatic moralism, although obviously Pinel's injunctions are comfortingly consistent with morality and convey an ubiquitous compassion, patience, and kindness.

Pinel thus appears, on the eve of the Revolution, as a physician of mature judgment, although of relatively little clinical experience, with a humane and humanistic view of somatic and psychological pathology.

In spring 1793, when the Revolution was in full swing and the Jacobin dictatorship solidified its hold on France, Pinel, at age 48 and at the height of his creative powers, was still unemployed. He had learned that the national Society of Medicine, in order to further the impending reorganization of medical education, had proposed the following topic for one of its prize competitions: "Determine the best method of teaching practical medicine in a hospital." He submitted a 33 folio-page manuscript. (This document has since remained in the archives of the Paris Academy of Medicine unpublished, untranslated, and forgotten.[53]) The three commissioners who judged Pinel's essay in February 1793 denied him the prize. In fact, they found all the essays unexciting and withdrew the topic. The commissioners had not found original, innovative ideas in the essays they scanned. Or perhaps they had not accorded Pinel's manuscript their undivided attention: Near their meeting place in the Louvre, the trial of Louis XVI was proceeding relentlessly toward the king's execution, while radical Jacobins fought moderate Girondists for control of the four-months-old First French Republic. Judging a medical prize essay contest attentively under these conditions may well have been impossible.

Despite this rebuff, Pinel was soon to reach prominence. Five months after he submitted the essay, he was appointed physician-in-chief at the Bicêtre Hospital; two years later he received a similar post at the Salpêtrière. Pinel also obtained one of the 24 initial professorships at the Paris Health School, the chair of Medical Physics and Hygiene (exchanged the following year for that of Medical Pathology). It is possible that one of the three judges in the essay contest intervened, namely Pinel's friend Thouret, soon to become Dean of the Paris Health School and a hospital commissioner for Paris. Or perhaps the other two commissioners, Pinel's friends Cabanis and Cousin, spoke in his favor. In attempting to explain Pinel's sudden rise to influence, it must also be recalled that Pinel had a political attribute that now made him a desirable candidate—he had always appeared as a patriotic scholar, uninvolved in party politics. And, in the intense partisan atmosphere of the Years I and II, many qualified candidates for important medical posts were unacceptable to one side or the other. In Pinel's own mind, the prize essay undoubtedly constituted a magisterial claim to professorial and professional appointments for which he was eminently qualified and that the elite of the Ancien Régime had hitherto denied to him.

Pinel's manuscript summarized his generation's most "enlightened" views on the urgent need for reform in medical teaching. In essence, the reformers advocated that medical students be instructed by full-time academic clinicians in special teaching hospitals. Under the professor's watchful guidance, the students would gradually assume responsibility for the treatment of their patients. But Pinel's 33 pages say much more: He also paid detailed attention to the measures and means by which young doctors and the hospital itself can help restore health. Patients in public hospitals did not, at the time, receive the solicitude and respect that Pinel advocated. Nor was it usual for a physician to demand a homelike atmosphere for the sickroom, frequent family visits, plentiful, nutritious food, and a minimum of medication as necessary therapeutic elements. Equally unusual was his insistence that patients should be urged to move about, that each sickroom be furnished with a comfortable chair, and that patients be encouraged to get up even when still extremely weak. "One must often fight courageously against the patient's inactivity and his tendency to stay in his bed." (fol. 19) A common room for convalescents would speed recovery through

> the pleasure of company, or conversation and of several innocuous diversions; but, as soon as the progress of recovery permits, patients should go out into a garden where plants are grown and take short walks or even do a little easy gardening or other movements designed to promote the play of muscles and favor the return of their strength. . . . [In fact, the hospital should provide a place where] physical exercises can be practiced and where a pool table, swings, *bocce,* or bowling games are available; there should be space enough to permit short walks, running, jumping

and other exercises that help electrify the limbs as soon as the patient's
strength allows it. (fol. 19)

Significantly, Pinel also advocated psychological therapy [*"remèdes mo-
raux"*].

> "During the years when I visited hospitals for my education," he ex-
> plained: and when I often learned what should have been done by seeing
> what was not done, I very often found that patients responded well to
> comforting words that reassured them about their illness. Frequently left
> to themselves, abandoned to dire thoughts about their fate, often isolated
> from their parents and all they loved, disgusted by the crudity and harsh-
> ness of the servants, often plunged into the blackest depression by the
> ever present thought of a real or imagined danger, they expressed the
> liveliest gratitude toward those who empathized with their sufferings and
> tried to inspire them with confidence in their recovery. What an excellent
> remedy it is to go to their bedside and ask how they are doing, express
> an interest in their suffering, encourage them to be patient and believe
> in a prompt return to health. I should also like to put a stop to the custom
> that forces seriously ill patients to receive extreme unction and surround
> themselves with the most lugubrious images. . . . I do not mean to deprive
> pious souls of the comforts of religion . . . that they crave . . . but one
> should not worsen the dark depression of a fearful patient who sees in
> the arrival of the priest a presage of his own imminent funeral. (fol.
> 19–20)

Given his concern for the patient, Pinel cannot have been unaware that
in a teaching ward the charity patient would in fact be used as subject
matter and example for lectures, examinations, and demonstrations.
The question worried him. True, he concurs in the consensus of progressive opinion that clinical teaching is essential for medical education and that the physician-administrator's primary objective must be
to have all interesting cases transfered to the teaching ward. But Pinel
asks how often and by whom this patient might be examined. In doing
so, he adduces precedents from Leyden, Edinburgh, Vienna, and
Pavia. He discusses in detail how Maximilian Stoll (1742–1787), whom
he greatly admired, organized his teaching ward at the *Wiener Allgemeine
Krankenhaus.* The best of Stoll's advanced students were put in charge
of one patient each and were responsible for presenting this patient
when the professor came on his daily rounds. S.A. Tissot (1728–1787)
at Pavia improved on this method, Pinel thought, since he assigned to
each patient one advanced and one beginning student, and let only
these two (and, if need be, the professor) examine this patient, "so as
not to expose him to tiring and repeated examination by a large num-

ber of students which may become dangerous in serious cases" (fol. 11). Pinel argued that France must emulate these examples.

In the context of this humane, psychologically sensitive attitude toward sickness and health and of his detailed views of medical education, Pinel's initial actions, when he became physician-in-chief at Bicêtre, acquire new meaning. Confronted with suffering, cruelty, filth, and mismanagement, he resolved first to achieve cleanliness and order. He sent syphilitic patients to the Venereal Disease Hospital and other dermatologic cases to the Hôpital St. Louis. Pinel also segregated the mentally ill and established a special infirmary for those afflicted with a somatic as well as a psychological illness.

It might be well to point out that Pinel, on the threshold of an influential career, was not yet a specialist in care for the mentally ill, and that others had given more thought to the reform of mental hospitals than he.[54] In Pinel's writings up to this time one detects a humane sensitivity to the psychological concomitants of somatic illness[55] and an interest in the psychological impact of the Revolution— but mental illness and even mental anguish were not yet the foci of his concern.[56] He was, however, undoubtedly acquainted with the humane and progressive methods practiced by the Brothers of Charity,[57] and may have known that Samuel and William Tuke at the York Retreat, Vincenzo Chiarugi in Florence, and Joseph Daquin in Chambéry had been experimenting with the release of mental patients from physical restraints.[58] (The persistent legend of Pinel being the first to strike the chains off the wrists and ankles of mental patients has a small factual basis in his intervention at the Salpêtrière where he freed 80 women in 1796.)[59] His only practical experience with mental patients, it will be remembered, derived from his employment at the Maison de Santé Belhomme in the 1780s, but Pinel reported frustration rather than enlightenment because the owner did not wish his paying guests to be cured.

The decisive influence upon Pinel came from Jean-Baptiste Pussin (1796–1811), keeper of the insane at Bicêtre since 1784. Pinel repeatedly insisted on his indebtedness to this unschooled but experienced administrator and also to Madame Pussin, both of whom taught him the practical management of mental patients. Pussin had created the conditions that the Duc de la Rochefoucauld-Liancourt, leading an investigative team from the Poverty Committee of the National Constituent Assembly, encountered in 1790, and which he described as follows:[60]

The insane housed at Bicêtre . . . are considered incurable and receive no therapy. They seem generally to be treated with kindness. Their quarters consist of 178 cells and a two-story pavilion where they sleep in single beds with the exception of three double-beds . . . an administrator ["gouverneur"—Pussin] and thirteen employes work in this division. The madmen are locked into their rooms or dormitories every night, but during the whole day they are free in the courtyards, as long as they are not violent. The number of these is small and varies with the seasons: only ten out of 270 were chained, the day of our visit.

If Pussin's methods confirmed Pinel's speculations of the 1780s, and Pinel was also elaborating a classification of mental illnesses, then this would help explain both the avid interest with which Pinel observed Pussin at work during Pinel's two years at Bicêtre (1793–1795) and the extraordinary spectacle of a learned doctor apprenticing himself to an unlicensed practitioner: It was as a student of Pussin that Pinel transformed himself into a psychiatrist.

From his two-year apprenticeship at Bicêtre, Pinel proceeded to the Salpêtrière over which he presided for 30 years. He found 542 gravely ill women when he arrived in 1795 and more than 600 mental patients "piled up without order, a prey to the rapacity and ineptitude of subordinate personnel." He obtained the transfer of Pussin "to introduce and maintain in this division the strictest regulations and the most orderly service."[61] Finding the water impure, he set his student C.J.A. Schwilgué (1774–1808) to analyze it chemically; wishing to teach, he organized a 30-bed clinical ward; wanting case histories written, he called upon his most outstanding disciple J.E.D. Esquirol (1772–1840). Pinel served as resident hospital director, physician-in-chief, professor of clinical medicine, and, with growing involvement and expertise, as psychiatrist.

The creation of psychiatry as a medical specialty profited decisively from Pinel's education and experience. His *Nosographie philosophique ou Méthode de l'analyse appliquée à la médecine* (1798) provided the framework to classify all his clinical observations. The *Traité médico-philosophique sur l'aliénation mentale* (1801) divided mental patients into four categories: melancholic, manic, demented, and defective. The successively enlarged editions of *La médecine clinique rendue plus précise et plus exacte par l'application de l'analyse ou Recueil et résultats d'observations sur les maladies aigües, faites à la Salpêtrière* (1802) publicized his psychiatric observations, diagnoses, and therapy.

Without the French Revolution, it is doubtful whether these three works would have been completed—surely not in their present form. For Pinel, the Revolution opened a career commensurate with his talents, a chance to test his abstract notions against reality in the nation's largest custodial institutions, to formulate and carry out reforms, and to teach talented younger men.

A particular concept of health and mental health remained the pivot of his therapeutic thought and teaching. For example, Pinel undoubtedly tried to simulate the "healthy," "normal" home situation when he requested that a hospitalized watchmaker's tools be sent to Bicêtre so that this artisan might resume his trade. Pinel sought to enlist the healthy part of the man's mind to help in the healing process.[62] Pinel is thus seen to progress from diagnosis determined by his nosographic categories, via minute and prolonged daily observation and conversation with the patient, to a therapy where the healthy part of the patient's personality is enlisted to aid recovery: This might require discipline for a soldier, gardening for a farmer, books for a scholar, or emphasis on the patient's lifelong habits, patriotic devotion, or conjugal relationships. To Pinel, health and mental health meant a sense of balance and well-being in the patient's own terms. "I feel impelled," Pinel wrote in 1797, "to voice high praise for [the patients'] moral qualities. Nowhere, except in novels, have I seen spouses worthier of love, fathers more tender, lovers more passionate, patriots more ardent and magnanimous than in the mental hospitals during the patients' rational and calm intervals."[63] The ability to work seemed a particularly important index to renewed health. "I can usually tell at a glance during my visit, the degree of progress made toward true convalescence," Pinel explained, "by the ardor and constancy for work."[64] This belief in the therapeutic powers of work corresponded to the conviction prevalent among eighteenth-century reformers that a man's self-respect hinged on his ability to support himself and his family.

Late in life Pinel discovered legal psychiatry, a new specialty just emerging from the reforms of the Revolution. With the Napoleonic civil and criminal codes well established, it was logical that modern legal definitions and criteria would be sought for mental illness. Pinel toyed with the project of writing a *Treatise on the Legal Medicine of Insanity.*[65] In a paper of 1816 he wrote:

Medical jurisprudence relating to insanity opens a vast field for research; I shall not attempt to define it. There is no doubt that its foundations are

little known and that the limits between the respective domains of jurisprudence and medicine are still vague. In seeking to understand them,
I have often been filled with doubts and perplexity, during the twenty
years that I have successively headed the mental hospitals of both sexes.

It is hardly surprising that at age 70 Pinel did not embark on this
venture. That the study of the connection between law and psychiatry
intrigued him further proves a lifelong effort to define the limits between ill and good health, maladjustment and adequate functioning,
the socially stigmatized and their sicknesses or crimes.

Pinel's broad training in the sciences and in medicine securely
anchored his perspective on mental illness as a variation that nature
plays on the theme of health—not as a frightening exception that must
be excommunicated from human society and, as Michel Foucault
would have us believe, controlled through silence, fear, and guilt.
There is a world of difference between using the form and discipline
of the asylum for therapeutic purposes and feeding bodies into a
"curing machine." It is not possible to make Pinel fit the description
that the so-called "anti-psychiatric movement"[66] nowadays draws of
the psychiatrist, as if vague knowledge, a malevolent drive toward
mechanization, the need to manipulate human beings, and a class-
conscious disdain for the poor motivated this medical discipline.[67] The
novelty of Pinel's contribution not only hinges on his "psychosomatic"
approach—he shared this with a generation of medical Ideologues,
who, like his friend Georges Cabanis, considered the moral and physical aspects of man as closely interrelated—Pinel's innovation consisted
in categorizing mental illnesses, focusing on psychological health, and
introducing this approach into the hospital. There, he applied to large
numbers of patients the classification and methodology developed
from the study of a few. But he never lost sight of the patient as a
suffering person, which is why the students called him *"ce bon Monsieur
Pinel."* He permanently enrolled the mentally ill among the patients
whom doctors must treat, and he permanently enlisted the medical
profession in the service of the mentally ill who could thus aspire to
benefit from the recently proclaimed "right of man" to care and thus
to the possible regaining of their health.[68]

Notes

Research for this paper was supported by a grant from the National Institutes of Health (NLM-EMP 1F13 LM 26,413) whose assistance is here gratefully acknowledged.

1. Many years ago, Marcel Fosseyeux and René Sand blazed a trail for these studies, and George Rosen wrote several thought-provoking articles. See, for example, M. Fosseyeux, "Les comités de bienfaisance de Paris sous la révolution," *Annales révolutionnaires,* 5 (1912), pp. 192–205, 344–358; and "L'Hôtel-Dieu de Paris sous la révolution, 1789–1802," *La Révolution française,* 66 (1913), pp. 40–85; R. Sand, *The Advance to Social Medicine* (London: Staples, 1952). See also: G. Rosen, "Hospitals, Medical Care and Social Policy in the French Revolution," *Bulletin for the History of Medicine,* 30 (1956), pp. 124–149; and "The Philosophy of Ideology and the Emergence of Modern Medicine in France," *Ibid.,* 20 (1946), pp. 328–339. Today the best work on this subject in France comes from the pen of Marcel Candille, for example, "L'humanisation de l'hôpital considérée du point de vue de l'infirmière," *L'hôpital et l'aide sociale à Paris,* 3 (1962), pp. 463–470, and "Evolution des principes d'assistance hospitalière," *Revue d'assistance publique,* 9 (1958), pp. 43–51. Important information can be gathered from P. Huard, *Sciences, médecine, pharmacie, de la révolution à l'empire, 1789–1815* (Paris: Dacosta, 1970); from E.H. Ackerknecht, *Medicine at the Paris Hospital, 1794–1848* (Baltimore: The Johns Hopkins University Press, 1967); from Marcel Reinhard, *La révolution* (Paris: Hachette, 1971); and from Jean Tulard *L'empire* (Paris: Hachette, 1970) in Nouvelle Histoire de Paris. Americans, apart from some diligent work in the military medical archives [D.M. Vess, *Medical Revolution in France, 1789–1796* (Gainesville: University of Florida Press, 1975)], have concentrated on the pre-revolutionary era. See, *e.g.* W. Coleman, "Health and Hygiene in the *Encyclopédie:* A Medical Doctrine for the Bourgeoisie," *Journal of the History of Medicine and Allied Sciences,* 29 (1974), pp. 399–421; T. Gelfand, "A Clinical Ideal: Paris 1789," *Bulletin of the History of Medicine,* 57 (1977), pp. 397–411; L.S., Greenbaum, "Jean-Sylvain Bailly, the Baron de Breteuil and the 'Four New Hospitals' of Paris," *Clio Medica* 8 (1973), pp. 261–284; C.C. Hannaway, "The Société Royale de Médecine and Epidemics in the Ancien Régime," *Bulletin of the History of Medicine,* 40 (1972), pp. 257–273. The best continuing bibliography of the French monographic literature is to be found in the *Bulletin* of the Société française d'histoire des hôpitaux, under the editorship of Marcel Candille.

2. M. Foucault, ed., *Les machines à guérir* (Paris: Institut de l'environnement: Dossiers et documents d'architecture, 1976), p. 11. See also the author's stimulating but controversial *Folie et déraison: Histoire de la folie à l'âge classique* (Paris: Plon, 1961), *Naissance dev la clinique* (Paris: Presses universitaires de France, 1972), and *Surveiller et punir: Naissance de la prison* (Paris: Gallimard, 1975).

3. J. Tenon, *Mémoires sur les hôpitaux de Paris* (Paris: Pierres, 1788), p. ii.

4. P. Pinel, *Nosographie philosophique, ou Méthode de l'analyse appliquée à la médecine* (Paris: Brosson, 1798; 2nd ed., 3 vols., 1802–1803; 3rd ed., 3 vols., 1807); P. Pinel, *Traité médico-philosophique sur l'aliénation mentale* (Paris: Brosson, 1801; 2nd ed., 1809); English tr. D.D. Davis (Sheffield: W. Todd, 1806); P. Pinel, *La médecine clinique rendue plus précise at plus exacte par l'application de l'analyse ou Recueil et résultats d'observations sur les maladies aiguës, faites à la Salpêtrière* (Paris: Brosson, 1802; 2nd ed., 1804; 3rd ed., 1815).

5. Americans are perhaps most familiar with Pinel as portrayed in G. Zilboorg, *A History of Medical Psychology* (New York: W.W. Norton, 1941), pp. 319–341, and W. Riese, *The Legacy of Philippe Pinel: An Inquiry into Thought on Mental Alienation* (New York: Springer, 1969). To see Pinel in appropriate context, the reader might consult M. Laignel-Lavastine et J. Vinchon, *Les malades de l'esprit et leurs médecins, du 16ème au 19ème siecles* (Paris: Maloine, 1930); L. Pezé, *Les précurseurs de Pinel en France au 17ème et 18ème siecles* (Paris: These médecine, 1922); and M.D. Alexander, *The Administration of Madness and Attitudes Toward the Insane in 19th-Century Paris* (Ph.D. Diss., Johns Hopkins University, 1976). Both Zilboorg and Riese rely heavily on René Semelaigne, *Les grands aliénistes français: Philippe Pinel, Esquirol, Ferrus, Falret, Voisin, Georget* (Paris: Steinheil, 1894) and *Aliénistes et philanthropes: Les Pinel et les Tuke* (Paris: Steinheil, 1912). But Semelaigne was the grandson of Pinel's nephew Casimir and the family has, for more than a century, been extremely protective of its famous ancestor. All the letters published by Casimir contain favorable evidence [*Lettres de Pinel* (Paris: Masson, 1859)]. Pinel's surviving private papers are still in family hands; his clinical entries on the ledgers of the Salpêtrière Hospital are preserved in a provincial depot of the Archives de l'Assistance publique in Paris.

6. The Ideologues are at last receiving the attention they deserve from a modern scholar; see Sergio Moravia, *La scienza dell'uomo nel settecento* (Bari: Laterza, 1970), *Il Tramonto dell 'Illuminismo: Filosofia e politica nella società francese, 1770–1810* (Bari: Laterza, 1968), and especially *Il pensiero degli Idéologues: Scienza e filosofia in Francia, 1780–1815* (Firenze: La Nuova Italia, 1974) and "Philosophie et médecine en France à la fin du 18ème siècle," *Studies on Voltaire and the 18th Century*, (1972): pp. 1089–1151. See also, F. Colonna d'Istria, "Ce que la médecine doit à la philosophie: Pinel," *Revue de métaphysique et de morale* 12ème année (1904), pp. 186–210; A. Guillois, *Le salon de Madame Helvétius: Cabanis et les idéologues* (Paris: Calmann Lévy, 1894); F. Picavet, *Les Idéologues: essai sur l'histoire des idées et des théories scientifiques, philosophiques, religieuses, etc. en France depuis 1789* (Paris: Alcan, 1891); W. Riese, "Philippe Pinel, His Views on Human Nature and Disease; His Medical Thought," *Journal of Nervous and Mental Disease*, 114 (1951), pp. 313–323; *idem*, "La méthode analytique de Condillac et ses rapports avec l'oeuvre de Pinel," *Revue philosophique*, 158 (1968), pp. 321–336; C. H. Van Duzer, *Contribution of the Ideologues to French Revolutionary Thought* (Baltimore: Johns Hopkins Press, 1935), and J. Kitchin, *Un journal "philosophique": La Décade, 1794–1807* (Paris: Minard, 1965).

7. See S. Moravia, "Philosophie et médecine . . . ," pp. 1089–1091.

8. G. Cuvier, "Eloge historique de Pinel, lu le 11 juin 1827 à l'Académie des sciences," Paris, Académie des sciences, *Mémoires*, 2nd series, 9 (1830), pp. ccxxvi–cclx. This *éloge* relied on a biographic sketch by Pinel's son Scipion that is full of errors, see G. Bollotte, "Documents sur Philippe Pinel," *Information psychiatrique*, 44 (1968), pp. 823–841. Scipion Pinel's "Vie de Philippe Pinel par son fils Scipion" can be found in the "Fonds Cuvier," Archives, Académie des sciences, Paris.

9. E. Pariset, "Eloge de Philippe Pinel, lu à la séance du 28 août 1827, *Histoire des membres de l'Académie royale de médecine*, 2 vols (Paris: Baillière, 1845), I, pp. 209–259.

10. See, for example, A. Cabanès, "Un grand médecin, qui fut un grand philantrhope," *Gazette des hôpitaux*, 84 (1926), pp. 1354–1356; H. Codet, "L'influence de Philippe Pinel," *Progrès médical*, 42 (1926), pp. 1562–1567; J. Noir, "A l'occasion de centenaire de la mort de Philippe Pinel," *Concours médical* (1926), pp. 2795–97. In contrast, see the excellent

brief summary by P. Huard and M.J. Imbault-Huart, "Philippe Pinel, idéologue, nosolo-giste et psychiatre," *Gazette médicale de France,* 82 (1975), pp. 2605–2607.

11. E. Woods, and E.T. Carlson, "The Psychiatry of Philippe Pinel," *Bulletin of the History of Medicine,* 35 (1961), pp. 14–25 and P. Marset, "Veinte publicaciones psiquia-tricas de Pinel olvidadas. Contribución al estudio de los origenes del *Traité sur la manie,"* *Episteme,* 6 (1972), pp. 163–195. See also the same author's medical thesis, *El punto de partida de la obra psiquiatrica de Pinel* (Valencia: 1972).

12. W. H. Lechler, *Philippe Pinel; seine Familie, seine Jugend- und Studienjahre 1745–1778: Roques, St. Paul Cap-de-Joux, Lavaur, Toulouse, Montpellier, unter Verwendung zum Teil noch unveröffentlichter Dokumente* (Munich: The author, 1959) and P. Chabbert, "Les années d'études de Philippe Pinel: Lavaur, Toulouse, Montpellier," *Monspeliensis Hippocrates* 3 (1960), pp. 15–23; see also the same author's "L'oeuvre médicale de Philippe Pinel," *Comptes-rendus du 96ème congrès national des sociétés savantes* (Paris: Bibliothèque nationale, 1971), pp. 153–61.

13. B. Chabbert, "Philippe Pinel à Paris jusqu'à sa nomination à Bicêtre," *Aktuelle Probleme aus der Geschichte der Medizin; Proceedings of the 19th International Congress of the History of Medicine* (Basel: Karger, 1966), pp. 589–595.

14. Chabbert had thought this student to have been George Coltman (1752–1828), but now tends to agree with A. Spencer Paterson (*Proc. Royal Soc. Med.,* 65 (1972), pp. 553–556) that it was probably Sayer Walker (1748–1826). The question is of some importance, since Pinel owed to this British student his knowledge of English and his acquaintance with British medical literature (letter from Dr. Chabbert to the author, here gratefully acknowledged).

15. P. Pinel, "Mémoire sur le talent qu'exige l'application des mathématiques au corps humain," *Mémoires de mathématique et de physique,* Société royale des sciences de Montpel-lier, 1 (1777), pp. 185–199; and "Des courbes que décrivent les extrémités de nos membres dans leurs divers mouvements," présenté le 5 juin 1777, MS. D 176, No. 38, pp. 1–16, Archives départementales, Hérault, Montpellier. (Both listed in Lechler, *op. cit.,* pp. 212–213.)

16. Chabbert has some doubts as to exactly which member of the family Pinel tutored. Cf. Chabbert, "Les années d'études . . . ," p. 21.

17. Quoted in Chabbert, "Philippe Pinel à Paris," p. 591. Chabbert finds no evidence for, and therefore discounts, other biographers' assertion that Pinel tried three or four times to pass the examination for *docteur régent.* But he does substantiate and document the story that Pinel had ghost-written the doctoral dissertation of his successful rival for the Diest prize, when Desmarescaux was preparing for the M.D. in Montpellier. P. Chabbert, "Un rival heureux de Pinel: Desmarescaux," *Monspellensis Hippocrates,* 4 (1961), pp. 17–23. The topic of this dissertation: "A Medical Essay on Horsemanship"!

18. R. Semelaigne, *Les grands aliénistes francais,* p. 52.

19. W. Cullen, *Institutions de médecine pratique,* trans. by Philippe Pinel, 2 vols. (Paris: Duplain, 1785); G. Baglivi, *Opera omnia medico-practica,* trans. and annot. by Philippe Pinel, 2 vols. (Paris: Duplain, 1788); and P. Pinel, *Abrégé des transactions philosophiques de la Société royale de Londres, 5ème–8ème partie* (Paris: Buisson, 1790–1791).

20. P. Pinel, "Mémoire sur l'application des mathématiques au corps humain et sur le mécanisme des luxations," read to the Société royale des sciences de Paris, published

in *Journal de physique,* 31 (1787), pp. 350–362; "Mémoire sur le mécanisme des luxations de l'humérus," *ibid.,* 33 (1788), pp. 12–24; "Mémoire sur le mécanisme des luxations des deux os de l'avant-bras," *ibid.,* 35 (1789), pp. 457–470; "Recherches sur l'étiologie ou le méchanisme de la luxation de la mâchoire inférieure," in A.-F. de Fourcroy, ed., *La médecine éclairée par les sciences physiques,* 3 (1792), pp. 183–192.

21.   P. Pinel, "Mémoire sur l'application des mathématiques," p. 358.

22.   *Ibid.,* p. 352.

23.   P. Pinel, "Nouvelles observations sur la structure et la conformation des os de la tête de l'éléphant," *Mémoires de la société médicale d'émulation,* 3 (1799–1800), pp. 253–277.

24.   P. Pinel, "Mémoire sur une nouvelle méthode de classification des Quadrupèdes, fondée sur les rapports de structure mécanique que présente l'articulation de la mâchoire inférieure," *Mémoires de la Société d'histoire naturelle,* I (1791), pp. 359–374.

25.   P. Pinel, "Observations sur les aliénés et leurs division en espèces distinctes," *Mémoires de la société médicale d'émulation,* 3 (1799–1800), pp. 1–26.

26.   Institut de France. Académie des sciences. *Rapport fait au nom de la commission nommée par la classe des sciences mathématiques et physiques pour l'examen de la méthode de préserver de la petite vérole par l'inoculation de la vaccine* (Paris: Baudouin, 1803). On this question, see also G. Rosen, "Problems in the Application of Statistical Analysis to Questions of Health: 1700–1800," *Bulletin of the History of Medicine,* 29 (1955), pp. 27–45.

27.   P. Pinel, "Résultats d'observations et construction de tables pour servir à déterminer le degré de probabilité de la guérison des aliénés," Institut national de France, *Mémoires de la classe des sciences mathématiques et physiques,* 1st series, 8 (1807), pp. 169–205.

28.   G. Cuvier, "Eloge . . .", p. ccxxxxvi.

29.   P. Pinel, "Mémoire lu à la Société d'histoire naturelle sur les moyens de préparer les quadrupèdes et les oiseaux déstinés à former des collections d'histoire naturelle," *Journal de physique,* 39 (1791), pp. 138–151. The words quoted appear on p. 138.

30.   R. de Saussure, *French Psychiatry in the Eighteenth Century,* p. 1235 and *passim.*

31.   On the "Maison Belhomme," see E.H. Ackerknecht, "Political Prisoners in French Mental Institutions," *Medical History,* 19 (1975), pp. 250–255, and A. Ferroni, *Une maison de santé pour le traitement des aliénés à la fin du 18ème siècle* (Paris Thèse: Medicine, 1964).

32.   "Indiquer les moyens les plus efficaces de traiter les malades dont l'esprit est devenu aliéné avant l'âge de Vieillesse." The unpublished *Plumitif* [minute book] of the Société royale de médecine indicates that, according to custom, Pinel's prize-winning essay was read aloud to the membership in the fall of 1792. (Académie de médecine de Paris. Archives, *Plumitif,* vol. 11 bis, folio 286 verso.) Pinel undoubtedly destroyed this essay since he wrote that the piece "does not seem to me worthy of publication in its primitive form; but it will be recast in a treatise on insanity that I am planning to write." P. Pinel, "Recherches et observations sur le traitement moral des aliénés," *Mémoires de la société médicale d'émulation,* 2 (1798–1799), p. 218, n. 1.

33.   P. Pinel, "Reflexions sur la buanderie, comme objet d'économie domestique et de salubrité, et application de ces principes à un établissement à l'île du pont de Sève," *La médecine éclairée par les sciences physiques,* 2 (1791), pp. 12–21.

34.   A. Garrigues, "Philippe Pinel, journaliste," *Concours médical,* 48 (1926), pp. 2294–2299.

35.   For stimulating recent comment on the subject, see J.J. Bylebyl, "Galen on the Non-Natural Causes of Variation in the Pulse," *Bulletin of the History of Medicine* 45 (1971), pp. 482–485; S. Jarcho, "Galen's Six Non-Naturals: A Bibliographic Note and Translation," *ibid.,* 44 (1970), pp. 372–377; L.J. Rather, "The 'Six Things Non-Natural': A Note on the Origin and Fate of a Doctrine and a Phrase," *Clio Medica,* 3 (1968), pp. 337–347.

36.   C. Pinel, *Lettres,* pp. 46, 48.

37.   *Gazette de santé,* 1784, Nos. 23, 29; 1785, No. 50.

38.   *Ibid.,* 1784, No. 36.

39.   *Ibid.,* No. 24.

40.   *Ibid.,* 1784, Nos. 36, 46.

41.   *Ibid.,* 1787, No. 32.

42.   *Ibid.,* 1788, No. 51.

43.   *Ibid.,*

44.   His wife, Jeanne Vincent, "that thrifty and sensible person," would bear him two sons, Scipion and Charles. C. Pinel, *Lettres,* 51.

45.   *Gazette de santé,* 1787, No. 25.

46.   *Ibid.,* 1787, No. 25.

47.   *Ibid.,* 1787, No. 2.

48.   *Ibid.,* No. 30.

49.   *Ibid.,* 1784, No. 31.

50.   *Ibid.,* 1788, No. 11.

51.   *Ibid.,* No. 16.

52.   *Ibid.,* 1787, No. 50.

53.   A critical, bilingual edition is now being prepared for publication. See P. Pinel, "Mémoire sur cette question proposée pour sujet d'un prix par la Société de médecine: Déterminer quelle est la meilleure manière d'enseigner la médecine pratique dans un hôpital." Autograph manuscript, 33 pp., Archives, Académie de médecine de Paris, carton 115. Recently, the French psychiatrist G. Bollotte published Pinel's notes for the above essay (though Bollotte did not recognize this relationship). They are a part of the Cuvier papers at the Paris Academy of Sciences. Bollotte assumes that the commissioners of the Royal Society never read Pinel's work because the archivist of the Paris Academy of Medicine found the seal on Pinel's essay unbroken in 1935. That seal in fact only closed the accompanying envelope [*"billet cacheté"*] covering the author's identity. The title-sheet of the manuscript carries the three commissioners' signatures and the notations *"lu."* See G. Bollotte, "Pinel et l'enseignement de l'art de guérir," *Atti del XXI Congresso Internazionale di Storia della Medicina* II (1968), pp. 1074–1079, and "Pinel et la réforme de l'enseignement de l'art de guérir," *Information psychiatrique* 46 (1970), pp. 657–668; see also M. Genty, "Un mémoire inédit de Pinel sur l'enseignement clinique," *Progrès médical,* 12 (1935), pp. 86–88.

54.   See, e.g., J. Colombier et F. Doublet, "Instruction sur la manière de gouverner les insensés et de travailler à leur guérison dans les asiles qui leur sont destinés," *Journal de médecine, chirurgie, pharmacie*, 44 (1785), pp. 529–583, and P. Carrette, "Tenon et l'assistance aux aliénés à la fin du 18ème siècle," *Annales médico-psychologiques*, 12th series, 2 (1925), pp. 365–386.

55.   One might cite as an example a paper on "Congenital Deformity of the Sexual Organs and Apparent or Real Characteristics of Hermaphroditism." In this paper, discussion of anatomical and physiological detail leaves Pinel little space for psychological remarks, and yet the paper is dated 1789! P. Pinel, "Sur les vices originaires de conformation des parties génitales et sur le caractère apparent ou réel des hermaphrodites," *Journal de physique*, 35 (1789), pp. 297–307.

56.   For Pinel's perception of the psychological impact that the Revolution exerted on contemporaries, see his curiously conventional letter to the editor entitled "Coup d'oeil d'un médecin sur les effets de la révolution opérée en France," *Journal de Paris*, January 18, 1790, reprinted in *L'Esprit des journaux*, 19 (1790), pp. 365–368.

57.   Dr. H. Bonnafous-Sérieux, *Une maison d'aliénés et de correctionnaires au 18ème siècle: La Charité de Senlis* (Paris: Presses universitaires de France, 1936); P.-A. Chatagnon, et A. Morel, "L'ancien régime et l'assistance aux malades mentaux," *Annales médico-psychologiques* 118 (1960), II, pp. 437–446; P. Sérieux, et L. Libert, "Documents pour servir à l'histoire de la psychiatrie en France aux 17ème et 18ème siècles: Règlements de quelques maisons d'aliénés," *Bulletin de la société de médecine mentale de Belgique* No. 172 (1914), pp. 209–250.

58.   See, e.g. F. Spezzaferri, "Chi per primo spezzo le catene degli alienati: Pinel o Chiarugi?", *Pagine di storia della medicina*, 6 (1962), pp. 44–48; G. Mora, "Vincenzo Chiarugi (1759–1820)—His Contribution to Psychiatry," *Bulletin of the Isaac Ray Medical Library* 2 (1954), pp. 51–104.

59.   Misinformation about this, as other, aspects of Pinel's life can be traced back to his son; see: Scipion Pinel, "De l'abolition des chaînes," *Mémoires de l'Académie de médecine de Paris*, V (1836), pp. 32–40; see also P. Pinel, [presented by René Semelaigne his nephew's grandson)], "Observations sur l'hospice des insensés de Bicêtre," *Bulletin de la société française d'histoire de la médecine*, 9 (1910), pp. 177–189.

60.   C. Bloch, et A. Tuetey, *Procès-verbaux et rapports du Comité de mendicité de la Constituante, 1790–1791* (Paris: Imprimerie nationale, 1911), p. 604.

61.   P. Pinel, *La médecine clinique*, 2ème ed., Introduction, xxv.

62.   P. Pinel, *A Treatise on Insanity*, D.D. Davis, trans. (New York: Hafner, 1962), pp. 26, 72.

63.   P. Pinel, "Mémoire sur la manie périodique ou intermittente," *Mémoires de la société médicale d'émulation*, 1 (1797–1798), p. 100.

64.   P. Pinel, "Résultats d'observations pour servir de base aux rapports juridiques dans les cas d'aliénation mentale," *Ibid.*, 8 (1817), p. 677.

65.   M. Laignel-Lavastine and J. Vinchon, "Pinel médecin-légiste," *Annales médico-psychologiques*, 85 (1927), pp. 58–68.

66.   P. Pinel, "Résultats d'observations pour servir de base," p. 682.

67. This term is used, *e.g.*, by Jean-Claude Guédon, "Michel Foucault: The Knowledge of Power and the Power of Knowledge," *Bulletin of the History of Medicine*, 51 (1977), p. 247.

68. See, *e.g.*, H. Baruk, "L'oeuvre de Pinel et d'Esquirol devant 'l'anti-psychiatrie'," *Académie nationale de médecine. Bulletin*, 155 (1971): 205–215 or G.N. Grob, "Rediscovering Asylums: The Unhistorical History of the Mental Hospital," *Hastings Center Report*, 7 (1977), pp. 33–41.

69. For the more general context of this problem, see D.B. Weiner, "Le droit de l'homme à la santé—Une belle idée devant l'Assemblée constituante: 1790–1791," *Clio Medica*, 5 (1970), pp. 209–223 and "Three Champions of the Handicapped in Revolutionary France," in *From Parnassus: Essays in Honor of Jacques Barzun* (New York and London: Harper & Row, 1976), D.B. Weiner and W.R. Keylor, eds., pp. 161–176.

German Jews, English Dissenters, French Protestants: Nineteenth-Century Pioneers of Modern Medicine and Science*

ERWIN H. ACKERKNECHT

The eminent role which German Jews played during the nineteenth century in medicine and science and which has been completely out of proportion to the size of this always small (less then one percent) German minority, has always been striking and puzzling. Thorsten Veblen for example, 60 years ago devoted a special essay "The intellectual pre-eminence of Jews in Modern Europe."[1] to this seeming anomaly. It is still more or less a matter of common knowledge confirmed by Nobel prizes in the twentieth century.

I would, nevertheless, prefer to present a few facts and names supporting this generalization, before discussing the matter. I hope that these lists of names will evoke in the reader meaningful associations, which may help him to overcome the boredom generally inherent in such unavoidable listings. As it is, these lists can be but selective and rather short compared to the existing evidence. They include less than one fourth of the more than 400 eminent German Jewish medical men listed by Kaznelson.[2] Microscopic anatomy in Germany profited from the work of two stars of the first order J. Henle and R. Remak; microscopic pathology from the work of J. Cohnheim and C. Weigert. In nineteenth-century physiology we find such first-rate men as G. Valentin, G. Magnus, M. Schiff, R. Heidenhain, J. Breuer, L. Hermann, R. Semon, J. Loeb; such biochemists as O. Meyerhof, R. Willstätter, Otto Warburg, G. Embden, K. Landsteiner. In bacteriology F. Cohn, A. Wassermann, H. Sachs, E. Freund excelled, as did O. Liebreich, O. Loewi, C. Koller, L. Lewin in pharmacology. The enormously important field of chemotherapy was created by Paul Ehrlich.

But German Jews excelled not only in the theoretical (and financially unrewarding!) disciplines. They shone also as clinicians. One thinks of such eminent names as L. Traube, H. Bamberger, S. Basch, L. Lichtheim, O. Rosenbach, J. Boas, O. Minkowski, A. Biedl, A. Mag-

86

nus-Levy, G. and F. Klemperer, the Zonde brothers, A. Goldscheider, and of pediatricians like E.H. Henoch, A. Jacobi, A. Baginsky, H. Finkelstein. Outstanding surgeons were Benedict Stilling, A. Wölfler, W.A. Freund, R. Nissen, A. Hoffa, J. Israel, J. Halban, M. Sänger, E. Wertheim. In neuropsychiatry we find M. Romberg, M. Benedikt, E. Hitzig, H. Oppenheim, L. Edinger, K. Goldstein, R. Bing, M. Bielschowsky, H. Liepmann, G. Aschaffenburg, O. Binswanger, P. Schilder, M. Sakl, S. Freud, and A. Adler. In ophthalmology let me mention H. Cohn and J. Hirschberg; in ears, nose, and throat A. Türck, A. Politzer, R. Barany, H. Neumann; in dermatology M. Kaposi, G. Unna, O. Lassar, A. Neisser, J. Jadasohn, B. Bloch, A. Buschke; in sexology M. Hirschfeld, I. Bloch, A. Moll. And what would German medical history have been without J. and W. Pagel, Max Neuburger, and August Hirsch? In the sciences we mention here only[3] such outstanding men as Heinrich Hertz, A. Michelson, A. Einstein, H. Minkowski, L. Meitner, N. Bohr, M. Born, W. Pauli, G. Hertz, J. Franck, R. von Lieben, Graf Arco, A. von Bayer, and F. Haber.

It is well known that the Jewish contribution in banking, commerce, and industry[4] after emancipation and simultaneously with the medical achievements was no less remarkable. Even today the names of nineteenth-century German bankers such as Rothschild, Mendelsohn, Bleichröder, Warburg, Fürstenberg, or of department-store organizers as Tietz, Wertheim, or Karstadt are well known. L. Loewe founded important weapon and tool producing establishments; W. Herz did the same for rubber, Hirsch for copper, E. Rathenau in electricity, F. Caro and Weinberg in chemistry, A. Ballin and W. Kunstmann in shipping. German Jews also played a significant role in other fields such as literature, music, and philosophy, but not comparable to the fields cited above. Their role was least prominent in politics—which did not prevent their being made the scapegoats for national disasters, like the defeat of 1918.

How can this medico-scientific preeminence be explained? The genetic explanation which comes first to mind is unlikely in view of the racial history of the Jews. Moreover, no one has ever assumed that the two groups to be discussed later, who played in many ways a very similar role in England and France, existed and behaved as the result of a dissenter or Protestant gene. Veblen, therefore, rightly discarded the genetic hypothesis.[5]

He also saw no connection between the Jewish intellectual, that is religious, tradition and modern science.[6] It must also be noted that most of the German Jewish doctors and scientists were highly assimilated.

Neither Veblen's explanation that Jews are "sceptics"[7] nor Bodamer's claim of an "innere Verwandtschaft des jüdischen Geistes mit dem Zeitgeist des 19. Jahrhunderts"[8] seem to give us a much better understanding. The only undeniable "spiritual" fact—the majority of the Jews were literate while the majority of their Christian brethren were not—does not seem of decisive importance.

The inventor of "scientific socialism," Karl Marx, claimed in his notorious antisemitic pamphlet of 1844 a "spiritual relationship" between Judaism and capitalism.[9] Werner Sombart defended the same thesis in a more scholarly and historical way in 1911, thus paralleling the derivation of capitalism from Protestant ethics by Max Weber (1904), a point to which we will return later. Not much uncontroversial substance has emerged from both hypotheses which have, nevertheless, produced mountains of discussion.[10] Neither the Calvinists nor the Jews, for the better or the worse, have apparently invented either modern science or modern capitalism. Italians of the late Middle Ages preceded them.[11] H. Lüthy[12] has rightly emphasized that it was the Counterreformation which stopped existing economic and scientific progress in many Catholic regions, while progress continued in Protestant areas (e.g., the Netherlands).

We would like here to venture a far more prosaic and partial explanation of our phenomenon: The Jews played the role of a typical minority. The years after the emancipation of the Jews in Germany (in Prussia in 1812) allowed the Jews, hitherto limited by law to money transactions and trade with used goods, to expand in several new directions. The positions valued more highly by the average Christian German—officer, judge, high bureaucrat[13]—were still closed to the unbaptized. But just at this moment, science developed explosively and became dominant in medicine and industry. And positions in medicine and science were less attractive to the Christian majority. Is it surprising then that the Jews, bursting with the energy of the newly liberated, and favored sometimes by their international and family connections, rushed into these fields, and that many of them became highly successful? What Herbert Lüthy has said of the Protestant French banker[14]—"he filled the functions which society abandoned to him"—is true of all minorities, the German Jews included.[15] The minority cannot afford to follow the way of its innermost choices, even if such choice should exist. The minority moves in those directions in which it is allowed to move. For the German Jews, a later statement of Herbert Lüthy is also valid[16]: "The role of dissenting minorities is quite unconnected with the form of their dissent. In each case theirs is a response to a challenge imposed by discrimination". I have long felt that this way of looking at the problem of the German Jews in medicine brings us closer to reality than former hypotheses of special "affinities," and I have been strengthened in this conviction by the history of two analogous nineteenth-century groups: the English dissenters and the French Protestants who with a different "ethical" background played a similar role.

It is at first perplexing that so many outstanding nineteenth-century English medical men and scientists (e.g. Th. Young, J. Dalton, Th. Hodgkin, D.H. Tuke, Lord Lister) belonged to the numerically minute Quaker sect. The test acts, however, barred *all* non-members of the Church of England between 1673 and the 1870s (that is *all* "dissenters": Quakers, Baptists, Congregationalists, Methodists, Unitarians, etc.) from public office and the universities of Oxford and Cambridge,[17] not to mention other forms of discrimination. Consequently, a situation similar to that of German Jews was created. Many dissenters were thus pushed into medicine and science—or industry and commerce.[18] Many studied at Edinburgh where dissenters were admitted and where, unlike at Oxford or Cambridge, science and medicine were seriously cultivated. It is characteristic of the situation that the four eminent scientists to whom Oxford gave honorary degrees at the first visit of the British Association for the Advancement of Science there in 1832—Dalton, Faraday, Brown and Brewster—were dissenters and would not have been allowed to matriculate there.[19] The physiologist Michael Foster, a Baptist, was as late as 1870 barred from a professorship at Cambridge because of his religion.

One small dissenting academy at Warrington (between Manchester and Liverpool), which existed only from 1757 to 1787, graduated several of the future leaders of the medical profession in England: Th. Percival, Caleb Hillier Parry, John Aikin, and J. Bostock. One of the professors (all Unitarians) was the great chemist and electrician Joseph Priestley, and another one of the disciples was Thomas R. Malthus.[20] Though the dissenters were never more than a rather small minority of the population (today about three percent),[21] of the 180 leading British scientists whom Galton analysed in 1874, *one third were not members of the established church.*[22] The Quakers alone had forty times their proportion among members of the Royal Society.[22a]

Dissenters became eminent in medicine and science as early as the seventeenth century (e.g., Sydenham, John Ray). The peak of their influence was reached in the late eighteenth and in the nineteenth centuries. It is amazing how many famous medical and scientific men were members of that small "Society of Friends" (Quakers). Let me mention only: J. Rutty, J. Fothergill (the friend of John Howard), Th. Dimsdale, J. Lettsom, R. Collinson, J. Ferriar, W. Philipps, J. Dalton, Th. Young, Th. Hancock, J.C. Prichard, T. Hodgkin, F. Galton, J. Lister, D.H. Tuke, J. Hutchinson, E.B. Tylor, R. Godlee, A.S. Eddington. But there are, besides Quakers, who are easier to trace, numerous other dissenters, as, for example, the above mentioned Warrington graduates Percival, Parry, Aikin, Bostock; the Methodists Davy and Marshall Hall, the devoted Sandemanian Faraday, the Baxterian Clerk Maxwell, the Baptist Michael Foster. Many of the very numerous pre-1870 English Edinburgh graduates[23] had gone north less for the excellence of this university, than because they simply would not have been admitted at Oxford or Cambridge. The somewhat exaggerated discretion of the Dictionary of National Biography in this respect does not allow one to check easily the religious affiliation of such Edinburgh graduates, but the probability that Charles White (the master of John Aikin), for example, or John Hope, W. Withering, and T. Fowler were dissenters, is very high. Virtually all the eminent Scotch and Irish medical and scientific men active in England during the eighteenth and nineteenth centuries were dissenters in the eyes of the Anglican Church.

English dissenters, like German Jews or French Protestants, participated in banking, commerce, and industry far out of proportion to their percentage of the population. We still remember the names of the Quakers W. Allen as a founder of the chemical industry, of D. Pease as a founder of English railroads, of J. Bright in the textile industry, Joseph Fry in chocolate, W. Cookworthy in porcelain manufacture, and R. Ransome in agricultural implements. Quakers promoted mining, especially in copper and lead. There would have been no English iron industry without the Quakers Darby, Rawlinson, Lloyd, and Hanbury. The names of the Quaker bankers Barclay, Lloyd, Gurney, and Backhouse loom large in the history of English banking.[24] About half of the political steering committee of dissenter MP's (not the Quakers) in 1800 were bankers.[25]

Such data seem to support the 1904 thesis of Max Weber about the causal role of the "Protestant (or more accurate Calvinist) Ethic" in the formation of capitalism, of its "spirit," a thesis discussed vigorously ever since. The thesis, however, has not resisted closer examination of Calvinism and time sequences,[26] and also the fact that the German Jews, with different "ethics," played the same role. Another parallel thesis—Protestantism has favored the genesis and spread of modern science—has done better. Alphonse de Candolle[27] demonstrated first the prevalence of Protestants (and especially the sons of Protestant clergymen) in Western science during the eighteenth and nineteenth centuries in his classic of 1873. Since 1938 R. Merton has defended with much talent the role of puritanism in the growth of English science.[28] J. Pelseneer has repeatedly insisted since 1946 on this role of Protestantism.[29] R. Hoykaas has summarised in a very well balanced and competent way the points on which science and Calvinism might contact.[30] Yet he leaves open the question whether religious or utilitarian motives came first in Protestant predilection for science, and admits even early opposition to science in groups as Quakers and Mennonites.[31] Merton sees the common ground between Protestantism and science in utilitarianism, individualism, rationalism, and empiricism.[32] Lüthy[33] feels that "in the liberation of man from spiritual submission lies the true connection, between Calvinism and modern industrial society, positive science and modern democracy."

There is no doubt of the special relations between Protestantism and modern science. Statistical research on Nobel prize men or "scientists starred in American Men of Science"[34] has confirmed de Candolle's results. But our knowledge of these special relations is still vague. *The connection between the medico-scientific contributions of the dissenters in England and their persecution and discrimination by another brand of Protestants, seems quite clear, however.*

There are other parallels between the dissenters and the other two minority groups, German Jews and French Protestants. For instance, the English dissenters were accused of being enemy agents, that is French agents during the Napoleonic wars.[35] There are "Quaker names" in England,[36] as there are "Protestant names" in France and "Jewish names" in Germany, evidence of the enforced or self-chosen extensive intermarriage in these groups. It is but natural that these persecuted and discriminated peoples should practice group solidarity and cohesion. A further parallel is the general literacy of these outsiders.

English dissenters resembled French Protestants in the eagerness of their political participation—much more than German Jews—and have, especially the Quakers, particularly cultivated the fields where politics and philanthropy overlap: the abolition of slavery, prison reform, sanitary reform, the Charter, peace movements.[37]

The French Protestants (Huguenots), unlike the German Jews or even the English dissenters, began as a very sizeable minority, evenly spread in all strata of the population, and as an important political factor. Around 1560 they probably comprised about 25 percent of the French population. By 1639 the civil war, the massacre of St. Bartholomew's Day, emigration, and reconversion had reduced them to about ten percent. The revocation of the Edict of Nantes in 1685, which forced the departure of about 500,000 refugees, and inaugurated new, cruel persecutions reduced them to a level which has never exceeded two percent of the population, that is to a minority position comparable to that of the German Jews and the English dissenters.[38]

The Huguenots had had some interesting scientists like G. Rondelet, B. Palissy, and Olivier de Serres. Among the exiles of 1685 and especially their offspring in Switzerland, Prussia, Holland, and Britain, there were very many outstanding scientists and doctors, listed carefully by de Candolle.[39] As there is no continuity between this group and the nineteenth-century group in France, we shall not discuss them here.

French Protestantism had a semi-legal existence among southern peasants and bourgeois until the Revolution liberated them, only to persecute them anew during the abolition of Christianity in 1793–1795. Napoleon eventually legalized them in 1802. The Protestants participated far beyond their population percentage in the revolutionary movement. Both Charlotte Corday and Marat were Protestants. Eleven of the fifteen southern deputies in the Constituent Assembly were Protestants and 20 (nine "pasteurs" among them!) of 29 in the Convention.[40] The parson Rabaud St. Etienne presided over both assemblies, but died under the guillotine. Peletier de la Lozère presided over the Convention and the Council of 500. Leading politicians like Cambon, Barnave, and Boissy d'Anglas were Protestants. Some parsons became famous administrators like Jeanbon St. André, or generals like Rapp.[41] As most Protestant politicians tended towards Girondism, Robespierre eliminated many. They returned under Napoleon, to fade again away under the Restoration. But the leading politician of the Orleanist era (1830–1848), François Guizot of Nîmes (also one of France's greatest historians), was an engaged Protestant. Other Protestants like Count de Gasparin played important political roles.

Lavisse[42] feels that, disappointed by politics in 1848, they transfered their affections to science. But while they were very active, indeed, in science, nothing could actually deter them from politics. Even under the clerical Second Empire (1852–1870), there were Haussmann, Pourtalès, and Fould in high places. They played a large role during the Third Republic when several premiers (e.g., Waddington, Fréycinet) were Protestants. In 1879, five out of nine Cabinet ministers were Protestants. J. Ferry used Protestants like F. Buisson, Steeg, and Pécaut in his educational ventures. Protestants founded *Le Temps*. They were important in the *affaire Dreyfus* (Picquart, Scheurer-Kaestner). Their political role continued between the Wars—G. Doumergue, André Siegfried, M. Sagnier, and M. Boegner.[43]

De Candolle has statistically demonstrated the pioneering role of French Protestants in science. Surveying the French members of the Royal Society in 1829 he found a 1:1 proportion of Protestants to Catholics; in 1869 it was even a little more favorable to the Protestants, this with a two percent of the population![44] This is not surprising considering that the leading French scientist around 1800, G. Cuvier was a Protestant who protected Protestants and for several years was even officially charged with administering them.[45] The elder Candolle, the four Réclus brothers, all geographers, the chemists Wurtz, Gerhardt, Friedel, and J.B. Dumas were Protestants. Here also the line extends to the twentieth century with Pierre Curie and Jacques Monod. Simultaneously, we find in medicine and surgery E. Littré, Davaine, and Brown-Séquard, Rayer, Lugol, Broca, S. Pozzi, G. Monod, Jaccoud, P. Réclus, P. Berger, and Jean Louis Faure.

Again, we find the parallel of Protestants pioneering not only in medicine and science, but also in banking, industry, and commerce. As to banking, we can refer to the masterful study of Lüthy *La banque protestante en France* (1959). As to industry we need mention only Oberkampf, Eichhoff, Phil. de Girard de Lourmarin, de Pressensé, Dan. Legrand, Delessert, and J.L. Le Grand.[46]

Our last group has also, like the two groups discussed above, been accused of responsibility for national defeats (1557, 1870). It, too, differed from the majority through its almost general literacy. Its character is also select: It is composed only of the descendants of a minority of original members, who have resisted the pressures and temptations to abandon the belief of their fathers. But it is hard to see how this could have predestined them to be pioneers in science and medicine. There is, as stated above, some so far ill defined connection between science and Protestantism. But here, again, the role of French Protestants in science and industry is easier explained by their minority role, a role, which has condemned them to centuries of persecution and suffering. Suffering does by no means always produce achievement. Yet it did in the case of our three groups.

Notes

*I owe thanks to my friends H. Schurer, London; F. Schiller, San Francisco; A. Bussard and J. Théodoridès, Paris, for help in finding documentation.

1.   Reprinted in *The Portable Veblen*, ed. M. Lerner (New York 1950), pp. 467–479.

2.   Kaznelson, S., *Juden im deutschen Kulturbereich* (Bern, 1959).

3.   Kaznelson, *l.c.*, pp. 386–450. Vogel, K. in Reinisch, L. ed. *Die Juden und die Kultur* (Stuttgart, 1961). Theilhaber, F. Schicksal und Leistung 1931.

4.   Zielenzinger, *Juden in der deutschen Wirtschaft.* (Berlin, 1930).

5.   Veblen, *l.c.*, p. 470.

6.   *Ibid.*, p. 473.

7.   *Ibid.*, p. 477.

8.   Bodamer, in Reinisch *l.c.*, p. 31.

9.   Marx, K., *Zur Judenfrage.* Reedit. (St. Grossmann, Berlin, 1919). "What is the secular basis of Judaism? Practical requirements, self-interest. What is the secular cult of Jews? Low trade. . . . We recognise thus in Judaism a general present day, antisocial element, which through a historical evolution in which the Jews have eagerly collaborated in this bad direction, has reached its present heighth" (p.42).

10.   Sée, H. *Les origines du capitalisme moderne* (Paris, 1930), p.47.

11.   Lüthy, H. "Once Again: Calvinism and Capitalism," in Eisenstadt, S. N. *The Protestant Ethic and Modernisation* (New York, 1968), p. 98. Andreski, St. "Method and substantive theory in Max Weber," *ibid.* p. 60.

12.   Lüthy, in Eisenstadt *l.c.*, p. 95.

13.   Candolle, A. de., *Zur Geschichte der Wissenschaften seit zwei Jahrhunderten* (Leipzig, 1911), p. 352.

14.   Lüthy, H. *La banque protestante en France*, 2 vol. (Paris, 1959), vol. I, p. 90.

15.   O.W. Hazeloff (in Reinisch *l.c.*, p. 60) has explained in a somewhat similar vein their role as psychologists by their minority position.

16.   Lüthy in Eisenstadt *l.c.*, p. 94.

17.   MacLachlan, H., *English Education under the Test Act* (Manchester, 1931).

18. Raistrick, A., *Quakers in Science and Industry.* London 1950, p. 43, 53. Singer, Ch., Holmyard, E.J., Hall, A.R. *History of Technology* (London, 1954), vol. V, p. 808. See also Halévy, E., *Histoire du peuple Anglais au 19e siècle,* 4 vols. (Paris 1923), vol. I, p. 563 ff. "The Sects and Science."

19. Singer, *l.c.,* p. 780.

20. Fulton, J.F., "The Warrington Academy (1757–1786) and Its Influence upon Medicine and Science," *Bull.Inst.Hist.Med.* I (1933) pp. 50–80.

21. Centr. Office of Information (London, 1962), pp. 204–205.

22. Galton, F., *English Men of Science* (London, 1874), p. 126.

22a. Raistrick, *l.c.,* p. 222.

23. Comrie, J.D. *A History of Scottish Medicine,* 2 vols. (London, 1927), vol. II, p. 715. A second place for dissenter medical graduation was Leyden, *e.g.,* Fothergill graduated in Edinburgh, his friend Lettsom in Leyden.

24. See Raistrick *l.c.*

25. Hunt, N.C., *Two Early Political Associations: The Quakers and the Dissenters Deputies at the Age of Walpole* (Oxford, 1961).

26. See Lecerf, A., *Études Calvinistes* (Neuchâtel, 1949); Lüthy, H., *l.c.* 1959 and 1968., Eisenstadt, *l.c.,* pp.4–8; Walzer, M., "Puritanism as a Revolutionary Ideology," in Eisenstadt, *l.c.,* pp. 109–134. Burrell, S.A. Calvinism, "Capitalism in Prerevolutionary England," *ibid.,* pp. 155–176.

27. Candolle, A. de., *Histoire des sciences et des savants depuis deux siècles* (Geneva, 1873), pp. 121–141.

28. Merton, R. K. *Science, Technology and Society in 17th Century England* (New York, 1970).

29. A summary of his work: "La réforme et l'origine de la science moderne," *Revue de l'Université de Bruxelles* (1954), pp. 406–418.

30. Hoykaas, R. "Science and Reformation," in Eisenstadt, *l.c.,* pp. 211–239.

31. *Ibid.,* p. 212, 223.

32. Merton, *l.c.,* p. 222.

33. Lüthy, in Eisenstadt, *l.c.,* p. 104.

34. *Science* 92 (1940), p. 310; Visher, S.S. (Baltimore, 1947).

35. Halévy, *l.c.,* vol. I, p. 525.

36. Jones, Rufus N., *The Later Periods of Quakerism,* 2 vols. (London, 1891), vol. I, p. 393.

37. Curteis, G.H. *Dissent in Its Relation to the Church of England* (London, 1874).

38. Leonard, E.G., *Le protestant Français* (Paris, 1953); McNeill, John, T., *History and Character of Calvinism* (New York, 1954).

39. Candolle, A. de., *l.c.,* pp. 131–134.

40. Lüthy, *l.c.* (1959), p. 782.

41. Stephan, Raoul, *Histoire du protestantisme Français* (Paris, 1961); Poland, Burdette, C., *French Protestantism and the French Revolution* (Princeton, 1957).

42. Lavisse, E., *Histoire de France contemporaine depuis la révolution,* vol. VI (Paris, 1921), p. 399.

43. Chazelin in Boegner, M. *et al, Protestantisme français* (Paris, 1945), pp. 77ff.

44. Candolle, A. de., *l.c.,* p. 122.

45. Lee, M., *Mémoires du Baron Cuvier* (Paris, 1833), p. 265.

46. Leonard, *l.c.* (1953), p. 108; Sée, H., *l.c.,* p. 120

Hospital, Disease and Community:
The London Fever Hospital, 1801–1850

W.F. BYNUM

The social character of medicine is also the result of the fact that in all medical actions there are always two parties involved: the medical corps, in the broadest sense of the word, and society; or, in its simplest form, physician and patient, whereby, however, the two meet not only as individuals but also as members of society with obligations toward it.[1]

Arrangements to provide for the needs of the sick have always been intimately linked with the varying economic, political, social, and cultural conditions that govern the life of man. Whether man lived in a city or on the land, whether he suffered scarcity or enjoyed abundance, how he saw his fellow men and how they looked upon him, the religion he practiced and the values he prized, the learning, arts, and sciences that gave shape to his society—all have affected the development of the hospital, the form it has achieved, and the services it offered. To be understood, the hospital has to be seen, therefore, as an organ of society, sharing its characteristics, changing as the society of which it is a part is transformed, and carrying into the future evidence of its past.[2]

To both Sigerist and Rosen, medicine was above all a social phenomenon. No interaction between a particular healer and a particular sufferer, no medical discovery or medical institution, can be properly understood apart from the wider economic, social, and cultural forces which have moulded those individuals and their ideas and institutions. Within this framework, it becomes possible to view broader issues through biography. Our present example is the biography of an institution, but I should like to use my brief narrative of the foundation and first few decades of the London Fever Hospital as a means of considering certain features of the medical, philanthropic, religious, and social responses to that peculiarly British revolution, beside which the American, French, and Russian Revolutions pale into relative insignificance.

I mean, of course, the Industrial Revolution. Britain was the first industrial nation, and the London Fever Hospital and similar institutions in the provinces were products of that complex but fascinating process whereby Britain became for two or three generations the workshop of the world. Significantly, 'gaol fever' and 'camp fever' were two names for the disease that these fever wards and fever hospitals were designed to combat. 'Institutional fever' would have been a more accurate term, and crowded institutions of all kinds proliferated in early industrial Britain. Not only jails, but also workhouses, prisons, barracks, factories, orphanages, infirmaries, asylums, and boarding houses, all became common features of the urban landscape. And in working-class areas all over Britain, four, five, six, or more families, along with assorted transients, could easily be found crammed into dwellings designed for a single family. It did not require a sophisticated epidemiologist to realise that, by and large, fever was a disease of poverty and of overcrowding.[3]

Indeed, the whole fever hospital movement was founded on the recognition of precisely that association between disease and poverty and overcrowding. By the time that Edwin Chadwick, Lemuel Shattock, and Rudolf Virchow were writing in the 1840s, the fever hospital movement was more than half a century old.[4] This is to deny neither the importance nor the originality of those leaders of what is generally reckoned the public health movement's heroic period. As we shall see, the partial failures and the qualified successes of the prior, but more limited, fever hospital movement, helped shape the nascent public health programs of the 1840s. Initially, the two movements were complementary, though public health and bacteriology eventually made fever hospitals unnecessary. The London Fever Hospital remained a hospital for infectious diseases until the 1946 National Health Service Act amalgamated it with the Royal Free Hospital group. Now, sadly, the rather distinguished, mid-Victorian buildings which were the London Fever Hospital are largely empty, as shifting urban populations and new disease patterns have made the hospital redundant.[5]

Although the London Fever Hospital no longer formally survives, its records do. These archives provide a reasonably complete chronicle of the hospital's 150-year history. They contain information about its foundation, its management committee, its finances, the behind-the-scenes squabbles of its governors, the activities of its medical committee, the comings, goings, and misdemeanours of its staff, its formal relations with various poor-law boards, parish guardians, and workhouse officials, and, after 1867, its relations with the Metropolitan Asylums Board, which was created to oversee the State's first systematic provision of fever hospitals.[6] As so often, the archives tell us rather less about the patients themselves than about those who looked after them and those whose donations of time and money supported the hospital. Nevertheless, there is one volume of case records from 1824 and early 1825 which contains the histories and hospital courses of about 130 consecutive female admissions. It confirms what contemporaries frequently stated: fever was a disease of young adulthood about two-thirds of these patients were between the ages of fifteen and 35. From this series we can sense the occupational and geographic range of the hospital's clientele. Not surprisingly, most of the women in employment were servants, though several nurses also became patients. Eight of the women were transferred from workhouses. Finally, the volume's tersely recorded histories and physical examinations remind us that eighteenth- and early nineteenth-century diagnoses of fever do not conform to any single modern diagnostic category. During our period fever was a disease in itself, rather than simply a sign of disease. And though it is undoubtedly correct to assume that many patients whom fever hospitals treated would today be diagnosed as having typhus, the recorded case histories are not sufficiently detailed either to confirm or to falsify that assumption.[7]

It was, of course, during the first half of the nineteenth century that fevers began to be separated accurately on the basis of more careful histories and physicals and systematic post-mortem examination. One of the earliest physicians to distinguish typhus from typhoid on these grounds was Sir William Jenner. He did that work at the London Fever Hospital, though Jenner is more intimately associated with University College Hospital, where he was for many years professor of pathological anatomy and clinical medicine.[8] Other distinguished physicians later in the century also put their associations with the London Fever Hospital to good use. Sir William Broadbent left some superb clinical studies of typhus and meningitis, and Charles Murchison's classic treatise on what he called the *Continued Fevers of Great Britain* was swelled by his experience as assistant physician to the Hospital.[9]

But the work of Jenner, Broadbent, and Murchison falls outside my temporal limits. Rather, I should like to look at some of the philanthropic and medical rationales behind the foundation of the Hospital, examine its therapeutic program in action, and then consider how that program slowly evolved over 50 years, as new medical staff brought new ideas to bear. To anticipate one of my conclusions, I shall suggest that the institution itself imposed a kind of form onto the activities of the individuals working there.

This meant that while the initial ideas were enormously important, subsequent actions were shaped by the force of institutional protocol. Like Tristram Shandy, institutions almost inevitably bear long-term marks of their conception and birth. For the London Fever Hospital, this was not a bad thing.

First, then, its foundation: it was established along the conventional voluntary hospital model, which had been initiated in London early in the eighteenth century, subsequently spread to the provinces, and provided a general framework for finance, management, and patient selection for most of the hundreds of hospitals established in Britain during the eighteenth and nineteenth centuries.[10] Nevertheless, certain differences existed between the two principle forms of hospitals: the *general,* all-purpose hospital, such as Westminster Hospital, St. George's, the Middlesex, the London, etc., on the one hand, and the profusion of *specialized* hospitals which began to increase in the late eighteenth century. General hospitals tended to be dominated by lay governors, whereas the smaller, specialized institutions, such as lying-in hospitals, hospitals for chest diseases, skin complaints, and venereal disease, were ordinarily established and subsequently dominated by the doctor or doctors who staffed them.[11]

The London Fever Hospital falls between these two basic patterns. It was of the general, voluntary type in the breadth of its lay support and in the composition of its management committee. But it differed from the general, voluntary pattern in several ways. First, the general management committee bowed to specific medical authority in many policy decisions. There was a medical sub-committee which oversaw aspects of patient care, hospital cleanliness, ventilation, etc. Second, patients did not need a letter from a hospital governor to be admitted. In ordinary voluntary hospitals, lay governors exerted considerable influence on admissions, but admission to the Fever Hospital required a letter from a *medical man,* stating that the patient was suffering from a contagious fever. In addition, the original hospital founders (largely laymen) appealed to a group of eminent London physicians for medical justification for the foundation of a hospital. At the organizational meeting on May Day, 1801, a letter from fifteen London physicians was read. The signatories included Richard Budd and John Latham of St. Bartholomew's, William Saunders and William Babington of Guy's, John Cooke and William Hamilton of the London Hospital, and Robert Willan and Thomas Murray of the Public Dispensary.

The letter is worth recording, since it outlines definite features which subsequently became hospital policy. It was dated London, April 19, 1801:

> Having been desired to state our sentiments on the situation of the Poor with respect to Contagion, we declare that Infectious, Malignant Fever is at all times prevalent among the Poor of the Metropolis, in whose habitations it has an instant tendency to diffuse itself more widely; that it often extends from them to the higher orders; that it derives its origin principally from neglect of cleanliness and ventilation; and that its communication from the person first attacked, to the other members of a family is an almost necessary consequence of the crowded state of the dwelling of the Poor. Although the present season of the year is not that, at which in general Typhus chiefly prevails,[12] yet we know that at this time many persons are daily suffering from its attacks. We are of opinion that the evils which result to individuals and to the Community from this circumstance are of such magnitude as to render it necessary that they should be immediately remedied. We believe that in many instances the infection of a family and neighbourhood is owing to contagion introduced by a single person, and would be prevented by his timely removal. We are therefore satisfied that the evils above mentioned would be in great measure obviated by the establishment of an institution which should have for its object—the removal of persons attacked by Contagious Fever from situations where, if they remain, the infection of others is inevitable, and the cleansing and purifying of the apartments, furniture and clothes of those, in whose habitations a contagious Disease has subsisted, or is likely to appear. We conceive that the present number of patients labouring under Typhus and other contagious Diseases in London, can only be estimated from numerous individual communications.[13]

Several points of interest might be stressed, such as the recognition of the association between poverty and fever, coupled with the fear that the higher orders were not infrequently endangered by the diseases of their inferiors. There was a specific statement of contagion and the important proviso that an epidemic could be started by a single infected individual. There was the emphasis on dirt and bad ventilation in the etiology of contagious fevers, and the complementary stress on cleanliness and fresh air in the prevention and treatment of the condition. Finally, the letter pinpointed the wider social significance of the proposed institution in *containing contagion* as well as for treating those already infected.

The specific stimulus for establishing the institution was the prevalence of fever in London during the previous two autumns.[14]

But, more generally, the notion of fever hospitals had already been elaborated in the provinces, and the London institution self-consciously took its cue from pre-existing fever wards and Houses of Recovery in Chester, Dublin, Manchester, and Liverpool. These and subsequent similar establishments in Leeds, Stockport, and elsewhere are sufficiently important to justify Miss Buer's label 'Fever Hospital Movement,'[15] the patron saints of which were James Lind and Sir John Pringle. Between them these two military physicians did much to raise public consciousness—medical and lay—about the connexion between dirt and overcrowding and the diseases of military and institutional life.[16]

In the 1770s, John Haygarth, (1740–1827), then practicing in Chester, became intrigued by the correlation between social class and diseases such as fever. Haygarth surveyed the town, noting that the more densely populated suburbs were less healthy than the more spacious and elegant center of Chester. Believing contagion to be associated with human effluvia, he found it unsurprising that the overcrowded poor should suffer most:

> . . . they want most of the conveniences and comforts of life: their houses are small, close, crowded, and dirty: their diet affords very bad nourishment, and their cloathes are seldom changed or washed. . . . The air they breathe at home is thus rendered noxious by respiration and putrefaction. . . . This noxious air is the most frequent cause of malignant fevers. In these poor habitations, when one person is seized with fever, others of the family are generally affected with the same fever in a greater or less degree. This dreadful consequence is naturally to be expected, as putrid steams arising from the diseased body are added to the other.[17]

Having stated his convictions in this article in the *Philosophical Transactions,* Haygarth went on to enunciate the corrolary upon which much of the early fever hospital movement was to be based: 'If a regulation could be universally adopted of immediately removing out of the family such of the poor people as are seized with fevers, it is evident that the most salutary consequences would follow.'[18]

Haygarth got the opportunity to put his proposals into action a few years later, when, during an epidemic of fever, he was permitted to turn a spare room into a fever ward for the Chester Infirmary. His program was based on the general principles enunciated in his earlier article, combined with his belief that, so rapid was the dropping off of infective air with distance, by placing the beds in his ward some six feet apart, with proper ventilation, hospital infections could be effectively contained: 'When the chamber of a patient ill of an infectious fever is spacious, airy and clean, few or none even of the most intimate attendants will catch the Distemper.'[19]

Haygarth himself would be worth a proper study as an example of a provincial physician with wide medical, philanthropic, and social concerns.[20] He was the friend of numerous other physicians associated with the fever hospital movement, such as John Ferriar, Thomas Percival, and James Currie. Currie of Liverpool was particularly significant for the early program of the London Fever Hospital, for he introduced two aspects of diagnosis and treatment which were adopted in London: the diagnosis of fever by the use of the thermometer, and the treatment of elevated body temperature by cold water baths. Currie's *Medical Reports on the effects of Water, cold and warm, as a remedy in Fever and other Diseases,* published in 1798, reported his own successes in using cold water to rid the patient—temporarily, at least—of excess body heat.[21] It is pleasant to read his case histories, where he stressed the symptomatic improvement which accompanied these periods of normal body temperature. During these periods, patients could eat and rest, something which clearly benefitted them more than the usual low diets with which physicians were prone to treat fevers. On the other hand, Currie saw his therapeutic regimen as countering the emphasis which William Cullen in Edinburgh had placed on *general debility* as the cardinal symptom of fever. Currie's use of cold water baths, Haygarth's emphasis on the cooling effects of ventilation, and James Hamilton's recommendation of purgation in fever,[22] were all reactions against Cullen's theory of fever. Since cold water, fresh air, and purgation were all widely used in most of the early fever hospitals, the movement can be seen as one indication that Cullen's influence was waning by 1800.[23]

This, then, is a brief account of the provincial background against which a group of individuals determined to establish a fever hospital in the capital. London medical men, of course, knew of the provincial aspects of the movement, but there was a further, lay relationship between London and the provinces, for the charitable organization behind the London Fever Hospital had vigorous connexions with the industrial north of England. This was the Society for the Betterment of the Condition of the Poor.[24] Several of its most prominent members —William Wilberforce, (Sir) Thomas Bernard, and Shute Barrington, Bishop of Durham—were instrumental in establishing the London institution. The Bishop of Durham took the chair at the inaugural, May

Day meeting, and he was one of five appointed to prepare the regulations for the new institution. The driving force behind the Society for the Betterment of the Condition of the Poor was evangelical religion —that fervent and active branch of the Anglican Church most intimately associated with Wilberforce's fight to abolish the slave trade, and ultimately, slavery itself in Britain and her dominions.[25] The Evangelicals combined a passionate hatred of the godless French under Napoleon with an aloof but genuine concern for what they feared were the increasingly godless working-classes of their own country. They carried the intense individualism so frequently found among evangelical Protestants into their social philosophies. Above all, the poor were to be helped to help themselves, through example, through innumerable useful tracts and pamphlets, through basic moral and practical education, and through institutions which could aid them in times of trouble. Among the literally hundreds of pamphlets distributed by the Society and other evangelical organizations, was one by John Ferriar, giving advice to the poor on cleanliness.[26]

The Evangelical's ideal, working-class individual had a pious mind in a sound body, so hospitals were obvious outlets for their charitable activities. In the specific case of the London Fever Hospital, aid was extended to each sick pauper and his family, through medical treatment, white-washing the walls of the infected dwelling, washing the clothes of each patient (and usually of his family as well), and general fumigation of infected houses with the nitrous acid solution which Carmichael Smyth popularized in the 1790's.[27] It was a program tailored to the notion of individual contagion, to the belief that fever epidemics could and did begin with a single person.

The May-Day, 1801 meeting approved the London Fever Hospital, so the management committee—with Wilberforce and Barrington among its vice-presidents—could look for accommodation. They deliberately chose a site near the densely-populated St. Giles, Holborn (the Rookery made famous by a subsequent vice-president of the hospital, Charles Dickens).[28] Their choice, a house in Constitution Row, Gray's Inn Lane, inevitably aroused local opposition, as did their third and final location in the Liverpool Road, Islington, in 1848.[29] To allay fears the Committee called upon its recently appointed medical committee—which included such men as John Coakley Lettsom and Sir Walter Farquhar—to assure the locals that 'From the experience of Chester, Manchester, Waterford, and other places' where fever hospitals had been established, 'the Number of Contagious Fevers has been greatly diminished, not only in the Town, but in the very Districts where the houses were situated.'[30] It is of interest to note that, five years later, the Hospital's physician Thomas Bateman could report that there had not been a single case of contagious fever in the immediate neighborhood of the House of Recovery, as it was called. The hospital itself had not been so fortunate, having lost a nurse, a porter, and its first physician, Thomas A. Murray, a young Edinburgh graduate who contracted a fatal fever within a year of his appointment—not, as the Committee was quick to point out, in the hospital itself, but in the house of a pauper family about to be admitted. The family—man, woman, child—went into hospital, and all recovered.[31]

We know virtually nothing about Murray, since he died so young.[32] But we do know that his two successors, William Dimsdale and Thomas Bateman, practised thermometry and the cold water treatment of Currie. Dimsdale married wealth and retired from medical practice after only three years at the hospital, but Bateman remained some 13 years, until ill health forced his retirement to Yorkshire.[33] Although no actual case records survive from Bateman's period, we can get some idea of his regimen from two works on fever which he published in 1818 and 1819.[34] By the end of his career, he had abandoned the use of both the thermometer and cold baths, stressing instead the similarity between contagion and inflammation, the treatment for which was blood letting, leaching, and aperients. In fact, though his regimen in 1818 appeals less to the modern reader than one which he described in 1805, he had merely shifted his emphasis, for Bateman still saw himself firmly in the tradition of Haygarth and Currie, combatting the teaching of Cullen and, above all, of John Brown. Brown insisted that even diseases of the sthenic variety (including fevers) almost inevitably produce asthenia via indirect debility.[35] According to Bateman, Brown's doctrines contravened the fundamental Hippocratic principle: *Contraria contrariis medentur.* As Bateman wrote, 'No appearance of languor or debility should induce a disposition to swerve from a steady pursuit of the antiphlogistic plan, in diet, regimen, and medicine.'[36] Bateman's abandonment of the cold water program was only gradual, because his clinical experience convinced him of its futility. Nevertheless, he continued to allow London Fever Hospital patients to be sponged with tepid water, as a means to temporary symptomatic improvement.

For the rest, Bateman saw little cause to change the general therapeutic and prophylactic program of the hospital. He continued to attribute the cluster of fevers with which he had daily contact to a contagion; his discussions of etiology stressed poor nutrition as the primary cause of contagious fevers, overcrowding in his opinion playing a secondary role.[37] Cleanliness and proper ventilation still featured in the hospital's ethos. The patients' own clothes were replaced on admission with specially designed, loose-fitting hospital attire; if they managed to survive the hospital stay, their clothes would have been laundered in the hospital's own laundry. Indeed, whatever the changing fortunes of the concept of contagion within the medical profession itself, the poor seemed to believe in it—and to believe that dirty clothes were powerful fomites. The job of laundress to the hospital appears to have been highly hazardous; fever was rife among the women who worked in the laundry, and it was one hospital position which the Committee had difficulty keeping filled.

Bateman himself never wavered from his belief in the specific contagiousness of fever, or in his conviction that a single person in a single dwelling could be the locus of a fever epidemic. The hospital maintained its policy of white-washing and fumigating the dwellings of its patients; indeed, it was said, had the Bishop of Durham had his way in the matter, the houses of the poor throughout England would have continually dripped with white-wash and reeked with nitrous acid. Nevertheless, we can discover in the hospital records the accumulating evidence belying the adequacy of this individualistic approach. The Committee kept good records of the geographical distribution of its patients. This practice was partially motivated by the necessity to remind appropriate parish guardians that they were expected either to pay two guineas for each pauper they sent to the hospital or to contribute a substantial annual sum to the hospital's exchequer. But one result of the Committee's geographical sensitivity was the recognition that despite all efforts at fumigation and white-washing, certain particularly notorious pockets of the Metropolis continued to supply a steady stream of patients. Spread Eagle Court, not far from the original hospital site, proved especially intractable, and more than once, the Committee asked the Governors and Directors of the Parish of St. Andrew, Holborn, to look into the matter.[38]

Workhouses provided another steady source of patients and another fascinating mixture of cooperation and conflict between hospital officials and workhouse guardians. Cooperation was the ideal, since the basic function of the hospital was to remove contagious patients before they could act as foci of spread. Conflict was all too frequent,

however, as the Committee complained that parishes were not uphold-
ing their share of the financial responsibility, and hospital physicians
complained that patients were often not received from the workhouses
until already moribund. Indeed, problems of timing constantly
plagued the hospital. It seemed obvious that early removal was necessary for the effective operation of both the therapeutic and the preventative aspects of the hospital's activity. But workhouse guardians resisted sending their infected inmates unless absolutely necessary
because of the expense, and the poor themselves resisted coming to
the hospital for a variety of reasons. The Committee had originally
adopted the name which Ferriar had coined—'House of Recovery'—
to counteract the reputation which hospitals had among their clients.
Inevitably, the historian is forced to come to grips with the 'gateway
to death' thesis.[39] Were hospitals places where more harm than good
was likely to come to patients? The Committee was certainly aware that
many paupers and medically indigent individuals had a dread of hospitals as the last stop along the road to death. Obviously, neither Committee members nor doctors believed it, or we may assume that—
barring some vicious middle and upper-class vendetta against their
social inferiors—they would never have supported the hospital with
their time and money. Within the Committee's own frame of reference,
it was precisely this lower-class fear of hospitals which fed the 'gateway
to death' reputation in the first place, for, as was frequently reiterated,
more than 40 percent of hospital deaths occurred within five days after
admission.[40] Patients, the doctors insisted, were waiting until they
were beyond the reach of medical help before seeking that help. Given
the doctrine of contagion, this was socially irresponsible as well as
individually dangerous. But, as the Committee sadly noted, tardiness
simply diminished hospital efficiency.[41]

On the other hand, hospital officials were convinced that the positive value of their endeavors was being gradually accepted by the
patients they served. At least, this was the interpretation they chose to
place on the impressive increase in applications for admission beginning about 1816.[42] By then, the London Fever Hospital had moved to
larger quarters adjacent to the Small Pox Hospital at Battle Bridge,
now the site of King's Cross Railway Station. Bed space increased from
fewer than 20 to between 60 and 70, though in the first decade of the
hospital's existence even the few available beds had rarely been filled.
It cannot be merely the increased hospital potential which caused the
number of patients treated to rise from 80 in 1804 to 760 in 1817.

Rising patient acceptance may have accounted for some of this increase, but of more importance was that epidemic fever—relatively
rare in London between 1805 and 1815—became common after a
serious epidemic in 1816.[43] By 1820, the hospital always filled up in
the autumn, and patients had to be turned away.

Since patients usually, though not inevitably, first presented themselves with a letter from a medical man, increased use of the hospital
probably reflects a significant change in medical policy rather than in
attitude among the poor of the districts the hospital served. Certainly,
mortality rates in the hospital did not improve. They varied significantly from year to year, ranging from eight percent to 16 percent.[44]
But the randomness of the yearly variation probably substantiates
Bateman's suggestion that the primary variable was the virulence of
the diseases, not any permutation in therapy. On the other hand,
Bateman was convinced that mortality outside the hospital for cases of
comparable severity was as much as 25 to 30 percent, in itself a potent
claim for the hospital's efficacy.[45]

Firm data either to verify or refute even the general tenor of
Bateman's assertion are tantalizingly difficult to find, since both statistics and disease categories are unreliable. From what we know of
hospital policy, it is reasonable to suppose that patients were considerably better off in hospital than in their overcrowded, ill-heated, and
ill-ventilated apartments. And the measures to prevent the spread of
contagion within the hospital were probably at least partially effective,
especially for the louse-borne typhus. Erysipelas, however, was not
infrequently acquired in the hospital; it complicated the ordinary fever
course, and was all too often the harbinger of death.[46]

The continuity of admissions policy, patient care, and wider community activity during the hospital's first quarter century is impressive.
In 1824, the election of Alexander Tweedie and Thomas Southwood
Smith as physicians to the hospital gave a stability to the medical staff
unknown during its earliest period. Between them, Tweedie and
Southwood Smith served for more than 70 years. It is perhaps appropriate that the hospital which had lost no less than three of its first eight
physicians to fever could have kept its physicians alive and more or less
well during this later period, when the doctrine of contagion was under
considerable medical attack. Tweedie, it might be added, continued to
uphold the doctrine. In his little volume of case studies of fever published in 1830, he admitted to a certain anxiety, since three of his
predecessors had been cut off in their prime by the disease the hospital

was supposed to cure. In fact, of the first eight physicians, only Bateman had escaped being attacked by fever, an observation which in Tweedie's opinion should have conclusively proved the disease's contagiousness. He further pointed out that in 1829 two resident medical officers, plus a medical pupil who assumed the duties after the medical officers fell ill, had all come down with fever. The medical student, having been taught the non-contagiousness of fever, remained unrepentant. As Tweedie remarked, 'I fear this almost fatal personal illustration has not convinced him of the contagious nature of fever.'[47]

This unnamed medical student and Southwood Smith belonged to the growing group of medical men who from the 1820's were increasingly critical of traditional doctrines of contagion. In a classic paper on anticontagionism, Erwin Ackerknecht has examined this phenomenon, which had strong social and economic reverberations.[48] Although the cholera epidemics of 1832 and 1848 provided the most urgent forums for debate, Southwood Smith's own concern with the matter flowed naturally from his experience with fever. In a series of articles for the *Westminster Review* and other periodicals, in his popular *Treatise on Fever* of 1830, and, most movingly, in his 1838 report on fever and poverty in two of London's worst areas, Whitechapel and Bethnal Green, Smith expounded his medical and social philosophy.[49] His presence as physician to the London Fever Hospital reminds us of a second major force moulding social reform in early nineteenth-century Britain: utilitarianism. Utilitarians and Evangelicals made strange bed-fellows, since they started from radically different assumptions about human nature. Nevertheless, they frequently found themselves working for the same cause and sitting on the same committees.[50] By the 1840's the public health movement wore utilitarian garb: Edwin Chadwick had been Jeremy Bentham's last secretary; Southwood Smith had been his last personal physician. Both had absorbed Bentham's utilitarian philosophy and his reforming zeal, and both came to believe that the permissive individualism underlying the London Fever Hospital's program had been proved inadequate in affairs touching the public's health.[51]

The London Fever Hospital continued to claim Smith's allegiance and energies, for, unlike Chadwick, he never lost his faith in the curative powers of medicine. But Smith's theories of what he called 'epidemic diseases' (including fever) required far more comprehensive social policies for their prevention than that provided by the fever hospital movement. Public health needed to acquire (in the memorable phrase of John Simon), 'the novel virtue of the imperative mood.'[52]

This shift from individual to community thinking was an essential feature of Victorian public health, but, as I suggested earlier, public health became an accretion to, rather than a displacement of, the programs of the fever hospital movement. Fever hospitals, moreover, served another important function, for they and other specialized hospitals brought together large numbers of patients suffering from similar or related diseases. And though Tweedie and Southwood Smith differed on the issue of contagion, they agreed on another important question concerning the essential nature of fevers. Were fevers local or generalized diseases? Both these physicians were aware of Broussais's work purporting to localize all fevers to the gastro-intestinal tract, and Henry Clutterbuck's equally fervent insistence that the primary manifestation of fever was inflammation of the brain.[53] They rejected these extreme localistic models, realizing at the same time that fundamental medical discoveries could be made in the post-mortem room. By the 1830's, physicians at the London Fever Hospital performed autopsies on almost two-thirds of their fatal cases. Indeed, by that decade, Tweedie and Southwood Smith were practising hospital medicine, with pathologico-clinical correlation of sign, symptom, and lesion. The local lesions of fever reinforced their belief in the disease's inflammatory nature, so neither modified the traditional antiphlogistic therapy of their predecessors. In the 1840's, just as 40 years before, a patient entering the London Fever Hospital could expect a low diet, blood letting, cupping, and aperients.[54]

What, by way of conclusion, do these hospital archives tell us about the relative importance of change and continuity during that crucial half-century of medical history, during which evolved what Ackerknecht has called hospital medicine, what Michel Foucault labelled the 'birth of the clinic,' and what Richard Shryock described as 'the emergence of modern medicine.'[55] Does our microcosm, the London Fever Hospital, reflect the macrocosm?

At one level, of course, the answer is yes. In so many of their professional attitudes, Tweedie and Smith were self-consciously modern, relying on their own observations and articulating a modern philosophy of medical science. By contrast, Haygarth and Bateman had deep reverence for medicine's past and saw themselves as still engaging in a Hippocratic debate.

At the level of ideas, vocabulary, and professional identity, then, a real contrast can be drawn between the men at the beginning of our period, and those at the end. But rhetoric changes more easily than practice, and when we examine what the doctors actually did, continuity rather than change becomes apparent. The basic features of the hospital's therapeutic and prophylactic program remained fixed for half a century and more. Both Management Committee and hospital staff justified their actions with a variety of new ideas; they treated their patients much the same. Until rather late in the nineteenth century, after all, there were only three principal approaches to the treatment of fever. It was conceived as a disease of debility (direct or indirect), which required building the patient up; it was thought to be a disease of inflammation or other condition of hyperactivity, which dictated lowering the patient's system; or it was a disease which nature knew best how to cure and that doctor served best who merely stood and waited. The British fever hospital movement was founded on the proposition that fever patients must be lowered, although cleanliness, fresh air, and loose-fitting hospital garments were as much a part of that picture as the purgative and the lancet. Perhaps more significantly, the movement was founded on the proposition that hospitals must be responsive to community needs, that hospital care must be extended to anyone who requires it, and that prevention is better than cure. By the end of our period, the movement had demonstrated its worth and its limitations. It had shown to a few people at least, that it takes more than hospitals to prevent disease. By 1850, Britain was slowly feeling her way towards social medicine.

Notes

The paper printed here is a slightly modified version of the first Henry E. Sigerist Lecture, delivered on April 4, 1977, at Yale University. My hosts at Yale were George and Beate Rosen, who with a number of other New Haven friends made the occasion a particularly happy one. In his remarks introducing the new series of Sigerist Lectures, George Rosen recalled how much Sigerist's friendship had meant to him. Nora Beeson, Sigerist's daughter, then gave a lively and affectionate account of her father.

This lecture was originally scheduled to appear in the *Bulletin of the History of Medicine*. Following George Rosen's untimely death, Lloyd Stevenson kindly released me from my obligation, so that the essay could appear in the present volume. It is altogether fitting that it should now be dedicated to the joint memory of Henry Sigerist and George Rosen.

I am particularly grateful to Dr. Edith Gilchrist of the Royal Free Hospital, London, for rescuing the archives of the London Fever Hospital and for generously making my access to them so easy. Most of the research for this paper was done at the Wellcome Institute for the History of Medicine, to whose staff I am indebted.

1. Henry E. Sigerist, *Primitive and Archaic Medicine* (New York, Oxford University Press, 1967), p.15.

2. George Rosen, "The Hospital: Historical Sociology of a Community Institution," in *From Medical Police to Social Medicine* (New York, Science History Publications, 1974), p. 274.

3. For explorations of various aspects of this large subject, see Arthur J. Taylor, ed., *The Standard of Living in Britain in the Industrial Revolution* (London, Methuen, 1975); Anthony J. Wohl, *The Eternal Slum: housing and social policy in Victorian London* (London, Edward Arnold, 1977); and George Rosen, "Disease, Debility and Death," in H.J. Dyos and Michael Wolff, eds., *The Victorian City: Image and Reality* (London and Boston, Routledge and Kegan Paul, 1973).

4. M.C. Buer, *Health, Wealth, and Population in the early Days of the Industrial Revolution.* (London, Routledge, 1926), esp. chapter 15; and George Rosen, *A History of Public Health* (New York, M.D. Publications, 1958), pp.182ff.

5. Two earlier buildings which housed the London Fever Hospital have long since disappeared.

6. Gwendoline M. Ayers, *England's First State Hospitals, 1867–1930* (London, Wellcome Institute of the History of Medicine, 1971).

7. A typical admission entry is the one for Francis Bristow, a seventeen-year-old servant from Wimbledon: "November 3. Was admitted yesterday with pain of head and back, heat, thirst and prostration of strength. Became ill on the 25th ulto.—but had been complaining a little two or three days before with headache, sickness, vomiting and pain of back, chills and heats. Knows no cause for her disease. Has headache, pain and tenderness of epigastrium. Slight cough; Pulse 86, full; skin hot and dry; Tongue furred and moist; has taken 3 gr. powder and half an ounce of oil which have operated 3 times. Bowels open from medicine before admission." This patient was dismissed cured on 30 November ("Mss. case book for 1824," f.154).'

8. Jenner became a member of the Committee of the Fever Hospital in 1848. He was Assistant Physician, 1856–1859, resigning when he became Holme Professor of Clinical Medicine at University College Hospital. His classic volume, *On the Identity of Non-identity of Typhoid and Typhus Fevers,* (London, Churchill, 1850), reprints articles which first appeared in 1848.

9. Many of Broadbent's more important papers are conveniently reprinted in W. Broadbent, ed. *Selections from the Writings, Medical and Neurological, of Sir William Broadbent* (London, Frowde and Hodder, 1908); and Charles Murchison, *A Treatise on the Continued Fevers of Great Britain* (London, Parker, 1862).

10. A general study of British hospitals in Brian Abel-Smith, *The Hospitals, 1800–1948* (London, Heinemann, 1964); of the numerous studies of individual voluntary hospitals, that by A.E. Clark-Kennedy is perhaps the best: *The London: A Study in the Voluntary Hospital System,* 2 vols., (London, Pitman, 1962).

11. The forthcoming work of M.J. Peterson should do much to clarify the uses to which doctors put the different kinds of hospitals in mid-Victorian Britain.

12. Autumn being the season when typhus usually was seen in epidemic proportions. An interesting parallel case is charted by Erwin Ackerknecht, "The Vagaries of the

Notion of Epidemic Hepatitis or Infectious Jaundice," in Lloyd G. Stevenson and Robert P. Multhauf, eds., *Medicine, Science and Culture* (Baltimore, The Johns Hopkins Press, 1968).

13.   "London Fever Hospital, Minutes of Committee Meetings, 1801–1815" (henceforth "Minutes, vol.I"), ff.1–2. The letter was published in *The Reports of the Society for the Bettering the Condition and Increasing the Comforts of the Poor*, 3 vols., 5th ed., (London, W. Bulmer, 1811), III: pp. 208–209. (Henceforth, *Reports*).

14.   Robert Willan, *Reports on the Diseases in London, particularly during the years 1796, 97, 98, 99, and 1800* (London, R. Philips, 1801).

15.   In the work cited (n.4).

16.   Pringle's life and work remain relatively unexplored, though one may consult Dorothea Singer, "Sir John Pringle and his circle," *Ann.Sci.* 6 (1948–1950), pp. 127–180, 229–261; and Sydney Selwyn "Sir John Pringle: Hospital Reformer, Moral Philosopher and Pioneer of Antiseptics," *Med.Hist.* 10 (1966), pp. 266–274. For Lind, see L.H. Roddis, *James Lind; Founder of Nautical Medicine* (New York, Schuman, 1950).

17.   John Haygarth, "Observations on the population and diseases of Chester, in the year 1774," *Philosophical Transactions* 68 (1778), pp. 131–154; 139–140.

18.   *Ibid.,* p.140.

19.   John Haygarth, *A letter to Dr Percival, on the Prevention of Infectious Fevers* (Bath, R. Cruttwell, 1801), p.38.

20.   Two useful examinations of his work are G.W. Weaver, "John Haygarth: clinician, investigator, apostle of Sanitation, 1740–1827," *Bull.Soc.Med.Hist.Chicago* 4 (1928–1935), pp. 156–200; and A.W. Downie, 'John Haygarth of Chester and inoculation against Smallpox,' *Liverpool med.Inst.Trans* (1964), pp. 26–42.

21.   Currie's *Medical Reports* went into its fourth edition in 1805.

22.   James Hamilton, *Observations on the Utility and Administration of Purgative Medicines in Several Diseases* (Edinburgh, C. Stewart, 1805).

23.   Cullen's place in British medical thought has never been adequately assessed.

24.   An idea of the range of the Society's interests can be obtained from *The Reports* (above, n.13). The best modern account can be found in J.R. Poynter, *Society and Pauperism: English Ideas on Poor Relief, 1795–1834* (London, Routledge and Kegan Paul, 1969), pp. 91–98.

25.   A brilliantly ironic study of Evangelical *mentalité* is Ford K. Brown, *Fathers of the Victorians: the Age of Wilberforce* (Cambridge, Cambridge University Press, 1961). More sympathetic is Ian Bradley, *The Call to Seriousness: the Evangelical Impact on the Victorians* (London, Jonathan Cape, 1976).

26.   John Ferriar, "Advice to the Poor," reprinted in *Reports* (n.13) II, pp. 271–276.

27.   James Carmichael Smyth, *The effect of the Nitrous Vapour, in preventing and destroying Contagion* (London, J. Johnson, 1799). In 1802, Parliament voted Smyth a reward of £ 5,000 for his work on disinfection with nitrous acid.

28.   Charles Dickens, "On duty with Inspector Field," in *The Uncommercial Traveller and Reprinted Pieces* (London, Oxford University Press, 1958), pp. 513–526.

29. Since the hospital's second site was adjacent the Small Pox Hospital, the locals apparently did not protest.

30. "London Fever Hospital, Committee Minutes," (1804–1815), ff. 34–35. The letter was transcribed in *Reports* (n.13), III, pp. 208–209.

31. "London Fever Hospital, Commitee Minutes," (1814–1815), f.52: "Dr. Willan reported that since the last Meeting of the Committee the Institution had sustained the heavy loss of their invaluable Physician Dr Thomas Archibald Murray by a Typhus Fever caught at the highly infected apartments of one Harris in Stone Cutters Alley Lincolns Inn Fields who with his wife and child were afterwards removed by the Doctor's direction to the House in Grays Inn Lane and there happily reovered." (Minutes for 26 March 1802).

32. An Edinburgh graduate, Murray apparently published only one item except for his M.D. thesis. This was a pamphlet entitled, *Remarks on the Situation of the Poor in the Metropolis, as contributing to the progress of Contagious Diseases.* (London, R. Noble, 1801).

33. [J. Rumsey], *Some Account of the Life and Character of the Late Thomas Bateman, M.D. F.L.S.* (London, Longman, 1826).

34. Thomas Bateman, *A Succinct Account of the Contagious Fevers of this Country* (London, Longman, 1818); T. Bateman, *Reports on the Diseases of London, and the State of the Weather, from 1804 to 1816* (London, Longman, 1819).

35. *cf.* G.B. Risse, "The Brownian System of Medicine: Its Theoretical and Practical Implications," *Clio Medica,* 5 (1970), pp. 45–51.

36. T. Bateman, *Succinct Account* (n.34), p. 102. More generally, *cf.* Peter Niebyl, "The English Bloodletting Revolution, or Modern Medicine before 1850," *Bull.Hist.Med.,* 51 (1977), pp. 464–483.

37. T. Bateman, *Succinct Account* (n.34), p.11: ". . . epidemic fever is unquestionably generated in the first instance by defective nutriment. . . ."

38. A typical deliberation about a pocket of infection is recorded in the minutes of 30 July 1802 ("Minutes," vol.I, ff. 66–67). Spread Eagle Court first came to Committee's attention in July 1803. (*cf.* "Minutes," vol.I, ff. 92–97).

39. On this contemporary debate, *cf.* E.M. Sigsworth, "Gateway to death? Medicine, hospitals and mortality, 1700–1850," in Peter Mathias, ed., *Science and Society, 1600–1900* (Cambridge University Press, 1972); John Woodward, *To Do This Sick No Harm: A Study of the British Voluntary Hospital System to 1875* (London, Routledge and Kegan Paul, 1974); and, as a critic of early hospitals, Thomas McKeown, *The Modern Rise of Population* (London, Edward Arnold, 1976); and T. McKeown, *The Role of Medicine: Dream, Mirage or Nemesis?* (London, Nuffield Provincial Hospital Trust, 1976).

40. Curiously, only four out of the 20 deaths recorded in the one surviving case book (above, n.7) occurred within five days of admission. In the *Annual Report* for 1829, however, 43 out of 79 deaths took place in the first week of hospitalization.

41. *e.g.,* "Minutes," vol.I, ff. 147–148 (Meeting of 26 April 1805). *cf.* Bateman, *Succinct Account* (n.34), pp.85–86.

42. As discussed, for instance, in the *Annual Report* for 1817, recorded in 'Minutes,' vol.II, Meeting for 24 April 1818. (Pages in this minute book were never numbered.)

43.   The annual printed *Reports* of the Hospital are a good source of regular information on the prevelance of fever in London. The 1816 epidemic is discussed in Bateman, *Succinct Account* (n.34).

44.   Bateman, *Succinct Account* (n.34), pp. 74ff. puts the mortality statistics of the London Fever Hospital into a national context.

45.   In fact Robert Willan, *Reports* (above, n.14), p.229, believed that epidemic contagious fever could have an out-of-hospital mortality of almost 50 percent.

46.   Although the Annual Reports give a separate breakdown for 'typhus' and 'scarlatina,' the surviving case-book suggests that patients admitted with a diagnosis of 'typhus' sometimes died with other infectious diseases.

47.   Alexander Tweedie, *Clinical Illustrations of Fever* (London, Whittaker Treacher, 1830), p.89.

48.   Erwin H. Ackerknecht, "Anticontagionism between 1821 and 1867," *Bull.Hist.Med.* 22 (1948), pp. 562–593.

49.   T. Southwood Smith, "Contagion and Sanitary Laws," *Westminster Review* 3 (1825), pp. 134–167, 499–530; *A Treatise on Fever* (London, Longman, 1830); "Report on Some Physical Causes of Sickness and Mortality," in *Fourth Report of the Poor Law Commissioners* (London, 1838), pp. 83–94. Although Smith is inadequately studied, F.N.L. Poynter, "Thomas Southwood Smith—the Man (1788–1861)," *Proc.roy.Soc.Med.* 55(1962), pp. 381–392, is an attractive short assessment.

50.   Neatly symbolized by the presence, on the 1848 Board of Health, of Chadwick the Utilitarian and Shaftesbury the Evangelical.

51.   On Chadwick, *cf.* R.A. Lewis, *Edwin Chadwick and the Public Health Movement, 1832–1854* (London, Longmans, 1952); and S.E. Finer, *The Life and Times of Sir Edwin Chadwick* (London, Methuen, 1952). There is also an excellent introduction by M.W. Flinn to the reprint of Chadwick's 1842 *Report on the Sanitary Condition of the Labouring Population of Great Britain* (Edinburgh, University Press, 1965).

52.   The phrase is Simon's description of the 1867 Public Health Act, quoted in Royston Lambert, *Sir John Simon 1816–1904 and English Social Administration* (London, MacGibbon and Kee, 1963), p.386.

53.   T. Southwood Smith, *Fever* (n.49), pp.10ff; A Tweedie, *Fever* (n.47), p.52; Henry Clutterbuck, *An Inquiry into the Seat and Nature of Fever* (London, J. Anderson 1825).

54.   Though by 1862, Tweedie had abandoned bleeding: A. Tweedie, *Lectures on the Distinctive Characters, Pathology, and Treatment of Continued Fevers* (London, Churchill, 1862), p.255.

55.   Erwin H. Ackerknecht, *Medicine at the Paris Hospital, 1794–1848* (Baltimore: The Johns Hopkins Press, 1967); Michel Foucault, *The Birth of the Clinic,* trans. by A.M. Sheridan Smith (London, Tavistock, 1973); Richard Shryock, *The Development of Modern Medicine* (New York, Knopf, 1947), chapter 9.

Florence Nightingale on Contagion:
The Hospital as Moral Universe*

CHARLES E. ROSENBERG

We prefer our heroes to be not only heroic, but consistent—consistent, that is, with our preconceptions, not necessarily theirs. Students are still taken aback to discover that Harvey's experimental studies of the circulation were influenced by a bewildering neo-Platonic concern with the body as microcosm, or that otherwise liberal statesmen could advocate a disquieting racism. One instance of such apparent inconsistency is the lack of understanding, even hostility, displayed toward the germ theory in the last third of the nineteenth century by certain individuals prominent in the mid-century movement for public health reform.[1]

None of these reformers is better known to posterity than Florence Nightingale. Her two most widely-read books, *Notes on Nursing* and *Notes on Hospitals* had an extraordinary vogue in the second half of the century; it would be hard to overestimate her influence in the shaping of modern nursing and the reordering of hospitals. Nevertheless, there is a curious gap in our understanding of her work. Though historians have told us a good deal about the dramatic events of Nightingale's life—her struggle to escape the stylized routine of upper-class life, her heroic work in the Crimea, her commitment to reforming army hospitals and bringing public health to India—almost nothing has been written about her medical ideas, concepts which informed and justified her well-known program of reform.[2]

Yet the content of these ideas tells us much about their appeal to many of her contemporaries. Florence Nightingale's medical views were based on a deeply internalized and little questioned view of the world and on a consequent model of relationship between behavior, individual responsibility, and disease. These views demand explanation for they are radically different from concepts of illness which have come to be accepted in the twentieth century. We must not allow the alienness of her ideas to blind us to their internal consistency, a consistency which bound together Nightingale's view of the world generally with her personal needs and career as reformer of hospitals and nursing.

116

The idea that disease could be induced by a specific contagion was anathema to Nightingale—denial of the filth, disorder, and contaminated atmosphere which seemed responsible for hospital fevers and infections. To assume the reality of contagion was, as she saw it, to deny the possibility of improving hospital conditions and perhaps even to question the need for the hospital's existence. The idea of specific particles causing disease also conflicted with an even more fundamental way of understanding the body, its functions, and their relationship to health and disease. Contagion seemed morally random and thus a denial of the traditional assumption that both health and disease arose from particular states of moral and social order. To understand Nightingale's medical views is to understand how a sanitarian of her generation could find both contagionism at mid-century and the germ theory a quarter-century later similarly uncongenial. Her ideas, finally, tell us something more general about perceptions of society in mid-nineteenth-century England.

Florence Nightingale's ideas on the hospital and of the nurse's role within it were based logically on a view of the body so familiar to educated Englishmen that its fundamental aspects needed little formal or systematic exposition. It was in essence an ancient view, but one whose very antiquity underlines its usefulness in explaining health and disease.

The body was visualized in terms of a central metaphor, one in which the organism was seen as a dynamic system constantly interacting with its environment.[3] Diet, atmosphere and ventilation, psychic stress, all interacted to shape a patterned but continuously reestablished reality. Within this framework of explanation, disease was no specific entity—even if local lesions characterized a particular ailment—but rather a general state of disequilibrium. Health, on the other hand, was synonymous with balance in the body's physiological state. Though physicians in the late eighteenth and early nineteenth centuries did tend to accept the specificity and infectiousness of smallpox and of a few other ills, these seemed at first atypical and only gradually helped undermine the plausibility of this older explanatory system. By mid-nineteenth century, however, changing views of pathology had begun to shift medical opinion toward a gradual acceptance of the assumption that most ills had a specific course, characteristic lesions, and—by implication—specific cause.[4]

But at mid-century such attitudes toward disease specificity were neither universally accepted nor thoroughly consistent. Most medical men still assumed that ailments could shift subtly from one form to another, that all reflected a basic underlying state. Nightingale, like many such physicians, emphatically disavowed the reality of specific disease states. Sickness, she contended, should be seen—in her own words—as an "adjective" not as a "substantive noun." It must, that is, be considered an aspect or quality of the body as a whole, rather than as an entity somehow separable from the state of a particular body at a particular moment in time. Nightingale left no doubt about the firmness of her commitment to this view. Some physicians, as she phrased it, taught that diseases were like cats and dogs, distinct species necessarily descended from other cats and dogs. But she considered such views misleading. Dogs did not change into cats, nor cats into dogs, while disease shifted its manifestations in precise response to environment. Not only had she seen disease arise spontaneously, without any possible contact with previous cases, she had also seen its characteristics change in response to altered environmental circumstances. She had seen filth produce remitting fever in a particular ward, a greater accumulation of filth change prevailing symptoms to those of typhoid, and, finally, still more dirt aggravate these symptoms into those of typhus.[5] Could she deny the evidence of her own senses? Or need she, at a time when sophisticated clinicians still found difficulty in distinguishing between some of the more common fevers? But Nightingale expressed an atypically strong aversion to the specificity of disease—a position far more categorical than that articulated by most of her medical contemporaries. Even smallpox, she believed, might emerge anew in an appropriately untoward environment. The stagnant air, for example, of a room long shut up could cause such sickness. "It is quite ripe," she warned, "to breed smallpox, scarlet fever, diptheria, or anything else you please."[6]

Disease must not be seen as response to a discrete external stimulus, but as an effort by the body to recover that normal state compromised by a particular set of unfavorable environmental circumstances or personal habits. Recovery could only be effected by the body's normal homeostatic processes. Disease, as she put it, was simply a "reparative process," and the same laws which maintained health in the well applied to nursing the sick.[7] Thus, the heat and sweating which characterized fevers could be seen as efforts by the body to rid itself of "excrementitious" matter through its normal channels. The same was true of discharges from the bowels in dysentery or the surface eruptions which characterized smallpox or typhus.[8] But in such natural patterns of recovery, Nightingale and many of her contemporaries believed, lay danger to the patient himself—and in a hospital to those unfortunate enough to occupy neighboring beds. A continued state of health and efforts to regain it depended alike on a careful monitoring of the body's intake and outgo and on the immediate removal of any discharged metabolic products. A hospital atmosphere contaminated not only with the undifferentiated filth resulting from inefficient house-keeping and shortsighted frugality, but with the peculiarly dangerous excretions and emanations of the sick, would certainly impede normal recovery—and in especially close conditions breed such ills as hospital gangrene, erysipelas, and puerperal fever. This explains her seemingly obsessive concern with the cleanliness of bedding and the regular emptying of chamber pots. The dangers she sought to avoid were not simply aesthetic. An unchanged bed, for example, means that a patient would have "re-introduced into [his] body the emanations from himself which day after day and week after week saturate his unaired bedding."[9]

> If you consider that an adult exhales by the lungs and skin in 24 hrs three pints at least of moisture, loaded with organic matter ready to enter into putrefaction; that in sickness the quantity is often greatly increased, the quality is always more noxious—just ask yourself next where does all this moisture go to? Chiefly into the bedding. . . . Must not such a bed be always saturated, and always the means of re-introducing into the system of the unfortunate patient who lies in it, that excrementitious matter to eliminate which from the body nature had expressly appointed the disease?

Adequate ventilation was similarly important. All those fevers and infections which seemed inevitably to infest the mid-nineteenth-century hospital's wards were preventable, Nightingale argued, through proper management; the very existence of such ills was a compelling argument for hospital reform.

Contagion and personal infection, on the other hand, seemed anti-social spectres, "affording to certain classes of minds, chiefly in the Southern and less educated parts of Europe a satisfactory reason for pestilence, and an adequate excuse for non-exertion to prevent its recurrence."[10] To entertain the possibility of personal contagion as the mode of transmitting hospital infection seemed, as Nightingale saw it, both to deny the need for improving hospital administration and nursing, and to replace the logic of personal responsibility with a fatalistic determinism which regarded fever and wound infection as inevitable in hospitals. This was simply unacceptable; Nightingale's emotions and intellect alike rejected such fatalism. On the contrary, she was convinced that controllable aspects of the environment, and especially the atmosphere, ordinarily caused hospital infection. "All my own hospital experience confirms this conclusion," she affirmed in emphasizing the ability of pure air alone to prevent infection. "If infection exists it is the result of carelessness, or of ignorance."[11]

The atmosphere, as Nightingale and many of her physician contemporaries believed, was the single most important medium for the transmission and creation of acute illness. The distinction between transmission and causation could not be truly meaningful for them; disease, they assumed, would inevitably develop in a sufficiently contaminated atmosphere, while that same atmosphere served as its mode of transmission. The only explanatory difficulty, an increasingly intractable one at mid-century, was whether a *specific* element in the atmosphere was needed to produce a specific disease. Nightingale could not accept such specificity. She endorsed the traditional and seemingly commonsensical notion that a sufficiently intense level of atmospheric contamination could induce both endemic and epidemic ills in the hospital's crowded wards (with particular configurations of environmental circumstance determining which). The lowered vitality, the fevers and infections which resulted from such contaminated states were morally compelling arguments for improving conditions within the hospital. Florence Nightingale was a formidable activist, and she marshalled a framework of medical doctrine which not only explained the cause of hospital infection, but indicated a possible and thus necessary mode of prevention. That sickness had always haunted the hospital's wards seemed to her hardly a justification for tolerating the conditions which seemed to breed it. "In what sense," as she put it, "is 'sickness' being 'always there,' a justification for its being 'there' at all?"[12]

As striking as the substantive aspects of this position was the language in which Nightingale expressed her arguments. They were based on the use of a special vocabulary and a series of related and emotionally compelling images. First, as has been suggested, Nightingale's etiology assumed a certain way of visualizing the body and its physiological processes—a vision structured around an ancient and accepted metaphor. Other specialized uses of language and related imagery helped communicate and legitimate her understanding of the hospital and the ills which infested it. One was the idea of "zymosis," the concept that infectious ills spread through a process analagous to fermentation; another was a peculiar use of statistics. The hospital itself, finally, was not only a dismaying reality, but in her writings was also a didactic microcosm illustrating the interdependence of health and order in the larger world.[13]

But a word of explanation seems unavoidable. I have been using the terms image, metaphor, and language loosely, although I hope usefully. Much of man's perception of the world and capacity to communicate that perception comes not through his capacity to see things afresh and with a value free neutrality, but to shape his perceptions through a repertoire of conventionalized images and emotionally charged language. Language is obviously affective as well as denotative, and Florence Nightingale was in her analysis of hospital infection more rhetorician than scientist. Her understanding of bodily function and of the nature of contagion bound together perceptions of particular realities—the sickness, the filth, the disorder of mid-nineteenth-century hospitals, the everyday realities of yeast rising or beer brewing —within a language of explanation which incorporated both the prestige of science and moral certainties of a more traditional sort. Her language also communicated the perceptions of a particular class and time. In such diversity of reference lies the key to Nightingale's contemporary appeal. She expressed herself in a language rich in layers of meaning—all emotionally if not logically consistent.

Since the 1840's, students of disease had, following the influential example of William Farr, England's Statistical Superintendent of the General Register Office, categorized epidemic and infectious ills as zymotic.[14] The logic of this usage and the etiological model it implied seem clear enough in retrospect. The scientific debate surrounding the nature and possible specificity of fermentation was still fresh in the minds of Florence Nightingale's medical contemporaries; even educated laymen could not have been unaware of this learned controversy.[15] Scientists had disputed energetically for a generation whether the process of fermentation was "chemical" or "vital"—whether some living organism was necessary to initiate the changes which constituted fermentation. But to Nightingale and to many of her medical associates, this distinction was of little practical moment; for the essential elements of the model seemed little subject to change whether the ferment should prove ultimately chemical or vital. Since the seventeenth century, at least some medical men had suggested that the phenomenon of fermentation provided a plausible explanation for the "portability" of infectious matter. As in the process of fermentation itself, a minute quantity of some "virus" seemed to be able to induce a particular change in a much larger volume of material. Thus, it explained how the atmosphere could serve as a medium for the transmission of disease; ubiquitous and necessary to man's existence, the air could become the source of illness through its very indispensability. Contaminated by a minute quantity of putrefying matter, it might transmit cholera or yellow fever; within the confined walls of a hospital or tenement house, a contaminated atmosphere might cause any one of a score of ills as the exhalations from human bodies acted as a kind of yeast in this vitiated culture medium.[16]

This explanation of the origin and transmission of disease seems to us speculative and, as I have suggested, in an important sense metaphorical. But, of course, it seemed anything but that to Nightingale and to many of her mid-century medical contemporaries. The very familiarity of fermentation underscored its relevance in explaining the unfamiliar and the threatening. The plausibility of this model was based in part on the very concreteness of the associations it suggested; anyone who had seen bread rise could understand how a deleterious substance might contaminate the atmosphere.

Let me suggest, moreover, that at the same time an even deeper and still more compelling dimension of meaning helped inform Nightingale's use of the fermentation metaphor: the idea of filth as contamination, as embodying an absolute moral otherness which implied the capacity to pollute absolutely. This antithesis added emotional immediacy to Nightingale's analysis of the hospital and of the generation of infection within it. She was hardly unique in feeling and articulating this attitude toward contagion. For example, a committee of the New Jersey Medical Society in 1864 explained the communicable quality of "hospital gangrene" as[17]

> like begetting like; the offspring of an unclean embrace that sullies the virgin purity of the blood by a detestable impregnation; a mysterious, propagable, depraved, terrible something, we know not what.

Even the smallest "impregnation" could initiate those linked changes which constituted disease.

Perhaps most fundamentally, Nightingale's conception of the hospital and the generation of disease within it emphasized the role of volition and behavior in the causation of infection. This applied not only to the hospital, but to society generally. If civic authorities, she suggested, were only to monitor carefully the atmosphere of school-rooms, Englishmen would hear no more of scarlet fever or of other seemingly unavoidable childhood ills. They would hear no more of "Mysterious Dispensations"—of disease being in the hands of God—when the responsibility lay squarely in man's own hands and brain. We must, she reiterated, look first to our own habits in seeking to explain disease.[18]

> God lays down certain typical laws. Upon His carrying out such laws depends our responsibility (that much abused word), for how could we have any responsibility for actions, the results of which we could not forsee—which would be the case if the carrying out of His laws were not certain. Yet we seem to be continually expecting that He will work a miracle—i.e., break His own laws expressly to relieve us of responsibility.

For hospital hygiene, the meaning was clear enough: if we allowed contamination of the very air patients breathed, then fevers and infection must inevitably result. Only hard work and careful planning could avert them.

Nightingale's belief in the primary role of the atmosphere in causing disease was far more than a plausible speculation, simply one among several intellectual options certified as respectable by the world of medical conjecture—it was a necessity. Her etiological views didactically underlined the connection between behavior, environment, and health; for, practically speaking, Nightingale's emphasis on atmosphere was an emphasis on environment—environment construed, so that hospital morale was as much a determinant of that atmosphere as was the placement of windows and fireplaces or the frequency with which walls and floors were scrubbed. Her explanation of disease causation in terms of fermentation was effective in emphasizing the polarity implied by the absoluteness of the gap between the original purity of God's atmosphere and the necessarily culpable role of man in polluting it. As compelling justification for the social activism demanded by her personality, the image of zymotic disease could hardly have been more appropriate. (Significantly, she used the image of putrefaction in parallel fashion. Like fermentation, it was a progressive change familiar to the senses, yet incorporating intense emotional and moral overtones. Consistently enough, Nightingale's use of images of fermentation and putrefaction are almost interchangeable.[19])

Nightingale's use of statistical arguments related closely—if seemingly paradoxically—to her use of the fermentation concept. No student of her work and of that of her contemporaries in mid-century sanitary reform can doubt the centrality of their appeals to "objective" statistical data.[20] (One thinks, for example, of comparisons between urban and rural mortality rates or of the comparative incidence of puerperal fever in different kinds of hospitals and in private practice.) But again, let me suggest that Nightingale's use of statistical description and analysis was as much rhetorical as it was instrumental. Despite her well-deserved reputation for tactical acuteness in the service of pragmatic reform, Nightingale's mind ultimately saw things not in additive terms, but instead in morally resonant polarities: filth as opposed to purity, order versus disorder, health in contradistinction to disease. Hospital infection was thus a consequence of disorder in a potentially ordered pattern. Statistics defined the place of a particular ward along the continuum shaped by these polarities. Given her unwillingness to accept the specificity of disease and her tendency to correlate incidences of fever and surgical infection with levels of atmospheric contamination, it was only natural for her to point with indignation to correlations between particularly untoward hospital conditions and atypically high levels of hospital infection.[21] Thus the aggregate incidence of zymotic disease served as a seemingly objective index of human failure. The strength of Nightingale's statistical arguments lay not simply in their form, but in the assumed and unspoken polarity between filth and cleanliness, sickness and health which they dramatized. They served, that is, to underwrite her ultimately moral understanding of disease causation.

The central image which at once communicated and legitimated her program of reform was a vision of the hospital itself; her picture of the hospital can hardly be described as figurative, for it incorporated a careful analysis of existing realities and a blueprint for consequent reform. On the other hand, it was hardly a value-free rendering of these realities. The hospital seemed to her quite literally a microcosm of society, every part inter-related and all reflecting a particular moral order. Just as order in the body and an appropriate physical and psychological equilibrium constituted health for the individual, so order in the hospital implied a low incidence of fever and wound infection for its inhabitants. Similarly, in society at large, ill-health, poverty, and depravity, all sprang from a sequence of remediable human acts. The hospital was a part of that society, a microcosm of the moral and social relationships which determined the individual's health, on the one hand, and that of society generally on the other. Within this framework, one could hardly distinguish between the moral and the material, the individual and the community of individuals. Social health and individual health were bound together by a similar set of moral relationships and responsibilities; life on the ward illustrated these truths with didactic clarity. If a man failed to obey the dictates of God immanent in the organization of his body, he could only expect disease; if a hospital were contaminated by filth, administrative irresponsibility, and immorality, the fevers and infections which arose were equally unavoidable.

And for Florence Nightingale the hospital of her day was indeed a place of disorder. No woman of her class and education could well have encountered that would-be healing institution without finding it menacing and alien. It is no accident that her new-model trained nurses were responsible as much for discipline as they were for overseeing proper diets or dressing ulcers. Indeed, the emphasis in Nightingale's etiological and pathological thought on the interaction of the patient as a whole with every aspect of his environment implied that the distinction between moral and physical well-being, between mind and body was hardly meaningful.[22] It was of little use in explaining the causation of disease generally and certainly not applicable in understanding hospital infection. The mid-nineteenth-century hospital was a lower-class institution in many ways, organized in theory according to the moral assumptions of its lay trustees and administrators, but dominated in reality by values and behavior antithetical to those Nightingale saw as the only appropriate basis for a moral society. Zymotic images were also ideal for describing the hospital's fermenting and disorderly life—a below stairs without an above stairs to control it. We need not be surprised to learn that Nightingale's model ward arrangements placed the nurse's room, so that she might observe all its inmates from a single vantage point.[23] It was equally logical that closets and stairwells where "skulking" might occur or where convalescents might "play tricks" must be avoided.[24] These were to be eliminated by the enlightened hospital architect, just as he avoided corners in which dust might accumulate or sewers which allowed dangerous fumes to escape.

Since her etiological views were, as we have emphasized, fundamentally holistic and since she was unwilling to accept the specificity of disease and the possible existence of specific causative agents, Nightingale saw the nurse's role as both multifaceted and indispensable. It was also fundamentally moral. Nightingale explicitly contended that a trained nurse's endowments must be ultimately spiritual; the technical abilities which she might acquire were, if not precisely subordinate to her moral powers, at least subsequent to and dependent upon them.[25] Not the least of these moral qualities was—and here Nightingale obviously made a personal plea—activism itself. As she put it, "patience and resignation" in a nurse "are but other words for carelessness or indifference—contemptible, if in regard to herself; culpable, if in regard to her sick."[26]

That same holistic pathology and hygiene which explained the incidence of health and disease also explained the numerous ways in which the nurse could help to effect the patient's recovery. Like many of her forward-looking mid-century peers, Nightingale wrote comparatively little of drugs and bleeding, of therapeutics generally; discreet enough not to antagonize physicians on seemingly marginal issues, she generally ignored their potential for therapeutic intervention. Medicine, she explained, was not part of the essential curative process.[27]

> Pathology teaches the harm that disease has done. But it teaches nothing more. . . . It is often thought that medicine is the curative process. It is no such thing; medicine is the surgery of functions, as surgery proper is that of limbs and organs. Neither can do anything but remove obstructions; neither can cure; nature alone cures. Surgery removes the bullet out of the limb, which is an obstruction to cure, but nature heals the wound.

All nursing could accomplish—and it was no small achievement—was to put the patient into the best possible condition for nature to effect its plan of cure. But although a hospital could not *cure,* it seemed self-evident to Nightingale that it could and must avert the spread of infection and more generally promote the body's internally directed efforts to regain health. At least a well-run hospital could prevent a patient from being poisoned by the emanations arising from his own excretions and those of his ward-mates. Drugs and bleeding were marginal in her ideal hospital.[28]

The possibility of effective hospital administration implied its necessity. Translated into behavior, Nightingale's point of view emphasized the certainty of improvement through carefully directed activity. It is not surprising that Florence Nightingale was so resolutely hostile to the idea of specific contagion, nor so sceptical of the existence of

specific disease entities. Hospital infection reduced itself to the consequence of untoward behavior. Poor planning of windows, slovenly
nursing, cold and ill-prepared foods, drains and sinks placed where
they might contaminate the atmosphere, inadequate ventilation,
chamber vessels unemptied for hours were all remediable, all consequences of incompetence or irresponsibility. Will and the assurance of
humane accomplishment were closely related in Nightingale's thought
as she at once explained the world she saw about her in the hospital
and justified the social role she sought to fill.

In this interrelated world of volition and pathology, contagion
seemed arbitrary, random in its moral implications. It was not simply
an inability to comprehend the germ theory which made her hesitate
to accept it, but its irrelevance—if not, indeed, its destructiveness—to
her complex way of visualizing the nature of disease and its relationship to environment and behavior. If chance alone determined
whether an individual should intersect with a disease-causing microscopic particle, then sickness was bereft of meaning; it could play no
monitory role in a world of moral order.

It is easy enough to feel removed from many of the seemingly
quaint arguments which characterized mid-nineteenth-century anti-
contagionism. How are we, for example, to regard the oft repeated
contention that a belief in contagion during an epidemic would make
nursing impossible, that the fabric of social obligation would be rent
were laymen to regard infectious disease as contagious? These arguments were reiterated by anti-contagionists in the first two-thirds of
the century. Yet they are more than examples of obsolete casuistry.
Such warnings vividly represented the dangers contagionism seemed
to pose to the carefully elaborated relationship between health, behavior, and social environment which had been so prominent in traditional medical thought and so central to mid-nineteenth-century public health advocacy. On a practical level, moreover, it threatened the
future of nursing as a profession; if prudence, proper regimen, and
good general health could not protect against contagion, then nursing
must be a perilous trade indeed.

As late as 1894, Florence Nightingale could still warn that a will-
ingness to look into drains was at least as important as a knowledge
of bacteriology in the mental equipment of a district health officer.
"Mystic rites," she had complained the year previously, such as "disinfection and antiseptics, take the place of sanitary measures and hygiene."[29] Nightingale's highly atypical quest for achievement in the

public sphere only exacerbated her need for an explanatory system which would justify her zeal and the program to which she had dedicated her life. It was a framework she had espoused with enthusiasm; she could not easily adapt to new and seemingly less relevant modes of explaining disease.

In outlining this interpretation of Nightingale's medical views, I have in some ways painted an overly stylized picture of an individual's search for social legitimacy, of the depiction of real pain, real filth, real infection in the form of symbol and metaphor, on the one hand, and of rationalistic speculation on the other. The problem, however, in emphasizing the rhetorical structure of her argument is our tendency to equate the use of figurative language with a denial of the real, with our tendency to assume a categorical distinction between the rational and irrational in social discourse. Yet Nightingale's medical views illustrate the difficulty of defending such distinctions. Her descriptions of the hospital are entirely consistent with much of the surviving evidence. Even the intensity and peculiarity of the mid-century hospital's smells seemed viscerally to endorse the accuracy of her atmosphere-oriented etiological scheme.[30] It is difficult to overstate the impact which the hospital's bleak precincts must have had upon a woman of her class and previous experience. Nightingale's use of statistics, her measured disquisitions on ventilation and heating provided an idiom which could not only communicate specific information, but promised control while creating a reassuring emotional distance. To label certain of her characteristic modes of assimilating and expressing experience as metaphorical is not to imply that they were arbitrary (except in so far as they were necessarily expressions of individual need and perception). They were that, of course, but the very power and plausibility of Nightingale's arguments arise from their multi-leveled interaction with a particular reality and their peculiar appropriateness to time and place.

Perhaps we have already overemphasized the characteristic mixture of scientific and more traditionally spiritual arguments and sources of authority in Nightingale's medical and administrative program. But this is hardly surprising; nor was this emotionally resonant amalgam of ideas and images peculiar to Nightingale. Changes in world-view are presumably always syncretic and gradual, not abrupt, self-conscious, and categorical. The arguments I have sought briefly to outline constituted indeed a characteristic aspect of a more general adaptive strategy congenial to the educated and articulate in mid-nineteenth-century England and the United States. In approaching a variety of social problems, intellectuals such as Nightingale incorporated in their discussions, both the legitimacy and characteristic verbal forms of two seemingly disparate realms of authority, that of traditional moral assumption and that of science as dispassionate analysis.[31] Nightingale's generation played in some ways a key transitional role in the shift from an older world-view based on the rationalization of a complex and textured relationship between behavior and its consequences—personal, spiritual, physical—of a world in which every event and relationship was tinged with moral significance, to a very different one which found impersonal and reductionist modes of social explanation more congenial and increasingly appropriate to an ever more specialized, impersonal, and bureaucratic society. Since at least the time of Marx, social thinkers have grappled with this problem of fit between social structure and world-view.

Ideas formally medical and scientific have played comparatively little role in such debates. In general, historians of science and medicine have tended to accept past medical and scientific ideas on their own terms—that is as self-contained, value-free systems of ideas. In medicine particularly, however, such formal and intellectualistic interpretations of past thought have in the past generation come to seem increasingly one-dimensional. It is difficult, for example, to draw a categorical distinction between science and imagination, between the heuristic use of metaphor and a seemingly distinct process of ordered, disciplinarily defined investigation. The more we understand about the development of biology and medicine in the West, for example, the less enlightening seem the distinctions so frequently made between scientific and non-scientific modes of thought. Substantive insights often result from the previous elaboration of an illuminating metaphor which organizes accumulated data in a novel way.[32]

Even the diffuse concept of zymotic etiology could play such a creative role in hands more disciplined—and discipline-oriented—than those of Florence Nightingale. Let me refer by way of illustration, to the case of John Snow, the mid-nineteenth-century English physician deservedly and securely installed in the pantheon of medical history for demonstrating that cholera was a water-borne disease. Snow showed extraordinary epidemiological ingenuity in demonstrating the role of water in spreading the disease. He not only traced individual cases to particular sources of contamination (most dramatically, a popular well), but revealed a striking differential in cholera incidence among subscribers to two different water companies (one of which drew its water from the Thames above London and the other from the river after it had been contaminated by the city's sewage). Snow's work seems in retrospect both elegant and systematic. Yet the inspiration for his empirical investigation was drawn from a previously enunciated—and generally unsupported—analogy between the way in which a specific ferment could predictably alter an enormous substrate through the inducing of a "continuous molecular change," and how a pathogenic material might effect a similar change in a city's water supply.[33] Is Snow's work an example of the empirical style or a creative use of metaphor? To formulate the question is to suggest the awkwardness of making such absolute distinctions.

There are endless difficulties in attempting to defend the categorical distinction between the rational and the irrational, the scientific and the intuitive. To return, for example, to Florence Nightingale's own work: many of her practical suggestions must have proved efficacious despite their basis in a formal rationale that we consider mistaken. Many of the goals she sought to achieve were entirely consistent with policies dictated a generation later by the implications of the germ theory. Certainly her influence pointed toward a cleaner and in general more humane hospital environment—toward better sanitation, adequate ventilation, improved diet, competent nursing. That we cannot share all of Florence Nightingale's convictions, that we may find some of them alien or even repellent should not obscure their power to motivate or the reality of the misery she sought to meliorate.

It must be confessed, in conclusion, that Florence Nightingale was hardly representative as an individual; indeed, her very prominence and her almost improbably melodramatic career as self-willed secular saint remind us of her very uncommon aspect. Though the term charismatic has been subject to much casual misuse, it does apply to a Florence Nightingale. But the specialness of her life does not imply a specialness for her ideas. Nightingale's very deviance and the intensity of her motivation—admittedly personal and idiosyncratic—made her all the more dependent on the articulation of a rationale broadly plausible to her educated and influential peers. Thus, a central aspect of her historical significance hinged upon her rhetorical ability, her skill in shaping a compelling montage of emotionally rich and intellectually plausible images and her use of these figures in the advocacy of new institutional forms. Nightingale's career is symbolic not only of woman's emergence from the strictures of traditional roles, or the parallel emergence of perhaps equally constricting but certainly more novel bureaucratic roles, but of a fundamental reordering of English society, of its forms and self-conceptions.[34]

Notes

*Research for this paper was supported by a grant from the National Library of Medicine (LM 02826–02) whose assistance is here gratefully acknowledged.

1. For a pioneering attempt to explain the unwillingness of such reformers to deal with the implications of the germ theory and experimental medicine (as manifested in vivisection), see Lloyd Stevenson, "Science down the Drain," *Bulletin of the History of Medicine,* 29 (1955), pp. 1–26, which contended that a strongly-felt "pietistic commitment" shaped the unwillingness of certain mid-century sanitarians to accept a range of novel ideas ranging from the germ theory to vivisection. The present author's feeling is that "pietistic" is perhaps too inclusive a category; the interpretation suggested in the following pages is closer to a reflection in a footnote in Stevenson's paper (p. 4n): "Possibly the unwillingness to break down the conception of filth, to acknowledge dirt to be the mere vehicle of pathogenic micro-organisms, was unconscious resistance to the recognition and analysis of a metaphor which gave satisfaction in the moral realm." A significant parallel argument emphasizing the "secularization" of the concept of infection was formulated by Owsei Temkin in 1953 in "An Historical analysis of the Concept of Infection," reprinted in *The Double Face of Janus and other Essays in the History of Medicine* (Baltimore and London: Johns Hopkins, 1977), pp. 456–471. See also Temkin's "Metaphors of Human Biology," in *ibid.,* pp. 271–283. For a useful introduction to the problem of hospital infection, see Erna Lesky, "Hospital-acquired Infections—a Historical Survey," *Hexagon-Roche,* 5 (1977), pp. 1–10.

2. For biographical details of Nightingale's life, Edward Cook's standard biography is in some ways still the most complete: *The Life of Florence Nightingale,* 2 vols. (London: Macmillan, 1913). More successful as a biography is Cecil Woodham-Smith's *Florence Nightingale 1820–1910* (London: Constable, 1950). Neither of these studies critically discusses her medical ideas and their relationship to those of her contemporaries. Indispensable for any student of Nightingale's work is *A Bio-Bibliography of Florence Nightingale,* compiled by W. J. Bishop with the assistance of Sue Goldie (London: Dawsons, 1962). For a recent attempt to interpret Nightingale in psychological terms, see Donald R. Allen, "Florence Nightingale: Toward a Psychohistorical Interpretation," *J. Interdisciplinary History,* 6 (1975), pp. 23–45.

3. For a more elaborate exposition of this argument, see Charles E. Rosenberg, "The Therapeutic Revolution: Medicine, Meaning, and Social Change in Nineteenth-Century America," *Perspectives in Biology and Medicine,* 20 (1977), pp. 485–506.

4. For a study of the context in which this took place, see Erwin H. Ackerknecht, *Medicine at the Paris Hospital. 1794–1848* (Baltimore: Johns Hopkins, 1967). Ordinary physicians, however, were still far more comfortable at mid-century with less specific disease concepts. See also, Owsei Temkin, "The Scientific Approach to Disease: Specific Entity and Individual Sickness," *Janus,* pp. 441–455.

5. Florence Nightingale, *Notes on Nursing: What it is, and What is Not* (New York: D. Appleton, 1861), pp. 33n, 32–33. "For diseases," as she put it, "as all experience shows, are adjectives, not noun substantives." Some years later Nightingale repeated this argument in an edition of her *Notes on Nursing* addressed to "labouring men": "Is it not living in a continual mistake to look upon diseases, as we do now, as separate things, which must exist, like cats and dogs? instead of looking upon them as conditions, like a dirty and a clean condition, and just as much under our own control; or rather as the reactions of a kindly nature against the conditions in which we have placed ourselves." *Notes on Nursing for the Labouring Classes* (London: Harrison, 1876), p. 33.

6. *Ibid.,* p. 13.

7. *Ibid.,* p. 8: "The reparative process which Nature has instituted and which we call disease, has been hindered by some want of knowledge or attention, . . . and pain, suffering, or interruption of the whole process sets in. If a patient is cold, if a patient is feverish, if a patient is faint, if he is sick after taking food, if he has a bed-sore, it is generally the fault not of the disease, but of the nursing."

8. Nightingale, *Notes on Hospitals,* third ed. rev. (London: Longman, Green, Longman, Roberts, and Green, 1863), pp. 15–17; *Notes on Nursing,* pp. 74, 79–80. Similarly, Nightingale could assure her close friend and associate, Sidney Herbert, dying of renal disease, that the protein in his urine might be a sign of Nature working out its healing course: "The presence of a large amount of albumen is not proof in itself, of anything but that Nature is getting rid of something which ought not to be there." Cited in Woodham-Smith, *Nightingale,* pp. 357–358.

9. *Notes on Nursing,* p. 80. Thus the seemingly obsessive emphasis by mid-century hospital reformers on ventilation as an all-sufficient goal. See, for example, John Watson, *Thermal Ventilation, and other Sanitary Improvements, Applicable to Public Buildings, and Recently Adopted at the New-York Hospital . . .* (New York: Wm. W. Rose, 1851). Even after tentative acceptance of the germ theory as explanation for hospital infection, most physicians still interpreted the role of germs as—in effect—an explanation of the mechanism through which the atmosphere could be contaminated and spread infection. The germ theory seemed to many such physicians in the 1870s and early 1880s simply another argument which emphasized the need for hygiene and cleanliness within the hospital—goals endorsed vigorously by Nightingale. For revealing examples of such positions, see Charles Langstaff, *Hospital Hygiene being the Annual Address to the Southampton Medical Society. February, 1872* (London: J. & A. Churchill, 1872); John Simon, "Contagion," in Richard Quain, ed., *A Dictionary of Medicine* (London: Longmans, Green & Co., 1883), I: pp. 286–294.

10. *Notes on Hospitals,* pp. 8–9. Nightingale's emphasis on the "primitive" aspect of belief in contagionism and its association with less "advanced" cultures is consistent with Erwin H. Ackerknecht's interpretation of anti-contagionism in this period: "Anti-Contagionism between 1821 and 1867," *Bulletin of the History of Medicine,* 22 (1948), pp. 562–593.

11. *Notes on Hospitals,* p. 22. In the first edition of her study of hospitals, Nightingale was similarly emphatic in dismissing the notion that contagion made disease inevitable among hospital workers. "Ignorance and mismanagement lie at the root of all such

presumed cases of 'infection.' " *Notes on Hospitals: Being Two Papers Read before the National Association for the Promotion of Social Science* . . . (London: John W. Parker & Son, 1859), p. 19.

12. *Notes on Nursing*, p. 29; Woodham-Smith, *Nightingale*, p. 258.

13. The use of the hospital or asylum as metaphor has a long and complex history. The connection between disease, dirt, and disorder is even more ancient and complex—as is the use of metaphor to communicate such beliefs. Since at least the work of Evans-Pritchard, anthropologists concerned with health and healing and the relationship of both to particular belief-systems have sought to evaluate such questions—but ordinarily in non-Western contexts. Historians of Western science and medicine have conventionally assumed that such anthropological perspectives apply only to Third World cultures. For a recent and influential discussion of the use of symbolic forms in the shaping of particular relationships between health and world-view, see the work of Mary Douglas, especially *Purity and Danger* (New York: Praeger, 1966) and *Natural Symbols: Explorations in Cosmology* (New York: Random House, 1972).

14. For important studies on Farr and his relationship to contemporary etiological ideas, see John M. Eyler, "Mortality Statistics and Victorian Health Policy: Program and Criticism," *Bulletin of the History of Medicine*, 50 (1976), pp. 335–355, and "William Farr on the Cholera: The Sanitarian's Disease Theory and the Statistician's Method," *J. History of Medicine*, 28 (1973), pp. 79–100. Eyler emphasizes Farr's ability to shift gradually to a hesitant acceptance of the germ theory, using the zymotic mechanism as a basis for this shift. In general, he emphasizes the consistency between the moral values endorsed by Victorian lay social reformers and the programme of medically trained sanitarians. "In short then, the environmental theories of disease causation and the social or political interpretation of morbidity and mortality provided the theoretical basis for agreement between segments of the medical profession and a more heterogeneous group of Victorian reformers," "Mortality Statistics," p. 339. Farr was an associate of Florence Nightingale and their exchanges reveal not always consistent attitudes. See Zachary Cope, *Florence Nightingale and the Doctors* (Philadelphia and Montreal: J. B. Lippincott, *c.* 1958), Ch. 8, and "Dr. William Farr, the Medical Statistician," pp. 98–107; Michael J. Cullen, *The Statistical Movement in Early Victorian Britain* . . . (New York: Barnes & Noble, 1975).

15. William Bulloch, *The History of Bacteriology* (London: Oxford, 1938), Ch. 3, on "Fermentation," pp. 41–63; Joseph S. Fruton, *Molecules and Life. Historical Essays on the Interplay of Chemistry and Biology* (New York: Wiley-Interscience, 1972), pp. 22–86. To contemporaries, "it was Liebig who first expounded the resemblance of contagious diseases to the process of fermentation. In both, an infinitely small germ gives rise to successive changes which propagate surprisingly the material produced—a circumstance which makes their virulence greater than that of material poisons." E. Mapother, *Lectures on Public Health* (Dublin: Fannin & Co., 1864), p. 245.

16. Charles E. Rosenberg, *The Cholera Years. The United States in 1832, 1849, and 1866* (Chicago: University of Chicago, 1962). When empirical evidence pointed toward the possible analogous role of water in the transmission of cholera and typhoid, contemporary epidemiological thought had little difficulty in transferring this zymotic process to water from its more familiar site in the atmosphere. For a brief discussion of a seven-

teenth-century use of the fermentation idea and something of its origins, see: L. J. Rather, "Pathology at Mid-Century: A Reassessment of Thomas Willis and Thomas Sydenham," in Allen G. Debus, ed., *Medicine in Seventeenth Century England* (Berkeley, Los Angeles and London: University of California Press, 1974), pp. 79–83.

17.   Cited in David L. Cowen, *Medicine and Health in New Jersey: A History* (Princeton, New York, and Toronto: D. Van Nostrand, 1964), p. 25. Owsei Temkin has emphasized not only the ancient origins of "infection" in the image of a dye polluting a much larger and previously unsullied substrate, but the moral dimensions as well. Temkin, "Concept of Infection," *Janus*, pp. 456–457.

18.   *Notes on Nursing*, p. 25n. for citation, see also pp. 17n., 26–27.

19.   In this casual confounding of the processes of fermentation and putrefaction, Nightingale was typical of many medical men at mid-century. The dangers implicit in the disintegration of once living matter were vivid, embodying not only a compelling moral meaning, but incorporating sensory experience. Whose senses had not been assailed by the offensive odors and sights of putrefaction?

20.   See, for example, the articles on Farr by Eyler cited previously. Eyler emphasizes the social and moral dimension of Farr's use of statistical evidence. "Medical statisticians assumed that disease phenomena were regular and orderly not only in the individual but also in their progress within a community. Health, disease, death, and physical and moral condition were believed joined in an indissoluble link." Eyler, "Mortality Statistics," p. 336. As Farr himself wrote in 1875: "There is a relation between death and sickness. . . . There is a relation betwixt death, health, and energy of body and mind. . . . There is a relation betwixt the forms of death and moral excellence or infamy." Nightingale employed statistical arguments frequently and prominently in her own works. In addition to her *Notes on Hospitals*, she participated forcefully in the contemporary debate on puerperal fever and the possible dangers of lying-in hospitals, a debate which turned to a significant degree on statistical evidence. *Introductory Notes on Lying-In Institutions. Together with a Proposal for Organising an Institution for Training Midwives and Midwifery Nurses* (London: Longmans, Green & Co., 1871).

21.   The first edition of her *Notes on Nursing* (1859), for example, begins with a discussion of the uses of mortality and morbidity statistics. Coupled with such habitual reference to statistics was a characteristically gratuitous precision of statement. When Nightingale suggested, for example, a distance of at least three feet between the beds of fever patients, she found it easy to explain: "Miasma may be said, roughly speaking, to diminish as the square of the distance. With good ventilation, it is not found to extend much beyond 3 feet from the patient; although miasma from the excretions may extend to considerably greater distance." *Ibid.,* p. 58.

22.   The unwillingness to distinguish between the psychic and physical was typical of medical thought at this time; Nightingale, however, integrated such assumptions into her analysis of the hospital and the nurse's role with extraordinary effectiveness.

23.   At this time it was still assumed that the ward nurse would sleep in proximity to her patients. Nightingale's concern both with the hospital's ventilation specifically and with the allocation of space more generally is entirely consistent with this interpretation of her moral and medical views.

24.   *Notes on Hospitals* (1863), pp. 49, 52, 114.

25. Woodham-Smith's discussion of Nightingale's training school policies emphasizes her minute concern for the probationer's moral health. *Nightingale,* p. 347 and passim.

26. *Notes on Nursing,* p. 93.

27. *Ibid.,* p. 133, and for parallel arguments, pp. 74, 131.

28. *Ibid.,* pp. 8, 13. Not surprisingly, Nightingale—as we have seen—emphasized that disease was a normal reparative process, one which could be aided but never directed or demanded.

29. Nightingale, *Health Teaching in Towns and Villages. Rural Hygiene* (London: Spottiswoode & Co., 1894), p. 21. The quotation is drawn from "Sick Nursing and Health Nursing," in John S. Billings and Henry M. Hurd, eds., *Hospitals Dispensaries and Nursing* (Baltimore: Johns Hopkins University, 1894), p. 449. This essay, contributed by Nightingale to the International Congress of Charities, Correction and Philanthropy, held in conjunction with Chicago's Columbian exposition in 1893 provides a remarkable capsule presentation of her views and their consistency over a half-century.

30. Contemporaries all agreed that there was a peculiar "hospital smell" which characterized the mid-century institutions' wards; it seemed obvious that it must be associated with a contaminated atmosphere. "All foul smell indicates disease," Nightingale warned working men. "Never live in a house which smells. Either don't take it, or examine where the smell comes from, and then put a stop to it; but never think of living in it until there is no smell. A house which smells is a hot-bed of disease." *Notes on Nursing for the Labouring Classes* (1876), p. 24.

31. For a more general statement of this position, see Charles E. Rosenberg, "Introduction: Science, Society, and Social Thought," *No Other Gods. On Science and American Social Thought* (Baltimore and London: Johns Hopkins, 1976), pp. 1–21 and 109–131.

32. "The use of metaphors," as Owsei Temkin argued as early as 1949, "in human biology is not an aberration from which even great men have failed to escape. On the contrary, by using metaphors which they believed to represent adequate and true concepts, Aristotle, Galen, Paracelsus, Harvey, Descartes, Virchow, and Helmholtz shaped concepts of human biology which conformed with their own thoughts and feelings and with the thoughts and feelings of their times." "Metaphors of Human Biology," *Janus,* p. 283. Though he does not employ the language of anthropology, Temkin's substantive understanding of this medical use of metaphor is consistent with the suggestions of such contemporary advocates of "symbolic anthropology" as Victor Turner and Mary Douglas. For parallel and more detailed interpretations of the role of metaphor in the shaping of early modern science, see Walter Pagel's important work: *The Religious and Philosophical Aspects of van Helmont's Science and Medicine. Supplements to the Bulletin of the History of Medicine* No. 2 (Baltimore: Johns Hopkins University, 1944); *Paracelsus. An Introduction to Philosophical Medicine in the Era of the Renaissance* (Basel and New York: S. Karger, 1958); *William Harvey's Biological Ideas* (Basel and New York: S. Karger, 1967).

33. John Snow, *On Continuous Molecular Changes, More Particularly in their Relation to Epidemic Diseases: Being the Oration delivered at the 80th Anniversary of the Medical Society of London. Published by Request of the Society* (London: John Churchill, 1853). This is con-

veniently reprinted with Snow's other major essay on cholera, a biographical mem-
oir by B. W. Richardson, and an introduction by W. H. Frost: *Snow on Cholera* . . .
(New York: Commonwealth Fund, 1936).

34. This essay has avoided the so-called "woman's question," a significant matter
in interpreting Nightingale's work and social impact, but one inappropriate for this
brief discussion.

"All According to the Constitooshun": Charles Dickens and Lead Poisoning

LLOYD G. STEVENSON

In December, 1868, and in February, 1869, Charles Dickens, great novelist and perceptive journalist, published two reports on lead poisoning. The first, sombre and disquieting—although flecked characteristically with humor, in this case of the Irish variety—was an account of a friendly call at the home of afflicted working people; in sum, it was a melancholy episode. The second, which by comparison was almost buoyant, recounted the story of his visit to a white lead factory and his conversations with two of the proprietors, described as "my two frank conductors." In the first paper, the women he met were either sick and recumbent or, if up and about, were giving expression to a sad, comical, fatalistic "philosophy"; in the second paper women were pictured clambering around cheerfully in an airy loft like light-hearted denizens of a seraglio. Yet a pitifully sick woman he had seen on his first expedition had worked in the same airy cock-loft, and his chief informant in the workers' home had learned from the same factory that serio-comic philosophy of lead poisoning—Dickens saw comedy in her Irish brogue—which she passed along to Dickens. Dickens adopted it.

Before we accompany the author of *Hard Times* and the portrayer of Coketown on his lead-poisoning tours, let us turn back for a moment to the beginning of the century and the beginning of labor legislation; and then let us return quickly through the decades to the 1860's and to Dickens.

The Apprentices Act (1802) of Sir Robert Peel, sometimes called "the first Factory Act," was concerned with the working hours and the education of apprentices, and with the lighting and cleanliness of workshops.[1] A wider law of similar purpose was introduced in 1819, aiming also to limit child labor in the textile mills. This bill had been drawn up by Robert Owen, but the act as eventually passed was very much watered down from Owen's draft and left enforcement in the hands of local Justices, rather than providing for the appointment of paid and qualified inspectors as Owen had urged. While Owen's agitation was afoot, Samuel Taylor Coleridge was writing to his friend

137

Crabb Robinson, a lawyer and a journalist, to learn "if there is not some law prohibiting or limiting, or regulating the employment either of children or adults or both, in the white lead manufactory?" He wanted to know if there were any other instances in which the legislature had interfered in any way with what was ironically called free enterprise "(i.e., Dared to prohibit soul murder and infanticide on the part of the rich, and self-slaughter on that of the poor)."[2]

This attitude, needless to say, was distinctly radical. The Act of 1819 and subsequent legislation for the welfare of the industrial worker were delayed in the House and weakened in their operation by the doctrines then prevalent among employers—that restriction of the hours of labor would endanger national prosperity and that industry could only look upon workers as "hands," being in no way responsible for their personal wellbeing. Employers were piously convinced of the sacredness of their unregulated power, entirely persuaded also that national prosperity and their own profits must rise and fall together. Much of the early legislation, fully in the tradition of the Enlightenment, was aimed at the education of factory children and the regulation of the morals of the workers. Health was a secondary consideration, or, when its care threatened to interfere seriously with business, a bad third.

The provisions of the Factory Act of 1833, which applied only to textile mills, were still related not only to hours but to education. This act nonetheless opened a new era, for it established the principle of factory inspection by full-time government inspectors, in place of Justices of the Peace. In 1844 certifying factory surgeons were added, cleanliness and sanitation were required, and the reduction of overcrowding was insisted upon for the first time. Women and children were excluded from employment in certain dangerous occupations, except under special precautions. This reform was due in part to the activity of Edwin Chadwick, for the famous Report of the Poor Law Commission on the *Sanitary Condition of the Labouring Population of Great Britain*, with a synoptical volume by Chadwick himself, had appeared in 1842.[3]

The Reports made in 1861 and 1862 by Sir John Simon, Medical Officer of the Privy Council, on the death rates from lung diseases in certain industrial occupations led their author to the well-known conclusion that "the canker of industrial diseases gnaws at the very root of our national strength." Various improvements were possible which had not been put into effect. Reform could be initiated by the voluntary action of employers, by the demands and insistence of work-people, or by the coercion of law.

The employers of labor were divided by Simon into three groups. He recognized that there were, from his viewpoint, certain well-managed factories:

> . . . and, in those establishments where the better conditions exist, this superiority denotes that means of improvement have been voluntarily adopted by enlightened and kind-hearted employers. On the other hand, in many instances, the employer seems not to have given any thought whatever to the matter. . . . Again, in a considerable number of intermediate cases the employer has attempted to mitigate the unwholesome influences under which his workpeople are suffering, and has failed through want of knowledge, as especially in the many unskilful endeavours which have been made to amend the ventilation of work rooms.

As for the workman's insistence on reforms, Simon was forthright: "He cannot exact his sanitary rights. He could not do so unless he were one in a combination of claimants; nor even then unless, further, he had sufficient knowledge to shape demands for definite remedies. These conditions do not seem in any degree likely to be realized."

And what of the law? Simon did not hesitate to declare that "no existing law is more than very imperfectly applicable to procure the mitigation of unwholesome industrial conditions."

This distinguished public servant complained of the confused situation with regard to lead poisoning, due to the lack of statistics on its morbidity and mortality in industry. Although he reported, in writing about the manufacture of white lead and lead acetate, a universal allegation "that progress has been made in diminishing the dangers of the occupation," he himself was unconvinced: "in my opinion it deserves more particular consideration than it has yet received, whether the processes which diffuse lead-dust, and which occasion the chief danger in this industry, are not processes which ought to be discontinued or modified."

Influenced, no doubt, by Simon's reports, the Factory Act of 1864 required that every factory should be ventilated in such a manner as to render harmless, so far as practicable, any gases, dust, or other dangerous impurities generated in the process of manufacture. This did not prove to be immediately practicable.[4] As we shall see, the Factory Act of 1878 would be more specific.

Among the hardships of the working populace which fell under

the compassionate eye of Charles Dickens were occupational injuries
and diseases. "The borders of Radcliffe and Stepney, eastward of
London" he found to be the scene of an "uncompromising dance of
death" due not only to utter poverty, insufficient food, and unwholesome living, but also to dangerous work. His observations on
plumbism did not pass unnoticed in governmental circles, for he was
quoted by Alexander Redgrave in the *Report of the Chief Inspector of
Factories and Workshops* (1879), the first report to mention lead poisoning. (This, however, was ten years later.) What Dickens had to say
reflects prevailing attitudes of the period and seems worth considering
in some detail.

The Uncommercial Traveller, visiting the East End of London,
knocked at a door. He was admitted to a room almost bare of furniture,
with only a few sticks of wood on the grate and with the most meagre
utensils. "It was not until I had spoken with the woman for a few
minutes, that I saw a horrible brown heap on the floor in a corner,
which, but for previous experience in this dismal wise," he might not
have suspected to be "the bed." There was something thrown upon
it, and he asked what that was:

> Tis the poor craythur that stays here, sur; and 'tis very bad she is, and
> 'tis very bad she's been this long time, and 'tis better she'll never be, and
> 'tis slape she does all day, and 'tis wake she does all night, and 'tis the
> lead, sur.
> The what?
> The lead, sur. Sure 'tis the lead-mills, where the women gets took on
> at eighteen-pence a day, sur, when they makes application early enough,
> and is lucky and wanted; and 'tis lead-pisoned she is, sur, and some of
> them gets lead-pisoned soon, and some of them gets lead-pisoned later,
> and some, but not many, niver; and 'tis all according to the constitooshun,
> sur, and some constitooshuns is strong, and some is weak; and her con-
> stitooshun is lead-pisoned, bad as can be, sur; and her brain is coming
> out at her ear, and it hurts her dreadful; and that's what it is, and niver
> no more, and niver no less, sur.[5]

The poor ignorant woman, here quoted at length, was setting
forth for Dickens an opinion and was making a declaration ("some
constitooshuns is strong, and some is weak") about plumbism which
had already been much debated by the doctors and which would be
learnedly reiterated in the second half of the twentieth century. Toward the end of the nineteenth century, there were lengthy and acrimonious debates in the French Chamber of Deputies over the question

of compensation for industrial disease, during which the claim was repeatedly advanced that not all of the exposed workers were subject to *les maladies de plomb*, that a predisposition was necessary, and that "the diseases" were not, therefore, solely the effect of working conditions. This argument was repudiated by (among others) M. Armand Després, who in 1893 declared plumbism to be *"tout à fait profession-nelle."*[6]

Individual variations in susceptibility have been much discussed ever since. Taking into account diet factors, disease states, including alcoholism, and various other conditions, individual idiosyncrasy is yet presumed by some to play a large part.[7] Certain Pavlovian studies were thought to indicate, about twenty years ago, a compensatory role for the cerebral cortex in lead poisoning and a difference in compensation reactions between "a dog with a strong nervous system" by Pavlov's classification and "a dog with a weak nervous system." Experiments showed that adaptation to lead poisoning occurs, but that on continued exposure, the various compensatory mechanisms are damaged, and more intense nervous activity results, leading to death.[8] Whatever the truth of the matter, these publications of 1957 demonstrate that certain twentieth-century investigators have shared the views about plumbism expressed to Dickens by an ignorant Irishwoman in 1868: " 'Tis all according to the constitooshun, sur, and some constitoo-shuns is strong, and some is weak." As we shall see presently, some of the hygienic physicians of the last century had a different explanation of individual variations in susceptibility to lead poisoning.

When Dickens himself visited the lead-mills in the East End, he received a quite different impression; the tone of his report underwent a marked change. Welcomed by "two very intelligent gentlemen, brothers, and partners with their father in the concern, and who testified every desire to show their works to me freely," he went over the entire plant, cheerfully "hopping up ladders, and across planks, and on elevated perches . . . uncertain whether to liken myself to a bird or a brick-layer." He described the Dutch process of making white lead, in pots containing lead and acid, under tan, in a "series of large cock-lofts," where

> strong, active women were clambering about them busily; and the whole thing had rather the air of the upper part of the house of some immensely rich old Turk, whose faithful seraglio were hiding his money because the sultan or the pasha was coming.

As in the case with most pulps or pigments, so in the instance of this white lead, processes of stirring, separating, washing, grinding, rolling, and pressing succeed. Some of these are unquestionably inimical to health. . . . Against these dangers, I found good respirators provided (simply made of flannel and muslin, so as to be inexpensively renewed, and in some instances washed with scented soap), and gauntlet gloves, and loose gowns. Everywhere, there was as much fresh air as windows, well-placed and opened, could possibly admit. And it was explained that the precaution of frequently changing the women employed in the worst parts of the work (a precaution originating in their own experience or apprehension of its ill effects) was found salutary. They had a mysterious and singular appearance, with the mouth and nose covered, and the loose gown on, and yet bore out the simile of the old Turk and the seraglio all the better for the disguise.

Although "the Uncommercial countenance withdrew itself, with expedition and a sense of suffocation, from the dull-glowing heat and the over-powering smell" of the ovens, the Uncommercial Traveller "made it out to be indubitable that the owners of these lead-mills honestly and sedulously try to reduce the dangers of the occupation to the lowest point." These owners clearly belonged to the first, and the admirable, group in the three-part classification of Sir John Simon. It remained appropriate, however, to classify the employees according to the severity of their plumbism. A very doubtful assertion about the women workers was swallowed whole by Dickens: "It is found that they bear the work much better than men: some few of them have been at it for years, and the great majority of those I observed were strong and active. On the other hand, it should be remembered that most of them are very capricious and irregular in their attendance." The facilities and the care provided—a washing-place, a lunch room, a female attendant, and even "an experienced medical attendant"—were incredibly good.

American inventiveness would seem to indicate that before very long white lead may be made entirely by machinery. The sooner, the better. In the meantime, I parted from my two frank conductors over the mills, by telling them they had nothing there to be concealed, and nothing to be blamed for. As to the rest, the philosophy of the matter of lead-poisoning and work-people seems to me to have been pretty fairly summed up by the Irish-woman whom I quoted in my former paper.[9]

That Dickens should have troubled to make this inspection is remarkable: the subject had attracted little general notice, and the first official reference to lead poisoning in the *Chief Factory Inspector's Report* was to be delayed another ten years. That he should have found such conscientious effort to minimize the danger is also remarkable: Dr. Alice Hamilton was to find worse conditions in some American lead-works half a century later (an ironic comment on his faith in American ingenuity).[10] But most remarkable of all is his conclusion. We are told that these are the same lead-mills in which the "poor craythur" of the Irish household had worked before her sickness overcame her.[11] Yet Dickens is convinced that nothing remains to be done, and the Uncommercial Traveller ("I travel for the great House of Human Interest Brothers") is content to sum up the whole question in the Irish-woman's fatalistic observations on "constitooshun." With a flourish of his arm quite worthy of Mr. Podsnap, he dismisses the subject from consideration. The fault, it appears, lies with the sufferers themselves, as constitutional inferiors; or rather, since nobody is really to blame, the trouble must be referred to fate. In any case there is no further hope, short of a new triumph of American machinery. The managerial statement that women endure the work better than men is accepted, like other managerial statements, without question.[12]

The precautions taken in this particular factory were remarkably good for the period, yet poisoning occurred. Dickens himself had pointed to the pressure of poverty as an operative factor: it was better to risk plumbism than to have no work. Since the manufacturer had taken every reasonable care, and since the general poverty could not be laid to his account, what remained to be said? Do away with white-lead pigments? No generally adequate substitute had been found. Better precautions? Who knew of any better? The elimination of susceptible workers? A poor solution in a time of unemployment—it was not clear that starvation was the better part. A remedy for unemployment and poverty? As well demand the moon. Large questions these, but the Uncommerical Traveller, remarkable for his active social conscience, did not ask them. Leaving aside his importance as an entertainer, his great social function was not to remedy evils but to point them out. In this case, however, basing his "philosophy" of lead poisoning on his observation of a single factory, he perhaps added his own mite to the maintainence of that social inertia which he otherwise deplored. Dickens' white-lead factory was as exceptional as the model textile mills which had been operated earlier in the century by Robert Owen. Most of the precautions that Dickens found observed there had later to be enforced generally by the power of law, not to mention the more exacting requirements soon to be made.

It is not yet known, perhaps, who was the first employer in a dangerous-substance industry to blame its ill-effects on the carelessness or the unclean habits of his workers; nor is it known who first observed that these ill-effects were not uniformly evident throughout the workforce and so joyfully proclaimed singularity of constitution to be the key. If not a careless, dirty rogue, the poisoned worker had to be considered an unfortunate freak of nature; not just singularity but something like aberration was to be blamed. But perhaps, after all, it was only bad luck. In any case, who could hold the employer responsible?

A rather astonishing mixture of many of these attitudes (together with certain informed and enlightened views) may still be seen late in the century in a good, comprehensive general outline of the hygiene, diseases, and mortality of all the principal occupations pursued in Great Britain, based on the Milroy Lectures delivered in 1889 at the Royal College of Physicians by Dr. J.T. Arlidge, which were expanded into a book and published in 1892—more than twenty years after the death of Charles Dickens.[13] Dr. Arlidge was, of course, an expert in occupational disease, and it is natural enough that at the end of his Preface, after he had acknowledged the help of fellow experts, he should have concluded thus: "I must also not fail to express my best thanks to those many manufacturers who accorded me the privilege of going over their factories, and witnessing the principal processes carried on. They will do me a further service by notifying me of errors in technical descriptions, where such errors affect conclusions arrived at."[14] No more than in Dickens' experience was there any atmosphere of confrontation; a good understanding did not quite preclude criticism. Now it is plain that Dr. Arlidge, when he was touring factories, was immensely more knowledgeable than Dickens had been. Yet it is permissable to ask whether his eye was sharper than the great novelist's, whether he himself was shrewder and more sceptical than the author of *Hard Times;* and if he was sceptical, was his scepticism pointed in the right direction?

The original Milroy Lectures had "allowed only of the consideration of diseases consequent upon the inhalation of dust,"[15] whereas the book was panoramic. Fortunately, however, Arlidge gave more attention to dust problems than his hygienic predecessors had done; but because it was not before his concluding chapter that he reached "Hygienic Provisions Against Diseases of Occupations," he had to be succinct when he described them.

Since Dickens' time the skill of engineers had been applied, sometimes with happy results, to the solution of these problems. The Act of 1878 had called for the use of exhaust fans. And now, a dozen years later, Arlidge could write: "For withdrawing dust nothing appears more efficient than the 'exhaust' fans which are fast coming into use in all factories of any magnitude where steam-power is available." For smaller factories without steam, he recommended gas engines and added, with satisfaction, "it will not be long before electricity will be available."[16] Gone, we may think, is the fatalism found in Dickens, and to a considerable extent this is true. What has become, we consequently ask, of the "constitution" story which apparently satisfied Dickens? "There must be cleanliness of person, of the working place, and of the clothes," declared Arlidge. "Proper regard had to this particular explains, to a great extent, the escape of one workman from the ills that waylay another engaged in the same trade; and often dispenses with the facile hypothesis of idiosyncracy to afford an interpretation."[17] And although we cannot today altogether dispense with idiosyncracy in thinking about lead poisoning,[18] it remains true that careful study of the circumstances is required before we resort to it. The hygienic physician undoubtedly was sceptical of the "constitooshun" ploy; at the same time, a little surprisingly, he looked harder at habit than at environment. Or did he?

In pointing to the need for cleanliness of person, of working place, and of clothes, Arlidge appeared to shift something like two-thirds of the responsibility to the worker. And it is here that we may compare him once again with Dickens. Arlidge summed up his views in three sentences:

> When human ingenuity and skill have done all that is possible to remove causes of illness present in machinery, in materials employed and in the methods of work, the consequences of exposure and carelessness consciously remain within the control of the employed. It has been pointed out that the frequent connection of recklessness and dangerous occupations, is largely owing to the inferior grade of society from which such occupations draw their recruits. Here amendment can only be looked for in the advance of civilisation, in improved moral tone, and in the spread of education and intelligence, and of orderly and temperate habits.[19]

Dr. Arlidge was not writing merely about lead poisoning here, but about occupational disease in general; certainly he was writing, however, about "causes of illness present . . . in materials employed and in the methods of work." Did "the frequent connection of recklessness and dangerous occupations" exhibit itself in the white lead industry by careless behavior or simply by breathing in one of the lead-mill cocklofts? Or was breathing careless behavior in itself? Perhaps it might be said that simply to take such a job showed a disposition to recklessness. Yet the Uncommercial Traveller probably came very close to expressing the true attitude of the women of the lead-mills: "Better to be ulcerated and paralyzed for eighteen-pence a day, while it lasted, than to see the children starve."[20]

And it would be altogether untrue to suggest that *The Hygiene, Diseases and Mortality of Occupations* laid the blame chiefly on the individual worker. About defects of ventilation and in working space he said: "These surpass in their disastrous effects on the health of the employed all other injurious conditions taken together. . . . In not a few instances defective ventilation and working space represent almost the whole of the conditions recognisable as prejudicial to health. . . ."[21]

We may very well feel that Charles Dickens, for his part, was a little bit too ready to accept at face value the assertions of his mill owners and to agree that nothing more, nothing whatever, could be done at that time—a little too quick to adopt as "pretty fairly summed up" by the Irishwoman and as encompassing the whole "philosophy of the matter of lead poisoning and work people" the inexorable creed, " 'tis all according to the constitooshun." After all, his lines had fallen, for once, in more or less pleasant places, and he had found himself among more or less model employers. As for the distinguished physician who, more than twenty years later, was expressing his faith in "improved moral tone, and in the spread of education and intelligence, and of orderly and temperate habits," he seemed to be indulging in a kind of cant of which Dickens was rarely guilty. Dickens, at any rate, found none of the factory troubles to be "largely owing to the inferior grade of society from which such occupations draw their recruits."

The Dickensian faith in machines had proven, at least in the short term, to be over sanguine. Pending the American millenium, however, the constitutions of the lead workers were already better protected than they had been in Dickens' day. Exhaust fans were beginning to whirl out the stuffy, sweetish atmosphere of the old lead-mills and to whirl in a new day. Dickens would not have been surprised.

The exhaust fans were, of course, far from providing a complete solution of the problem. Wise legislation, employers of good will, employee education, and medical expertise were all necessary, as were additional technical innovations. But an informed public opinion was to provide the backing for all the needed changes. And informed public opinion grew from sound, stimulating journalism of a kind which Charles Dickens, at his best, so memorably supplied.

Notes

Most aspects (medical, industrial, political, labor) of the industrial hygiene problems of early nineteenth-century Britain are dealt with lucidly if briefly by A. Meiklejohn, *The Life, Work and Times of Charles Turner Thackrah, Surgeon and Apothecary of Leeds (1795–1833)* (Edinburgh and London: E. & S. Livingstone Ltd., 1957). The great work of C. Turner Thackrah was *The Effects of the Principal Arts, Trades and Professions . . . on Health and Longevity* (London, 1831, 2nd ed. 1832) which was reprinted by Meiklejohn in 1957. The principal authority on Dickens is of course Edgar Johnson, *Charles Dickens: His Tragedy and Triumph*, 2 vols. (New York: Simon and Schuster, 1952). My unpublished doctoral dissertation, "A History of Lead Poisoning" (Johns Hopkins University, 1949), has supplied most of the source material for the first two parts of the present three-part essay (supplemented by other, more recent work), whereas the third part is based on a fresh reading of Arlidge and a review of the recent literature.

1. Stevenson, "A History of Lead Poisoning," pp. 339 ff.

2. *The Diary, Reminiscences and Correspondence of H. Crabb Robinson*, ed. Thomas Sadler (London, 1869), II, pp. 93–95.

3. Stevenson, *op. cit.*, pp. 340–342. On the special hazards of women *cf.* below, n. 12.

4. *Ibid.*, pp. 342–345.

5. Charles Dickens, "A Small Star in the East," *All The Year Round*, n.s., vol. I, no. 3, Dec. 19, 1868; *cf. The Uncommercial Traveller*, ed. by Charles Dickens the Younger (New York: MacMillan and Co., 1896), pp. 276–277.

6. Stevenson, *op. cit.*, p. 388.

7. Irene R. Campbell and Estelle G. Mergard, *Biological Aspects of Lead: Annotated Bibliography. Literature from 1950 through 1964.* (Research Triangle Park, N.C.: U. S. Environmental Protection Agency, 1972), Part II, p. 922.

8. Ingher, I. et al: [Experiments on compensation reactions in lead poisoning] *Igiena* 6: 115, 1957. Idem: [Experimental studies on chronic lead poisoning] *Minerva Medica* 48, No. 31: 1361–4, 1957.

9. Charles Dickens, "On an Amateur Beat," *All The Year Round*, n.s., vol. I, no. 13, Feb. 27, 1869; *cf. The Uncommercial Traveller*, ed. cit., pp. 300–304.

10. In a 1932 government *Report*, Bridge observed: "Though we cannot yet say that it is practicable for white lead to be made entirely by machinery, direct pulping of white lead in oil, eliminating the drying and grinding processes, has been in the last decade the prime factor in the reduction of lead poisoning." Bridge, J.C., in *Annual Report of the Chief Inspector of Factories and Workshops* (London, 1932), p. 45.

11. Dickens, *l.c.* (n. 9 above), p. 300.

12. Dickens' reception by the managers is in marked contrast to Thackrah's experience. *Cf. The Effects of Arts, Trades and Professions*, etc. (2nd ed., London, 1832) p. 103: "We were not permitted personally to inspect the process, though we examined the men." *Cf.* Bridge, *l.c.*, p. 52: "The employment of women in white lead works and the potteries was the subject of much inquiry by the woman Inspectors in 1896. [Women were first appointed Inspectors in 1893.] . . . The exclusion of women from lead processes was continually urged, and the incidence of still-births among women pottery workers was emphasised."

13. J.T. Arlidge, *The Hygiene, Diseases and Mortality of Occupations* (London, 1892).

14. *Ibid.*, p. x.

15. *Ibid.*, p. vii.

16. *Ibid.*, pp. 566–567.

17. *Ibid.*, p. 568. The zealous sanitarian is revealed in Arlidge's astonishing assertion, on the same page, that "even where dust is the sole cause of illness the cleanly careful operative escapes, whilst his negligent neighbour succumbs to it."

18. *Cf.* n. 7 and n. 8 above.

19. Arlidge, *op. cit.*, p. 565.

20. Dickens, *l.c.* (n. 5 above) p. 277.

21. Arlidge, *op. cit.*, p. 565.

Isaac Ray:
"The Greatest Amount of Good
with the Smallest Amount of Harm"*

JACQUES M. QUEN

In 1860, Oliver Wendell Holmes observed: "The truth is, that medicine professedly founded on observation, is as sensitive to outside influences, political, religious, philosophical, imaginative, as is the barometer to the changes of atmospheric density. Theoretically it ought to go on its own straightforward inductive path, without regard to changes of government or fluctuations of public opinion. . . . [Actually there is] a closer relation between the Medical Sciences and the conditions of Society and the general thought of the time, than would at first be suspected."[1] It was not until a century later, in 1964, that Norman Dain resurrected this statement as a particularly apt framework for understanding the history of American psychiatry.[2]

Psychiatry, earlier, and more than any other branch of American medical practice, was almost totally dependent upon formal government support. As a result, an accumulation of legislative decisions, actions, and inactions defined the real world in which the nineteenth-century American psychiatrist had to treat his patients. In the late nineteenth and early twentieth centuries, neurologists, rebelling against the inadequacies and abuses of institutional treatment of the insane, introduced the outpatient treatment of the mentally ill.[3] While the more optimistic may have believed that this practice would free the interaction of psychiatrist and psychiatric patient from political control, it now appears that psychiatry is facing a probable repetition of its own history. The major difference seems to be that the stage for this drama has shifted from the municipal and state levels to the federal arena.

The chain of connecting links between legislative actions and the specific internal conditions of individual hospitals is a long, complex, and complicated one. The historian's task of understanding the development of these hospitals becomes easier, superficially, by viewing them as autonomous, individual fiefdoms under the absolute control of a sociologically and politically homogeneous group of superintendents acting in concert. While exceptions to this general tendency are found in the studies of the Worcester State Hospital[4] and the Eastern State Lunatic Asylum,[5] they remain infrequent. One popular author, unwittingly perpetuating the fiefdom fallacy, recently observed of the decline of American asylums in the last half of the nineteenth century: "Officials abandoned a high risk, high success operation for a minimum risk, minimum success one. Rather than rest the future of the asylum on an ability to rehabilitate the mentally ill, they assumed the failure-proof task of caring for the chronic."[6] Later, this author modified his view to characterize the superintendents as having "accepted with general complacence the change to custodial care without doing battle on behalf of therapeutic institutions."[7]

Superintendents, in fact, did fight many of these changes, winning occasional battles, but losing the war. Their defeat was partly caused by their political naiveté and their political impotence. There were, admittedly, other powerful forces, both obvious and obscure, that affected and will continue to affect the outcome of conflicts about proper care for the mentally disabled. Economic prosperity or depression are among the more obvious, while the social values, and personal, family, or economic situation of political and community leaders are among the more obscure factors determining the treatment of the mentally ill.

In the late nineteenth century in Philadelphia, Isaac Ray, a founder of the Association of Medical Superintendents of American Institutions for the Insane, fought to improve the care of the insane in the Philadelphia Almshouse. The Almshouse, a county institution, was one of the two American insane asylums singled out in 1876 for severe condemnation by John Charles Bucknill, the British psychiatrist.[8] The history of Ray's efforts in this incident are less important for what was accomplished than for what was attempted; his lack of success, is as significant as it was predictable.

Isaac Ray was characterized by Winfred Overholser, Sr., as "the most forceful" of the original thirteen founders of the American Psychiatric Association, "if not the giant among them all."[9] Born in Beverly, Massachusetts in 1807, Ray published his classic *A Treatise on the Medical Jurisprudence of Insanity* when he was a 31-year-old general practitioner in Eastport, Maine.[10] Three years later, Ray had his first institutional experience with the insane as the medical superintendent of the Maine Insane Hospital at Augusta. His predecessor had only lasted a year. After four years, Ray accepted the appointment as superintendent of the yet-to-be-built Butler Hospital in Providence, Rhode Island, where he remained until 1867, when he resigned and retired to Philadelphia.

In Philadelphia, Ray continued to lead an active professional life. In 1869 he was a charter member of the Philadelphia Social Science Association and a member of its Committee on Public Health. In 1870 he was appointed by the Supreme Court of Pennsylvania to Philadelphia's Board of Guardians of the Poor, the governing body of the Philadelphia Almshouse. Immediately upon joining the board, Ray was appointed to its three-man Committee on the Insane Department. He was the only member with practical experience in the care of the insane.*

Ray's first move was to take stock of the insane department and its functioning. On February 27, 1871, he submitted a careful evaluation from his committee. The tone and substance of the report make it clear that Ray found the condition of the asylum entirely unacceptable: "If the patients ever recover, it must be in spite of, and not in consequence of their surroundings, for we can imagine no conjunction of circumstances more calculated to exasperate the disease."

In pointing out the gross overcrowding of the asylum and its lack of space for exercise, farming, and other outdoor activity, he suggested that it was time to move the asylum out of the city and into the countryside. "But the present deplorable condition of the insane department does not entirely result from want of room—Much of it is attributable to arrangements that have no other excuse than a misplaced economy."

Ray particularly objected to the tradition of requiring indigent former patients of the hospital "to serve the Almshouse for a few weeks as a quasi compensation for the care and support they have themselves received." He wanted to dispense with these attendants whom he regarded as worse than useless. The almshouse had twelve paid attendants for the insane, whose responsibilities included overseeing the work of the pauper attendants. Ray suggested that 23 more paid attendants be hired. In the report, he pointed out that: "In our State hospitals for the Insane the proportion of attendants to patients ranges from one in ten to one in twenty—At the latter rate

*The following quotations are from the Minute-books of the Board of Guardians of the Poor of Philadelphia, which are located in the Philadelphia City Archives. Particular thanks are due to the staff for generous, helpful, and thoughtful assistance.

our number should be forty." He asked, however, for only 35.

Ray was worried about the inadequate diet of the insane patients. He objected to the fact that they were served meat only four times a week, and then always boiled. "We have no hesitation in saying that their dietary should be equal to that required by the average sane workman—That is to say, it should embrace animal food at least once a day, some vegetables, besides bread, and tea or coffee twice." Ray was also concerned about the inadequate facilities for washing the clothes of the patients; they often went without a change of under-clothing for as long as three weeks.

He closed the report by presenting the costs to the asylum of implementing his suggestions: $5,888 a year for the added paid attendants; $12,480 for the food; another $475 for a roaster, some furniture, and farming tools—$18,843 in all. While the report was accepted and copies were ordered to be printed, no action was taken on any specific suggestion.

In a separate statement at that same meeting, Ray reported that the committee "would inform the Board that it is now considered best to prohibit promiscuous visiting to the [insane] department, and that hereafter those only be admitted who have relatives and friends in the institution, and those who come from philanthropy and science."

For the remainder of 1871 and 1872, Ray's activities at the board meetings, as recorded in the minutes, were generally restricted to the management and administration of the insane department. These included housekeeping details, hiring watchmen, arranging to have water pumped to the patient's quarters, providing an adequate wash-house, and other such practical matters. On December 23, 1872, Ray made three motions that suggest that much had been going on at the asylum that incurred his strong displeasure. First he moved that visitors not be admitted on Sundays except in case of death or extreme sickness, the only other exception being clergymen. His second motion was that "any person in the service of this Institution, who shall strike, beat, kick, choke or otherwise abuse a patient, shall be arrested and prosecuted according to the law, and it shall be the duty of the Steward to take suitable measures for the enforcement of this rule,— It is also the duty of every employee of the Institution on becoming acquainted with any instance of abuse, to inform the Steward thereof." The minutes record that this was referred to the Committee on Revision of Rules.

Ray's third motion that day, obviously aimed at the members of the Board of Guardians, was "Believing it to be the duty of the Board of Guardians to protect the Insane committed to their charge, from unnecessary exposure of their infirmities, and knowing that [in] all other Hospitals for the Insane, such exposure is never permitted, therefore, *Resolved* that the practice of allowing company to witness the balls and other exhibitions of the Insane, is subversive of the feelings of delicacy, which should mark our care of the unfortunate and helpless class of our fellow man and trust that it will hereafter be discountenanced by every member of the Board." This was referred to the Committee on the Insane Department.

Two months and two meetings later, the Committee on the Insane Department reported that "believing that the purpose of the above resolution would be sufficiently accomplished by restricting the present privilege of admitting visitors to the Almshouse, would offer the following resolution as a substitute for the above: Resolved—That in future in giving permits to visit the Almshouse, the Guardian shall state clearly the number of persons allowed to enter on the strength of any one permit is limited to five." The story must be read between the lines. The committee consisted of Isaac Ray and two other members of the board. It is clear that Ray's original resolution was totally unacceptable and that the two committee members adamantly refused to support the abolition of this traditional prerogative of the board members. What motivated this strong opposition? What benefits could have accrued to the members of the board from this prerogative? A parallel in modern-day business practice is the providing of passes or tickets to popular plays or ball-games for potential clients or customers.

The following month, Isaac Ray presented a paper at the annual meeting of the Philadelphia Social Science Association titled "What shall Philadelphia do for its paupers?"[11] Ray reviewed the conditions of the entire Almshouse, indicting its management with facts, figures, and measurements. He did not mince words, charging that the Almshouse was one of the most life-endangering institutions of its kind. Ray's review included the pauper and insane departments, the lying-in hospital, the children's asylum, and the general hospital, later to become the Philadelphia General Hospital.

Ray opened his address with two sentences that remain remarkably relevant: "To provide public support for its poor—those who are unable to support themselves—is now generally recognized as an imperative duty of society. How best to discharge this duty so as to accomplish the greatest amount of good with the least amount of harm, has become one of the most interesting questions in social science." He continued: "In regard to the first requisite in any system of public support, that of rigid economy, or, more properly speaking, of a small expenditure, certainly no fault can be found with the Philadelphia almshouse. For the year 1872, the average cost was $1.77 per person per week." With his not uncharacteristic Yankee sarcasm, Ray observed that "Suspicion arises at first thought, that economy has been carried too far for the best interests of all concerned."

Ray's first major target was the insane department. He pointed out that the six-by-ten-foot rooms, originally designed to accommodate one person, usually slept two and frequently three. [This might be contrasted with the cells of the coeval Philadelphia penitentiary, also designed for one person, that were eight-by-twelve-feet.][12] He proceeded to observe that "There can be few more pitiable spectacles than that witnessed every day, of hundreds of men overcharged with nervous excitement, whose restless movements are confined to the limits of a narrow hall, and of as many more, silent and depressed, crouching down in corners and by-places—all of them worrying one another, and speedily losing from sheer inaction whatever of mind their disease may have left." He made a strong plea for moving the asylum out of the city to a site where 400 acres of land might be provided for the insane to have the outdoor recreation and farming demanded by moral treatment.

Another reason for moving the asylum out of the city was that "the close proximity of our hospital to a large city exposes the patients to a multitude of people who, as loafers, idlers, or sight-seers, are always ready to bestow their leisure upon others. They take up the time of employees, they give the patients what they ought not to have, such as money, tobacco, matches; . . . Some, bent on a higher degree of iniquity, break into the building, through doors or windows."

Of the general hospital, he said, "Of all places in the world, a hospital should be that in which the sick should find the most chances for relief, and yet not unfrequently, it presents the least. In this particular, the Philadelphia hospital is remarkably faulty. The patients do not readily recover after severe operations, the mortality on such occasions being exceedingly large. Indeed, not unfrequently the surgeons refrain from operating on that account, even though the patient may be suffering under a mortal disease, sure to destroy life." Contributing to this situation was the crowded state of the general hospital, "with a capacity for about five hundred patients, it now has under care nearly one thousand. . . ."

Ray next turned his attention to the lying-in hospital: "It is understood and admitted by medical men that the death rate in lying-in hospitals is larger on the whole than it is in private practice. Their statistics show a vast difference among them in particular, some of them showing a mortality much less than that of some private practice. During the last five years the average mortality at the Blockley has been one in twenty-two. Of the twenty-one hospitals, the statistics of which I have examined, not one shows so great a mortality as this, while in several the mortality has been less than one in two hundred." The Children's Asylum was, Ray charged, even more inimical to life. Here, he relied on a paper presented two years earlier to the Social Science Association by a Doctor Parry to document that "while about thirty per cent of all the children in Philadelphia, two years old and under, died, the mortality of the corresponding class in the asylum was over seventy-three per cent. During the last two or three years the death rate has lessened, but still it is much higher than it is in common life."

Ray closed his talk with a detailed consideration of conditions in the insane department: "To continue this crowding together of the insane, as is still being done at Blockley, is simply to perpetrate a great crime against humanity. To ignore the fact and to be reckless of the consequences, is no better in point of morals, than it would be for a railway company to use a bridge after it had been found defective and dangerous."

A heated discussion followed this presentation with at least two other members of the Board of Guardians participating from the audience. John M. Whitall, then president of the board, made several statements in defense of the Almshouse. Perhaps the most significant was his comment that "I was very much surprised to hear from Dr. Ray —I suppose there is no doubt, but that he is correct—that the mortality was so very high among the children, and in the lying-in wards. I do not say it is not so, but I was very much surprised to hear it."

At the following meeting of the board in April, Ray introduced a resolution that may have been sparked by Whitall's surprise. He proposed that "a committee be appointed by the president to revise the Table now in use for reporting the census of the house, so that the information sought to be obtained, shall be given in a correct and intelligible shape." The motion was adopted, and Ray was one of the three appointed to the committee.

At the following meeting, Ray introduced another resolution: "Whereas the number of patients in the department of the Insane being now 953 which is far beyond the capacity of the House, therefore Resolved that the Steward is directed to receive no more for that department until the number falls below 900 and to keep it as near that figure as possible." The motion was tabled and Ray followed it with a proposal for a statement from the Board of Guardians to the city's Common Councils on the same subject: "It is incumbent on every Christian community to provide for its pauper insane in the manner best calculated to promote their recovery and comfort, and Whereas the Insane of Philadelphia now in the Almshouse are not so cared for, but rather in a manner calculated to produce great discomfort and prevent recovery, for the reason that the Hospital is now, and has been for several years, excessively crowded, the present number 953 being twice as many as it can properly accommodate, whereby the patients disturb the rest and endanger the lives of one another at night, and because in consequence of the want of land on which they might labor, they are confined to the halls or narrow yards, enjoying none of the benefits of exercise and occupation in the open air, therefore, Resolved, That the Councils of the city be requested by the Board of Guardians of the Poor, to take measures immediately for erecting a Hospital of suitable capacity where the requisite amount of land can be obtained at a convenient place, at some distance from and unconnected with any other part of the Almshouse." This was adopted and a copy was forwarded to the City Councils and published.

At that same meeting, Ray proposed that a request be sent to the Governor to prevent the removal of the general hospital of the Almshouse to "some distant place." He enumerated seven reasons for the Governor to support the stand of the Board of Guardians. This too was adopted by the board and a copy sent to the Governor.

Isaac Ray's last act as a member of the Board of Guardians was to prepare and distribute at the meeting of June 23 (the last meeting he attended) the new table that he had suggested following his presentation to the Philadelphia Social Science Association. On August 25, after Ray had left the board, his resolution to limit admissions and to keep the census at a maximum of 900 was voted down; the board explained that they had no authority to close the doors of the Almshouse for any reason.

Isaac Ray was not reappointed to the Board of Guardians. John Charles Bucknill, a leading British psychiatrist who visited America in

1875 said: "Dr. Ray has been, I found, one of the Governors of the Philadelphia Almshouse and asylum, but for some reason which I failed to comprehend, he had been routed out from his office, wherein by Knowledge, benevolence and assiduity he had done all the good possible under the circumstances. Dr. Ray was ejected from his office for political reasons . . . although I should have thought that all politicians would at best have agreed upon the duty of duly providing for the needs of the destitute sick and insane."[13] Later, in his *Notes on Asylums for the Insane in America,* Bucknill characterized the Insane Department of the Philadelphia Almshouse as "thoroughly discreditable" to the community.[14] He reported that, at the time of his visit in 1875, Ray told him that the asylum, designed to accommodate 500, had 1,130 patients.

Isaac Ray died of tuberculosis in March, 1881. In a memoriam prepared for the College of Physicians of Philadelphia, Thomas S. Kirkbride, Superintendent of the Pennsylvania Hospital for the Insane, referred to Ray's removal from the board with uncharacteristic anger. While the details of his removal are not known to us, it is clear that contemporaries saw it as an act specifically directed against Ray as a professional concerned with the welfare of the insane.

In December, 1881 the Common Council of Philadelphia passed a resolution authorizing a committee of five to "investigate the entire management of the Almshouse and the Board of Guardians of the Poor."[15] The committee reported its findings on June 12, 1882: "The cruelty permitted towards old paupers and the insane and the death of *all* [emphasis in original] foundlings brought to the place is difficult to write of with calmness. It is in evidence and not disputed—indeed Mathew McNamara, a witness called by the Guardians, testified that he was whipping from eight to ten people a day, when he suddenly went to Ireland in April, 1880, there being a great many complaints against him. He said that his stick was his best friend, that it had a large nail in the end of it. Richard Penn, a policeman, who in 1880 was an attendant in the insane department, testified that he had seen a man named Michael Houten, who was in charge of the sixth ward, frequently knock down old insane people. He said he complained . . . but no improvement was made, and he . . . was finally discharged for making complaints."[16]

It would be difficult not to see this as the kind of incident that must have sparked Ray's strongly worded motion of December 23, 1872, regarding "any person . . . who shall strike, beat, kick, choke, or otherwise abuse a patient." The report of 1882 documents the continued decline of other deficiencies in the Almshouse that had disturbed Ray: "That such barbarous cruelty should be allowed in any civilized community is almost incredible, and yet the Superintendent of this Institution and the President of the Board of Guardians find nothing in regard to which they desire a change, unless it is in the smallness of the appropriations. There can be no right feeling person in this community who does not feel that he himself will in some degree be responsible for the continuance of such outrages, and it is the earnest hope of this committee that, whatever action Councils may take on this report, they will at least take such measures as will render impossible, in any of the institutions of this City, the beating of the poor, the crippled and the afflicted, and the abandonment of helpless infants to die for want of ordinary care."[17]

One year after the death of Isaac Ray and almost ten years after his exposure of the realities of the Philadelphia Almshouse, a legislative investigation revealed that the conditions that Ray had protested had become worse. That Ray failed, does not imply that he did not hope to win. Despite the persistent efforts of the Philadelphia Social Science Association, it was many years before the changes were made that transformed the Blockley into the nationally respected Philadelphia General Hospital.

One might also observe that the Philadelphia Almshouse merely reflected the problems of caring for the insane at the county level. In 1915, Florence L. Sanville reported the results of the Public Charities Association study of the Pennsylvania insane under county care.[18] Conditions at that time paralleled those described by Ray in 1873. Albert Deutsch's *Shame of the States*,[19] in the mid-twentieth century, demonstrated that the disgraceful conditions had merely been transferred from the county to the state level.

Oliver Wendell Holmes was correct: There is a closer relation between the medical sciences and social thought than one might at first suspect. Norman Dain was also correct: This is a particularly apt framework for understanding the history of American psychiatry. Finally, it appears that Isaac Ray, too, was correct: How best to discharge society's obligations to the disadvantaged "so as to accomplish the greatest amount of good with the smallest amount of harm, has become one of the most interesting questions in social science." It was of pressing relevance then, and it remains so today.

Notes

*The research for this paper was supported by a grant from the National Library of Medicine (RO1 LM MH 02591-01) whose assistance is here gratefully acknowledged.

1. Oliver Wendell Holmes, *Currents and Counter-Currents in Medical Science* (Boston: Ticknor and Fields, 1861), pp. 7–8.

2. Norman Dain, *Concepts of Insanity in the United States, 1789–1865* (New Brunswick, N.J.: Rutgers University Press, 1964), p. xv. See also Gerald N. Grob, *The State and the Mentally Ill. A History of Worcester State Hospital in Massachusetts, 1830–1920* (Chapel Hill, N.C.: The University of North Carolina Press, 1966), p. 3.

3. Jacques M. Quen, "Asylum psychiatry, neurology, social work, and mental hygiene: an exploratory study in interprofessional history," *Journal of the History of the Behavioral Sciences*, 13 (1977), pp. 3–11.

4. Gerald N. Grob, *op. cit.,* fn.2.

5. Norman Dain, *Disordered Minds. The First Century of Eastern State Hospital in Williamsburg, Virginia. 1766–1866* (Williamsburg, Va.: The Colonial Williamsburg Foundation, 1971).

6. David J. Rothman, *The Discovery of the Asylum. Social Order and Disorder in the New Republic* (Boston: Little, Brown and Company, 1971), p. 282. See also Jacques M. Quen, "Review of *The Discovery of the Asylum,*" *Journal of Psychiatry and Law*, 2 (1974), pp. 105–122.

7. David J. Rothman, "Review of *Mental Institutions in America,*" *Journal of Interdisciplinary History* (1976), pp. 533–536; p. 535.

8. John Charles Bucknill, *Notes on Asylums for the Insane in America* (London: J. & A. Churchill, 1876).

9. Winifred Overholser, "The Founding and Founders of the Association," in J. K. Hall *et al*, eds., *One Hundred Years of American Psychiatry* (New York: Columbia University Press, 1944), pp. 45–72; p. 45.

10. Isaac Ray, *A Treatise on the Medical Jurisprudence of Insanity* (Boston: Charles C. Little and James Brown, 1838).

11. Isaac Ray, "What shall Philadelphia do for its paupers?," *Penn Monthly* (April, 1873). Also in the *Papers of the Social Science Association of Philadelphia* in the Collection of the Historical Society of Pennsylvania. The only record of the discussion following the presentation is in the latter reference.

12. Jacques M. Quen, "Historical reflections on the sesquicentennial of the founding of the Boston Prison Discipline Society (1825–1854)," *Bulletin of the American Academy of Psychiatry and the Law*, 3 (1975), pp. 132–133.

13. John Charles Bucknill, remarks in "Proceedings of the Association of Medical Superintendents," *American Journal of Insanity*, 32 (1876), pp. 267–404; pp. 287–288.

14. John Charles Bucknill, *Notes on Asylums for the Insane in America* (London: J. & A. Churchill, 1876), pp. 40ff.

15. Charles Lawrence, *History of the Philadelphia Almshouses and Hospitals From the Begin-*

ning of the Eighteenth to the Ending of the Nineteenth Centuries, etc. etc. (No location [Philadelphia]: Charles Lawrence, 1903), p. 297.

16.   *Ibid.,* p. 305.

17.   *Ibid.,* p. 306.

18.   Florence L. Sanville, "Straight-jackets muffs and cages and the whole eighteenth-century mental attitude of the so-called sane toward the insane, as it survives in the county institutions of twentieth century Pennsylvania," *Survey,* 34 (1915), pp. 7–12.

19.   Albert Deutsch, *The Shame of the States* (New York: Harcourt, 1948).

School Buildings and the Health
of American School Children
in the Nineteenth Century

JOHN DUFFY

The history of American school health essentially begins in the early nineteenth century with the rapid expansion of the public schools. No serious attempt at mass education was made during the colonial period, and hence the nineteenth-century pioneers in large-scale public education had only a limited experience to draw upon. Schools of the eighteenth century bore little resemblance, either in form or function, to those of today. Often lessons were given in the home of the teacher where the physical environment was reasonably good. Where permanent buildings existed, however, they were usually overcrowded and dingy. Discipline was strict and school hours long, for it was well known that the devil found work for idle hands. Save for an occasional voice here and there, little was heard of school health. In this period life expectancy was short. Almost half the children died from the ever-present sicknesses, and those who survived the chronic gastro-intestinal disorders and malaria of infancy were often swept away by periodic plagues such as smallpox, measles, diphtheria, and yellow fever. Moreover, the amount of schooling was limited. Under the circumstances, no widespread interest in school health could be expected.

In the nineteenth century the movement for democracy with its emphasis upon equality proved a powerful stimulus to the building of public schools, and the 1830's and 1840's saw their numbers rise rapidly. As the lower economic groups began playing a decisive part in American government, the old principle of free schools, a concept going back to earliest colonial times, gradually widened to include free and compulsory schooling.

A high birthrate and the demands for capital on the widening American frontier, however, created serious difficulties in supplying the growing need for schoolhouses. Cities, towns, and rural communities alike were constantly outgrowing their public buildings, and, while virtually all Americans supported free education in principle, voting

161

taxes to pay for it was another matter. A Boston historian in 1851 reported that the greatest defect in the Massachusetts system of public schools was the failure to require school officers to report on the conditions of the schools. In every school district, he said, the tendency was to keep school appropriations—and taxes—at a minimum.[1] Despite resistance to taxation, compulsory schooling gradually spread throughout the American states. Since schools were almost exclusively under local control, the condition of the buildings and the quality of instruction varied widely, although where strong leadership was provided at the state level, standards tended to be higher.

The status of public or school health depended then as now upon the state of medical knowledge, and in the early nineteenth century medicine was still preoccupied with epidemic diseases, still desperately seeking the cause and cure of the perennial plagues and pestilences, and still searching for a rationale which would explain the nature of sickness and disease. Of the various theories set forth to explain the spread of disease, the most widely accepted was the miasmatic thesis, which postulated that a gaseous substance emanating from dirt, filth, and putrefying matter was responsible for sickness. It is, therefore, not to be wondered that the nineteenth century was preoccupied with proper ventilation for school buildings. No other single aspect of school conditions aroused as much debate or interest, and the creation of open-air classes in the twentieth century was a logical culmination of the fight for fresh air.

Nearly all writers on early American education agreed that the condition of public schools in the early nineteenth century was deplorable. Horace Mann wrote bitterly of the Massachusetts school system: "The school-houses in the state have a few common characteristics. They are almost universally contracted in size, they are situated immediately on the road-side, and are without any proper means of ventilation." In 1837 the State Board of Education declared of the schools in Salem, Massachusetts that they "excited vivid ideas of corporal punishment, and almost prompted one to ask the children for what offence they had been committed." A year later the Board of Commissioners of Common Schools of Connecticut reported that 73 out of 104 schoolhouses "were out of repair" and that 100 of them had no playground but the highway.[2]

From other sections of the United States came similar comments. The superintendent of the Ohio schools asserted: "At the present time, the aggregate amount of human suffering inflicted on children in unsuitable and poorly furnished schoolhouses is greater than the whole amount of punishment inflicted upon all the criminals in the State." The overcrowding of classrooms was dramatized even more vividly in the report of a Michigan superintendent on a visit to one of his schools. The air was so fetid, he said, that "we all got sick, and the candles went almost out."[3]

In New York State conditions were no better, and they may have been worse—but then the New York superintendents seem to have been an unusually articulate lot. From Steuben County one reported in 1843: "The lonely, bleak situation of our schoolhouses; their desolate and forlorn appearances, and their still more wretched internal arrangement, all indicate a want of attention to this subject." The superintendent of Madison County presented an equally discouraging picture: "The exterior is dreary, desolate and uninteresting, the interior is dark, gloomy and comfortless; in the old ones the fierce winds of winter rush in through every crack and crevice, in floor, casement, door and window, requiring a constant change of position of the inmates, to keep up an equilibrium of temperature, and in the new ones, the confined and poisonous air lulls the inmates to drowsiness, enshrouds their energies in a morbid, deathly stupor, and implants in them the seeds of premature death." The following year the State Superintendent spoke for all of New York—and, indeed, for all of the United States—when he summarized his impressions of the public schools: "And it is in these miserable abodes of accumulated dirt and filth, deprived of wholesome air, or exposed without adequate protection to the assaults of the elements, with no facilities for necessary exercise or relaxation, no convenience for prosecuting their studies; crowded together on benches not admitting of a moment's rest in any position, and debarred the possibility of yielding to the ordinary calls of nature without violent inroads upon modesty and shame; that upwards of two hundred thousand children scattered over various parts of the State, are compelled to spend an average of eight months during each year of their pupilage!"[4]

Some schools provided desks, but if they did, the desks were of a standard size, too small for a third or more of the pupils, and too large for another third. Benches were the standard form of seating. One of the county superintendents in New York asked rhetorically why it was that children should be forced to sit upon benches with neither arms or backs. "I have seen," he wrote, "the child confined to a seat, from which he could not touch the floor, and behind a bench, over which he could not see. . . ." In some of the rural schools, complaints were made of splintered benches, a serious hazard to the squirming mass of children packed upon them.[5]

The same buildings which became almost insufferably warm and fetid in the summer proved equally uncomfortable during cold weather. Heat was usually supplied by a glowing stove in the center of the schoolroom. The stove pipe, instead of leading to the roof, frequently was directed to one of the walls, and the teacher, forced to walk around the hot stove, stumbling over the feet of his pupils, and banging his head on the stove pipe whenever he failed to stoop low enough, was in danger of life and limb. The students close to the stove were uncomfortably warm, while those to the rear shivered from the icy blasts coming through the chinks in the walls and around doors and windows.

In the 1840's a large number of schools were still built of logs. For example, as of 1843 New York State had a total of 707 log schools. As late as 1852 the superintendent of the Wisconsin school system noted that log cabins constituted 778 of the state's 1,730 schools. The high percentage of log buildings may also account for one of the worst features of the schools, the lack of toilet facilities.[6] In 1844 a New York County superintendent complained that, for want of privies, one side of the schoolhouses "or in some instances the doorstep, if there be any, [was] rendered a scene more disgusting to sight and smell than the filth of the pigsty." Four years later the Education Superintendent of Connecticut, in speaking of that half of the state's schools which had outhouses, declared that these were generally so filthy as to be virtually useless.[7] The Illinois Superintendent of Education reported in 1860 that 4,600 of the State's schools were "destitute of outhouses." Similar conditions were described in other states. For example, in 1857 only 32 of the 276 school buildings in Erie County, Pennsylvania had privies, while in New Jersey, out of 1,423 school districts replying to a questionnaire sent out in 1860 by the State Superintendent of Schools, no less than 513 schools were devoid of all toilet facilities.[8]

In commenting on the lack of privies in 1848, the Connecticut superintendent made a rather significant observation. "Who can duly estimate," he wrote, "the final consequences of the first shock given to female delicacy from the necessary exposure, to which the girls in the public schools are inevitably subjected: and what must be the legitimate results of these frequent exposures during the school going years of youth." He then asked, ". . . may not the disinclination, the aversion of large numbers of families, of mothers especially, to sending their daughters to the public schools, have been created by the sufferings they themselves have endured, from the above cause . . .?" Discounting female delicacy, a subject which preoccupied the English-speaking peoples in the nineteenth century, it is easy to understand the reluctance of sensitive girls to put up with the atrocious conditions generally to be found in the schools. It is interesting to speculate whether this factor had any bearing on the relative numbers of boys and girls in the public schools.[9]

As state superintendents of education began to publish annual reports in the late 1830's and 1840's, a recurrent theme, as noted before, was the subject of ventilation. Whether discussing the construction of school buildings, the health of the students, or the welfare of the teachers, the problem of ventilation always arose. Teachers and pupils apparently became inured to the odors of the schoolrooms, but the occasional visitor was overwhelmed by the stench. Dr. Edward Jarvis asserted in 1846: "In the course of my official duty, I find it one of my greatest sufferings to enter these halls of learning (I might call them little dens of suffering) and breathe with the little sufferers, their polluted atmosphere."[10]

In response to a questionnaire distributed by the American Medical Association in 1849, Dr. James Wynne reported from Baltimore that on his visits to the schools he invariably found them "loaded with an atmosphere so unpleasant as not only to be sensible to myself, but painfully manifest to the teachers, who universally complain of headache, after two or three hours' confinement." According to the report of the School Committee of Groveland, Massachusetts, a member visited one of the schools "and upon opening the door, involuntarily stepped back and suppressed his breath. The air was actually fetid. A half hour spent in it gave him an intolerable headache, and spoiled that day."[11]

Dr. John H. Griscom of New York City blamed the poor health of school children upon crowding and "the absence of a scientific method of ventilation." The only fresh air in schools and other public buildings in Philadelphia, reported Dr. Isaac Parrish, came from the "casual opening of the windows and doors," a situation which also held true for Concord, New Hampshire. The one bright spot was Cincinnati where the respondent noted that the schoolrooms were "large, well-aired, with a good pitch of ceiling." A rather cryptic reply came from Dr. J.T. Gilman of Portland, Maine who wrote of the classrooms: "The

number of pupils varies from 50–150, in each room; each pupil, however, having sufficient space both for *moving* and BREATHING."[12]

To anyone studying school reports for the years before the Civil
War, the wonder is that the children learned anything. The majority
of them were jammed into dirty and dilapidated buildings, deprived of
toilet facilities, and only rarely provided with playground space. Under
these conditions teaching had to be either a dedicated profession or
else a refuge for the desperate and the worthless. A superintendent in
Adams County, Pennsylvania, must have been describing one of the
latter group when he wrote that he had found one of his teachers in
the classroom "without coat or jacket, his pantaloons low down on his
hips, and worse than all, *barefooted!*"[13] Schoolroom furniture consisted
largely of benches and a blackboard, and even these were occasionally
in short supply. The Boston School Committee in 1843 found that the
school rolls contained 934 more pupils than there were seats in the
public schools. The problem was not as grave as it might appear if the
conditions in Boston were similar to those in New York. The New York
superintendent complained in 1843 that from one-third to one-half of
the children were constantly absent, which he attributed to the large
number of schoolhouses which were "wholly unfit places for education."[14]

It is not easy to explain why the schoolhouses should have been
so bad. In 1848 the Connecticut Superintendent noted that even
schoolhouses "in large and wealthy districts [were] objectionable in
every particular." Conditions improved in the succeeding 13 years, but
many inadequate school buildings still remained. "In a portion of
these districts," the Superintendent explained, "the influence of a few
men of wealth has prevented the erection of proper buildings, but
more frequently, the great hindrance to educational progress has been
the want of interest of the professed friends of the cause. . . ." Frequently, educators contrasted the dilapidated appearance of the
schoolhouses with the barns and outbuildings of the surrounding
farms. In 1862 the Maine Superintendent noted that barns were clean,
well ventilated, painted, and decorated, while the schools were old,
dingy, and dirty.[15] Whatever the explanation for the deplorable school
conditions, it is clear that many of the more substantial citizens in the
communities resented being taxed to provide education for the children of the presumably dissolute poor.

The continuing westward expansion of the United States, the
burgeoning population, and the rise of the city combined to aggravate

the school health situation in the immediate postwar years. While an awareness of health needs was developing, the influx of children into the schools was too rapid to permit an orderly development of school systems. Consequently, old school buildings remained in use long after they should have been torn down; houses, stores, and warehouses were rented as temporary quarters only to serve for many years; and when new buildings were erected in the crowded cities, the notorious graft and corruption meant that little value was received for the money spent.

The grim conditions of the 1840's persisted during the next 30 or 40 years—the fetid air, the paucity of furniture, the lack of toilet facilities, the overcrowding, and the filth all were described in detail in school reports and in eye-witness accounts. Yet the picture was not one of unrelieved gloom. The few voices raised so fruitlessly during the early years were augmented after the Civil War and found numerous hearers as a rising standard of living was combined with a growing social awareness. By the end of the century, notable progress was made in many sections of the country, and everywhere, save for the worst slums and the most backward rural areas, the appeals for reform brought some action.

Illustrative of the gloomy reports in the immediate postwar period was that of a Pennsylvania superintendent who wondered why parents who tenderly nurtured their children at home would send them for six hours a day "to schools kept in houses at once so ill-constructed, so badly ventilated, so imperfectly warmed, so dirty, so instinct with vulgar ideas, and so utterly repugnant to all habits of neatness, thought, taste or purity."[16] The appalling conditions to be found in Tennessee caused the first State Superintendent, John Eaton, Jr., to wax eloquent. In the annual report for 1869, he first commented that school sites were always in the worst possible location, and then he turned to the buildings, which, he said, were "rendered more disagreeable to the beholder by the absence of doors and windows." The roof and walls, he continued, vie with the latter in their "capacity to admit light, air and rain." "Alas, the furniture!" he went on, "Desks rare; . . . seats rude, without backs, . . . Floors too often miry with dirt and tobacco, and walls and ceilings hardly less so." As for the outhouses, he concluded, where they do exist, they are often "utterly unfit for children to visit."[17]

In 1884 John Billings, in a book on heating and ventilation, said that "there are no good schools, although some are worse than others." His words were echoed by William B. Ruggles, Superintendent of the New York schools, who declared that no aspect of the school system stood "in more urgent need of radical and substantial improvement" than the sanitary condition of the school buildings. He praised an amendment to the school law setting certain minimum standards for new school buildings, but declared that it would not affect the 11,914 schoolhouses already erected, "nor can it remedy, in respect to new buildings constructed thereafter, the evils of improper seating, impure water, filthy and indecent outhouses, unhealthy sites, insufficient drainage and surrounding nuisances."[18]

In the rural state of Texas in the late 1880's, most districts had no school buildings. Out of 8,826 school districts, 3,286 had their own buildings, and only about half of these were reported in good condition. In over 5,500 school districts, the children were housed "in neighborhood churches, vacant barns or outhouses, and such other buildings as [could] be obtained for a nominal rental." "In many counties," one state superintendent asserted, "the value of the common jail exceeds that of all the school property in the county."[19] At the turn of the century, a New Hampshire doctor, writing in a State Board of Health report, summarized general school conditions when he remarked ironically: "Not a few of our schools, even in the principal cities boasting of their refinement and culture, are filthy and unhealthy, and in so far as uncleanliness goes give reason for the accusation made at times that they are ungodly."[20]

It should be borne in mind that most of those who described the atrocious school conditions were reformers at heart and not averse to hyperbole. Moreover, good schools seldom aroused comment. By the 1870's there was a general recognition of health needs, and an increasing number of directives from school boards ordering more attention to be paid to sanitation. In New Orleans, which had a relatively good school system, the Board of Health kept a close check on the buildings and general conditions, and it is evident from the annual reports of the inspectors that no serious defects existed.[21] In 1880 an inspector for the Massachusetts State Board of Health found many schools relatively clean and equipped with water closets. An officer of the Pennsylvania State Board of Health noted that in one high school he visited he "found much to commend" although some of the classrooms were too small and poorly lighted.[22]

By this time the flood of students into public schools had increased enormously. In 1882, for example, of the 1,681,161 children in New York State, 1,041,089 were attending the public schools. The annual school report pointed out, moreover, that many of the 644,000 not in public schools were either attending private schools or were youths under age 21 who had completed their schooling. The following year the Iowa superintendent mentioned the responsibility of caring for some 450,000 children enrolled in the Iowa school system.[23] When one considers the immigrants pouring in from Europe and the highly prolific families of native origin, it is readily apparent why serious crowding occurred in the school systems.

Despite some progress, toilet facilities in most American schools remained almost indescribably bad for much of the nineteenth century. In 1868 the Kansas Superintendent of Public Instruction circulated a questionnaire among his school districts and discovered that most schools had no privies, a few had one, and only rarely were there separate facilities for the two sexes.[24] In New York, a state which probably typifies conditions in the Northeast, an early school law permitted trustees to expend on repairs "a sum not exceeding $20 in any one year" for each schoolhouse. In 1867, when most schoolhouses still had no privies and the local voters consistently refused to vote taxes to erect them, the legislature amended the act to allow trustees to spend up to $50 to build outhouses. State Superintendent William B. Ruggles wrote later that this provision worked fairly well until a second amendment in 1875 added the phrase, "upon a vote of a district meeting." The net effect was to nullify the original amendment. Superintendent Ruggles noted with regret in 1884 that many district schools were still without privies and that neither the voters nor the trustees seemed anxious to provide them.[25]

In the cities water closets were gradually replacing privies, but their numbers were often too small and the design poor. An observer in Brooklyn schools described urinal troughs which in some cases were "so high that the smaller boys can scarcely peep over the edge. . . ."[26] In 1887 the New York legislature once again took action, this time passing the "Health and Decency Act," which required separate water closets or privies for boys and girls and made the trustees responsible for keeping them "in a clean and wholesome condition." Neglect of this duty could bring forfeiture of office or the withdrawal of state school aid. While considerable improvement was noted, for many years a lack of health inspectors prevented effective enforcement of the law.[27] By the end of the century, a nation-wide movement to improve school sanitation was underway, and state after state passed basic school sanitary codes.

The general interest in sanitation and toilet facilities also aroused an interest in school water supplies. An Iowa Board of Health Report asserted that almost all school wells were either contaminated or suspicious, "surrounded as they usually are, by privies, stables, and filthy back alleys of adjoining lots."[28] In Chicago, where the city water supply was seriously contaminated, the Health Department in 1898 shut off the water to the 230-odd public schools, very effectively drawing attention to the need for overhauling the water system. In Philadelphia school authorities, at the suggestion of the Board of Health, decided in 1898 to furnish "each pupil in the elementary departments with a drinking cup"—a dubious step, considering the habits of most young children.[29]

The rising awareness of environmental factors in school health was further indicated by the emergence of fire prevention measures. In 1879 the President of the Baltimore School Board requested that inspectors check the schools for safety, since in several recent fires the students and teachers had had difficulty escaping from the single school entrance. Three years later the Baltimore school system introduced fire drills.[30] Even earlier, in 1877, the Philadelphia City Council had passed an ordinance requiring schools, along with other public buildings, to be equipped with fireproof stairways. Subsequently, a Pennsylvania state law required all school buildings of more than two stories to have exterior fire escapes.[31] Difficult as it was to secure good laws, it was even more difficult to enforce them, and the fire laws were often honored in the breach. Nonetheless, the enactment of these laws was a major step in the right direction.

Ventilation continued to be of major interest as the nineteenth century drew on. In early public health journals, such as *The Sanitarian* and the *Annals of Hygiene,* articles frequently appealed for better ventilation in public buildings and gave technical instructions for installing fresh air systems. Dr. A.N. Bell, editor of *The Sanitarian,* declared in 1875: "A pure atmosphere is the first need of the school-room, without it none of the vital functions can be sustained in health." In a subsequent issue, doubtless carried away by enthusiasm for his cause, he declared in an article entitled "Schoolroom Stunting" that lack of ventilation and light leads to a "generation of dwarfs, a stunted progeny."[32] The American Public Health Association and the *Journal of the American Medical Association* also advocated better ventilation. In 1888 a writer in the latter journal spoke of the "very faulty" ventilation systems in American schools and declared that the "schoolroom is a propaganda of contagion." A United States Bureau of Education pamphlet in 1891 explained that children were able to survive the "vitiated air of the Schoolroom" only because of frequent recesses and the ability of the child's system to habituate "itself to throwing off the poison. . . ."[33]

The Northeastern states with their large urban concentrations led the way in the attempt to solve ventilation problems. In its first annual report for the year 1866, the New York City Health Department declared that after "viewing only the causes of preventable disease and their fatal results, we unhesitatingly state that the very first sanitary want in New York and Brooklyn is VENTILATION. . . ." The following year the Health Department specifically mentioned ventilation and overcrowding as "prominent evils" in the city schools. It noted, however, that the Board of Education had been provided with funds to hire additional buildings and that another $450,000 had been allocated for the erection of new buildings.[34] In the succeeding years the departmental reports continued to dwell on the need for more and better ventilated school buildings. In 1873 health inspectors made a study of schoolroom air and found that the concentration of carbonic acid varied from 9.7 to 35.7 parts per 10,000. During this same study, they noted that the temperatures of schoolrooms ranged from 47 to 70 degrees.[35] Gradually, the movement for better ventilation spread throughout New York, and the State Board of Health began to disseminate information and investigate conditions. By 1886 it was able to report that it was taking steps to remove many unsanitary conditions.[36]

In Massachusetts, a leader in education and public health, the State Board of Health from its inception in 1870 took a keen interest in the ventilation question. One of its first steps was to have a Massachusetts Institute of Technology professor investigate the air in the Boston schoolrooms. As with the New York investigators, emphasis was placed upon determining the temperature of the air and the relative amount of carbonic acid.[37] In the ensuing years some progress was made, and by 1878 the State Board could report that at least in the cities new schoolhouses were being "built with a supply of flues to carry the foul air from schoolrooms." Nonetheless, the *Report* added, in Boston ventilation "is very generally said to be poor." Nine years later, in discussing ventilation of schoolrooms heated by stoves, the Board declared that 90 percent of the rooms depended upon doors and windows for fresh air. Approximately one-fourth, however, had special appliances to direct the flow of air upwards and thus avoid direct draughts upon the children. The following year, 1888, the State Legislature passed a measure providing for proper ventilation in the public schools.[38]

In 1889 the *Boston Medical and Surgical Journal* took sharp issue with the Board of Health. As a result of "extravagantly worded articles" appearing in the daily press, its editor wrote, the Board of Health had made a survey of 163 Boston Schools and concluded that 146 of them were "without any modern or efficient means of ventilation." The editor roundly condemned the report, pointing out that it was possible to achieve good ventilation even without "heated shafts or fans."[39] The position of the medical journal was probably correct about those buildings designed as schools, but too often rented buildings simply did not have enough windows, or else a school building designed for 300 children had an enrollment of 600. Whatever the case, in 1889 the State Board of Health reported that all public school houses had been "examined and re-examined" and their defects brought to the attention of the superintendent of public buildings. In many instances, the report noted, drainage and ventilation had been improved.[40]

In Pennsylvania progress was both slower and more sporadic. In 1871 one of the county superintendents of schools declared that there was not a single well-ventilated schoolhouse in his jurisdiction and that he suspected there were "but few in the State." Three years later the State Superintendent noted that almost half of the 12,000-odd schools in the state were badly ventilated and over a third had no suitable privies.[41] In the succeeding years, health and education reports and articles continued to denounce the deplorable lack of ventilation in schoolrooms; the very violence of the attacks showed that they were intended to awaken the public conscience and to effect what was felt to be a much needed reform. The first significant innovation in ventilation in Pennsylvania seems to have been made in the town of Chester, where a new high school building was erected in 1885–1886 which included a complete system of ventilation designed to change the air in the classrooms three times each hour. In 1891 the State School Superintendent, responding to the general interest in fresh air, called for a state law requiring adequate ventilation for all school buildings. He pointed out that legislation had been passed to protect workers in the mines and factories, but that little had been done for students, although there were "more people in our public schools than in all our factories and mines." By the close of the century, school boards in

Philadelphia and in other cities and towns were slowly eliminating the overcrowded and poorly constructed schools, and the newer buildings were incorporating the best ventilation systems available.[42]

With occasional variations the ventilation pattern for the rest of the country followed that of the Northeastern states. For example, Chicago was compelled to rebuild its schools after the great fire of 1871. The old school buildings were no great loss to the cause of education—indeed, the descriptions of many schools indicate that other cities might well have benefitted from such a catastrophe. In any case, the Chicago Board of Health reported in 1873 that all but two of the public schools had been destroyed by the fire in October 1871. Since then they had all been rebuilt in a new and better design. Two-story structures had replaced the old three-story buildings, and the architects had made adequate provision for ventilation. Private schools in the city, however, had not recovered from their losses, the Board noted, since most were overcrowded and many were located in basements which were "dry but illy ventilated."[43]

Among the Southern states, Louisiana made the initial attempt to oversee sanitary conditions in the schools. After a series of yellow fever epidemics, the Louisiana State Board of Health was established in 1855, the first of its kind in the United States. Because this agency was designed primarily as a quarantine board and its health activities were restricted largely to the New Orleans area, historians have tended to disregard its efforts, but the Board's officers concerned themselves with a wide range of health problems, including school conditions. Sanitary inspectors appointed by the Board made yearly inspections of all schools within their districts, and their reports often led to effective action. Partly as a result of the Board of Health activities, the State Superintendent of Education notified all teachers in 1870 that they must "attend carefully to the ventilation and temperature of their school rooms." Principals were informed that they were to have general supervision over the grounds and buildings and would be held responsible "for any want of neatness or cleanliness on the premises."[44] Through the joint efforts of public health and education officials, the education superintendent was able to state in 1878 that henceforth all new schools in New Orleans would include provisions for "abundant light and ventilation." Subsequently, the reports of the sanitary inspectors indicate that the New Orleans schools had no real ventilation problems.[45] It should be pointed out, however, that the warm climate which enabled doors and windows to remain open for much of the year and the high ceilings in most Southern buildings obviously were favorable factors.

Elsewhere the state health and education reports generally showed deplorable conditions in the 1870's. For example, Kentucky's Superintendent of Education reported in 1874 that the schools were "full of foul air and feculent odors," and a survey by the Wisconsin Board of Health in 1879 showed that only 23 of 600 schools examined were properly ventilated.[46] On the other hand, a school hygiene committee for the Tennessee Board of Health reported that 60 percent of the schools answering a questionnaire had indicated satisfactory ventilation conditions.[47] Conditions everywhere seem to have improved around 1900.

As might be expected in these years, along with a concern for school buildings, the need for adequate school furniture received considerable attention. An extensive literature on the subject had already developed in Europe, and American educators were quick to apply the observations of Europeans to American conditions. The Michigan State Board of Health Report for 1874 quoted several European studies to the effect that school desks and the cramped writing positions of pupils were the prime causes of the spinal distortion to be found among children.[48] In 1875, in its first annual report, the Georgia State Board of Health summarized the findings of a committee on school hygiene. In describing school seating arrangements, the committee, no doubt hoping to make its report more effective, declared: "The torture of occupying such a seat daily, for five or six more hours equals a moderate appliance of the thumb-screw or the rack."[49] As state health boards were created and began to investigate school health problems, the subject of school furniture came increasingly to the fore. Medical journals, too, took occasional note of the matter.[50] For example, the *Maryland Medical Journal* carried an article criticizing the cramped desk space and narrow aisles in the Baltimore schools.[51] Unlike early protests, these criticisms bore fruit, and the end of the century saw considerable improvement in the quality of school furnishings.

By 1900 most of the states had made some provision for the inspection of school buildings and furnishings and had placed responsibility for ventilation and sanitary conditions upon either the local school board or the local board of health. At the community level enough interest had been generated to eliminate many of the worst abuses, and new designs in school construction were gradually solving many of the former problems. As was true of public health generally, large cities led in enacting school sanitary laws. For example, the New York City Health Department passed an ordinance requiring schoolmasters to take reasonable precautions with respect to "the safety or health of any scholar [or] pupil" and to "the temperature, ventilation, or cleanliness, or strength" of the school room or school building.[52]

In 1888 Massachusetts passed a well-written law setting up a sanitary code for school buildings, and other states rapidly followed suit. The Connecticut law, for example, provided for a system of inspection and established a fine of up to $100 for non-compliance. Typical of the new state laws was Vermont's enacted in 1896 which ordered local boards of health to conduct a sanitary survey of all schoolhouses in their districts and to report conditions both to the state board and to the local town meeting each spring. The law also established minimum standards with respect to ventilation, lighting, heating, and other sanitary arrangements for all new schools.[53] In 1897 the Health Officer for the District of Columbia, in noting that much progress had been made in heating and ventilation, summarized the rapid changes which were taking place in American school construction when he asserted that the new buildings stood "in as great a contrast to the old style buildings as daylight to darkness."[54]

By 1900 the entire face of America was changing; public health had become institutionalized, and local and state health boards were widespread; a rising standard of living had led to improved housing and better public buildings; and state supported education was universal. To contribute further to better school conditions, a start had been made in school medical inspection and school nursing. The growing presence of these health professionals in the schools during the twentieth century provided further assurance of continuing progress in providing a relatively decent physical environment for schoolchildren.

Notes

1. Emerson Davis, *The Half Century* (Boston, 1851), pp. 50–51.

2. Secretary of the Massachusetts Board of Education, *Report . . . on the Subject of School Houses* (Boston, 1838), pp. 6–7; Massachusetts Board of Education, *Second Annual Report of the Secretary, 1838,* quoted in Horace Mann, *Life and Works* (Boston, 1891), II, p. 498; Henry Barnard, *School-House Architecture* (Hartford, 1842), p. 2.

3. Ohio, Superintendent of Common Schools, *Second Annual Report, 1838* (Columbus, 1839), p. 11; Michigan, Superintendent of Public Instruction, *Annual Report, 1847* (Lansing, 1848), pp. 116–117.

4. New York State, Superintendent of Common Schools, *Annual Report, 1843* (Albany, 1843), pp. 352, 232; *ibid., 1844* (Albany, 1844), p. 10.

5. *Ibid., 1844* (Albany, 1844), pp. 316–317.

6. *Ibid., 1884* (Albany, 1884), p. 13; Wisconsin, Superintendent of Public Instruction, *Annual Report, 1852* (Madison, 1853), pp. 6–11.

7. New York State, Superintendent of Common Schools, *Annual Report, 1844* (Albany, 1844), p. 318; Connecticut, Superintendent of Common Schools, *Third Annual Report, 1848* (New Haven, 1848), p. 64.

8. Illinois, Superintendent of Public Instruction, *Third Biennial Report, 1859–1860* (Springfield, 1861), p. 84; Edgar B. Wesley, *NEA: The First Hundred Years* (New York, 1957), p. 10; New Jersey, Superintendent of Public Schools, *Annual Report, 1860* (Trenton, 1861), pp. 10–11.

9. Connecticut, Superintendent of Common Schools, *Third Annual Report, 1848* (New Haven, 1848), p. 64.

10. Edward Jarvis, "On the Necessity of the Study of Physiology," *American Institute of Instruction, Lectures* (Boston, 1846), p. 138.

11. James Wynne, "Sanitary Report of Baltimore," *Transactions of A.M.A.,* II (1849), p. 570; Massachusetts Department of Education, *School Committee Reports, Twenty-First Annual Report, 1858* (Boston, 1859), p. 9.

12. *Transactions of A.M.A.,* II (1849), pp. 446, 452, 457, 474, 500, 620.

13. Pennsylvania, Superintendent of Common Schools, *Report, 1860* (Harrisburg, 1861), p. 18.

14. Boston School Committee, *Annual Report, 1858* (Boston, 1859), p. 8; Elise G. Hobson, *Educational Legislation and Administration in the State of New York from 1777 to 1850, Supplementary Education Monographs,* No. 13 (Chicago, 1918), pp. 64–65.

15. Connecticut, Superintendent of Common Schools, *Third Annual Report, 1848* (New Haven, 1848), p. 63; *ibid., 1861* (New Haven, 1861), p. 4; Maine, Superintendent of Common Schools, *Ninth Annual Report, 1862* (Augusta, 1863), p. 22.

16. Pennsylvania, Superintendent of Common Schools, *Report, 1866–67* (Harrisburg, 1868), pp. 6–7.

17. Tennessee, Superintendent of Public Instruction, *First Report, 1869* (Nashville, 1869), p. 25.

18. John Billings, *The Principles of Ventilation and Heating,* 2nd ed. (New York, 1884), p. 159; New York State, Superintendent of Public Instruction, *Thirtieth Annual Report, 1884* (Albany, 1884), pp. 49–50.

19. Texas, Superintendent of Public Instruction, *Sixth Biennial Report, 1887* and *1888* (Austin, 1888), p. 22.

20. D. E. Sullivan, "School Hygiene and Sanitation," New Hampshire State Board of Health, *Sixteenth Report, 1899–1900* (Manchester, 1901), p. 203.

21. Foster J. Flint, *An Historical Study of School Health Education in Massachusetts,* Ph.D. dissertation, Boston University, 1954, pp. 114–119; Wilson G. Smillie, *Public Health, Its Promise for the Future* (New York, 1935), p. 426; Louisiana State Board of Health, *Annual Report, 1879* (New Orleans, 1880), pp. 51–70.

22. Massachusetts State Board of Health, *Lunacy and Charity, Second Annual Report— Supplement, 1880* (Boston, 1881), pp. 111–147; Pennsylvania State Board of Health, *Fourth Annual Report, 1888* (Harrisburg, 1889), p. 335.

23. New York State, Superintendent of Public Instruction, *Thirtieth Annual Report, 1884* (Albany, 1884), p. 14; Iowa, Superintendent of Public Instruction, *Biennial Report, 1885* (Des Moines, 1885), pp. 147–148.

24. Kansas, Superintendent of Public Instruction, *Eighth Annual Report, 1868* (Topeka, 1869), pp. 40–41.

25. New York State, Superintendent of Public Instruction, *Thirtieth Annual Report, 1884* (Albany, 1884), pp. 55–56.

26. Philo, "Brooklyn School-Houses," *The Sanitarian,* IV (1876), p. 447.

27. New York State, Department of Health, *Twenty-Fifth Annual Report, 1904* (Albany, 1906), pp. 696–711.

28. Iowa, State Board of Health, *Fifth Biennial Report, 1889* (Des Moines, 1889), p. 81.

29. Chicago, Department of Health, *Bureau and Division Reports, July, 1898* (Chicago, 1898), p. 4; Pennsylvania, State Board of Health, *Fourteenth Annual Report, 1898* (Harrisburg, 1899), p. 70.

30. Baltimore, Board of Commissioners of Public Schools, *Fifty-First Annual Report, 1879* (Baltimore, 1880), p. xv; *ibid., Fifty-Fourth Annual Report, 1882* (Baltimore, 1883), p. xxxix.

31. Philadelphia, Board of Public Instruction, *Sixty-First Annual Report, 1880* (Philadelphia, 1880), pp. 23–24.

32. A. N. Bell, "Brain Culture in Relation to the School-Room," *The Sanitarian,* II (1874–75), pp. 433–442; III (1875–76), p. 413.

33. J.A. Larrabee, "The Schoolroom a Factor in the Production of Disease," *J.A.M.A.,* XI (1888), pp. 613–614; Albert P. Marble, *Sanitary Conditions for Schoolhouses,* U. S. Bureau of Education, Circular of Information, No. 3 (Washington, D.C., 1891), p. 8.

34. New York City, Metropolitan Board of Health, *Annual Report, 1866* (New York, 1867), p. 154; *ibid., Second Annual Report, 1867* (New York, 1868), pp. 37–38, 136.

35. H. Endemann, "Chemical Examination of the Air of Various Public Buildings," New York [City] Board of Health, *Third Annual Report, 1872–1873* (New York, 1873), p. 301.

36. Report on the Condition of the Public Schools Throughout the State," New York State Board of Health, *Seventh Annual Report, 1886* (Albany, 1887), pp. 503–506.

37. Massachusetts, State Board of Health, *Second Annual Report, 1871* (Boston, 1871), pp. 400–405.

38. *Ibid., Ninth Annual Report, 1877* (Boston, 1878), pp. 231, 250; *Nineteenth Annual Report, 1887* (Boston, 1888), p. 316; Flint, *op. cit.*, p. 143.

39. *Boston Medical and Surgical Journal,* CXXI (1889), pp. 394–395.

40. Massachusetts, State Board of Health, *Twentieth Annual Report, 1889* (Boston, 1890), p. 421.

41. Pennsylvania, Superintendent of Common Schools, *Report, 1870–71* (Harrisburg, 1871), pp. 11–12; *ibid., Report, 1873–74* (Harrisburg, 1875), p. x.

42. Pennsylvania, State Board of Health, *Second Annual Report, 1886* (Harrisburg, 1887), pp. 320–324; Pennsylvania, Superintendent of Common Schools, *Report, 1890–91* (Harrisburg, 1891), p. v.

43. Chicago, Board of Health, *Report for the Years 1870, 1871, 1872, and 1873* (Chicago, 1874), p. 139.

44. Louisiana, State Superintendent of Public Education, *Annual Report, 1870* (New Orleans, 1871), pp. 155–156.

45. *Ibid., 1878,* p. 15; *1882,* pp. 390–396.

46. Moses E. Ligon, "A History of Public Education in Kentucky," *Bulletin of the Bureau of School Service,* University of Kentucky, XIV, No. 4 (Lexington, 1942), pp. 135–136; T. W. Chittenden, "Our School Houses," Wisconsin, State Board of Health, *Fourth Annual Report, 1879* (Madison, 1880), pp. 43–49.

47. E. M. Wight, "Report of Committee on School Hygiene," Tennessee, State Board of Health, *First Report, 1877–1880* (Nashville, 1880), p. 147.

48. Reverend J. S. Goodman, "The Relation of School to Health," Michigan, State Board of Health, *Second Annual Report* (Lansing, 1875), p. 71.

49. C. B. Nottingham, "Report of Committee on the Hygiene of Schools," Georgia, State Board of Health, *First Annual Report, 1875* (Atlanta, 1876), p. 119.

50. For example, see T. W. Chittenden, "School Furniture," Wisconsin, State Board of Health, *Tenth Report, 1886* (Madison, 1887), pp. 147–166.

51. E. M. Schaeffler, "Certain Sanitary Needs of Our City and its Public Schools," *Maryland Medical Journal,* XXXIII (1895), pp. 83–87.

52. New York City, Metropolitan Board of Health, *Annual Report, 1866* (New York, 1867), p. 406.

53. Connecticut, State Board of Education, *Report, 1893* (Hartford, 1893), p. 364; Vermont State Board of Health, *Thirteenth Report, 1900* (Rutland, 1902), pp. 36–37.

54. District of Columbia, Health Officer, *Report, 1897* (Washington, D.C., 1897), p. 74.

Dyspepsia: The American Disease?
Needs and Opportunities for Research

GERT H. BRIEGER, M.D.

At the 1966 annual meeting of The American Association for the History of Medicine, George Rosen delivered his presidential address which was a challenge to us all. Published as "People, Disease, and Emotions," Rosen urged his colleagues to shift their angle of vision because this frequently reveals new facets of a subject:

> By taking the social character of medicine as a point of departure, the history of medicine becomes the history of human societies and their efforts to deal with problems of health and disease. By placing and examining medicine within this broader context, it raises new questions and problems. This may be illustrated by calling attention to a characteristic of iatrocentric history. Physicians practice, teach, and write about their experiences; surgeons operate, invent new operations and techniques—but the patient for whom presumably all this is done rarely appears on the scene, that is, as far as the awareness of the medical historian is concerned. But certainly the patient deserves a more prominent place in the history of medicine.[1]

In attempting to meet this challenge, one of many that George Rosen has left us, I believe it is time that historians of medicine pay attention to an extraordinarily prevalent disorder, yet one neglected by almost all of us. It is indeed a puzzle why dyspepsia, so commonly written about in the period 1800–1920 has escaped the medical historian's ever-widening net. Dyspepsia serves as a convenient example of a subject that requires for its historical understanding an analysis of people, disease, and emotions.

Dyspepsia, according to the *Oxford English Dictionary*, is difficulty or derangement of digestion, or simply put, indigestion. It is applied to various forms of disorder of the digestive organs, especially the stomach, usually involving weakness, loss of appetite, and depression of spirits. If we are to believe the OED, the words dyspepsia and dyspeptic were first used in the seventeenth century. The idea of disordered or improper coction, of course, is an ancient one.

Dr. Tinsley Harrison's widely used textbook of medicine includes functional dyspepsia under disorders of the alimentary tract. "The

179

genesis of functional symptoms," Harrison states, "is poorly understood, but by definition they reflect disturbances of gastro-intestinal function. These undoubtedly are affected by psychogenic factors as well as physiologic, hormonal, . . . electrolyte factors, and nervous system influences. Functional symptoms are the leading reasons for which patients seek medical advice. The two most frequent functional syndromes in the gastrointestinal tract are flatulent dyspepsia and the irritable colon."[2] Thus, Harrison in the present day medical literature ventures an opinion and assessment of everyday medical practice that finds considerable confirmation in the nineteenth-century literature on dyspepsia.

Whether dyspepsia is a disease or a set of symptoms, and what are its causes, we will have some difficulty in deciding.[3] But that it was, and continues to be, a very common malady, I believe we will readily agree. Medical historians have responded to this ambiguous ailment by ignoring it. The word does not appear, for instance, in either number of the index to the *Bulletin of the History of Medicine* and is infrequently cited in the Wellcome Institute's *Current Work in the History of Medicine.*[4]

Recent books devoted to Charles Darwin's fifty-year battle with gastro-intestinal symptoms also curiously enough do not include dyspepsia in the index, yet nevertheless discuss it in the text. Two physicians, Dr. George Pickering and Dr. Ralph Colp, did not apparently like the term sufficiently to deem it worthy of an index entry. J.H. Winslow, a non-medical author, on the other hand, entitled two chapters in his monograph on Darwin's malady, "Victorian Dyspepsia and Its Authors" and "Some Famous British Dyspeptics."[5]

Behind all this, there lies an interesting tale. Before delving into the story of the disease, it might be well to return to Dr. Harrison's term of functional symptoms or functional illness. That even in the atmosphere of the highly vaunted medical sciences as they are now taught in our modern medical centers there is some confusion, or at the very least some imprecision, in the use of the medical language was very well illustrated in a paper in *The Journal of Medical Education* in 1956.

Joseph E. Bogen, then a medical student, asked his classmates to supply him with a definition of "functional" as in functional bleeding. The responses varied greatly. To some functional meant idiopathic. Others applied the term whenever the etiology was believed to be controversial. Physiological disturbance without demonstrable pathological changes was a frequent definition. And many students applied the term functional to those disorders in which patients suffered from multiple, poorly defined symptoms, none of which seemed to be life-threatening. Closer questioning of his friends revealed to Bogen that a functional disorder was any aberration from what was considered normal, and that when extended to its logical (but hardly workable) conclusion, there were no diseases that were not functional. Thus, some applied the designation to any disease or disorder of unknown cause, others to psychogenic in contrast to organically caused disease, and some to any normal variation that could not properly be classified as a disease or symptom of a disease. Needless to say, we all assume that we know what we mean, but our definitions and usages are far from precise.[6]

An anonymous reviewer of five books on gastro-intestinal disorders in the *Southern Review* of 1829 began his 34-page essay by telling his literary audience: "If the universality of a disease can render an investigation into its nature and cure proper in a journal of this kind, we know of none which is entitled to precedence over Dyspepsia. It is not the malady of the rich or the poor; the ignorant or the learned; the young or the aged; the virtuous or the vicious; of one sex or one condition; but the disease of all."[7]

As to the causes for this universal prevalence, this author believed firmly that the modes of life of an advanced state of civilization were in many respects inimical to those which nature prescribed. Our ancestors, he guessed, must surely have been troubled with dyspepsia, but it was only within 20 or 30 years, that is since about 1800, that it had become so familiar a form of distress. "It is only of late that luxury has affected, directly and indirectly, the whole mass of society, and scattered the seeds of this pestilence over the face of the land. . . . Our modes of life are entirely changed from what they formerly were in this country, as well as in Europe. We are less exposed to the open air, take less exercise, are more intellectual in our pursuits, and fare more sumptuously every day than formerly, when there were few carriages, few books, plain food and little wine."[8] In one way or another, similar sentiments appear throughout the nineteenth century and into our own. This author had a number of practical rules for healthy living. His tenth and last rule summed it up well: "Be regular in your habits, keep the feet warm, the head cool, and the bowels open."[9]

Because this study of dyspepsia is still very much a work in progress, I can only begin to establish a few points. We can come to some general agreement about what dyspepsia was in the eyes of nineteenth-century physicians, more rarely in those of their patients. We might begin to approximate its frequency. And finally, we might discuss briefly how the study of dyspepsia can influence our general interpretation of nineteenth-century medical practice.

In 1896 an Ohio physician entitled his paper on dyspepsia, "The American Disease." "In the distribution of diseases among nations," he wrote, "the English got gout, the French syphilis, and the Americans dyspepsia. But our friends, the pathologists, tell us there is no such disease as dyspepsia. As a pathological entity, it does not exist; as a clinical condition, we meet it almost every day of our lives."[10] In the same year that inimitable physician-entrepreneur from Battle Creek, Michigan, John Harvey Kellogg, began a book on the stomach and its disorders with this vignette:

> Some years ago, while calling upon a professional friend in London, a leading English practitioner, he remarked, 'I suppose that in American you have chiefly to deal with dyspeptics.' In reply, I could not but acknowledge that Americans enjoyed the unenviable but nevertheless deserved reputation of being a nation of dyspeptics; but added that the treatment of invalids in America was by no means so monotonous as might seem the case, for the reason that the general physical deterioration and vital derangements occasioned by dyspepsia give rise to a vast number of varied and complicated ailments which tax to the utmost the skill and ingenuity of the practitioner.[11]

After reading many articles and numerous textbooks on dyspepsia, I will vouch for Dr. Kellogg's assessment of an extremely varied clinical condition. There are, of course, a number of constant or frequently encountered symptoms, supposed causes, and therapy, no matter whether one reads the 56-page chapter in Trousseau's *Clinical Lectures,* the English physician Thomas Watson's *Principles and Practice of Physic,* or the very popular American textbook by Austin Flint.

While there is some disagreement as to nomenclature, the clinical picture of the typical patient is easily recognizable. Flint's description will serve as a handy guide:

> The disorder is manifested by a sense of weight, fullness, or pain in the epigastrium; nausea and perhaps vomiting may occur, or, after a time, looseness of the bowels ensues; some febrile movement may be induced, with pain in the head and general malaise. Succeeding these symptoms are loss of appetite, coating of the tongue, an unpleasant taste, with more

or less uneasiness referable to the digestive organs for several days. Such cases are sufficiently common.[12]

A number of words came to be associated with this somewhat vague constellation of symptoms. These include biliousness, or bilious attack, indigestion, and sick headache. Dr. A.K. Bond of Baltimore described it all much more picturesquely when he divided the forms of indigestion into the repleted stomach, the tired stomach, the starved stomach, the painful stomach, the hurrying stomach, the acid stomach, the bitter stomach, and last, but not least, the windy stomach.[13]

The supposed causes of dyspepsia, then, are as varied as they are a fascinating indication of what doctors and their patients believed to be inimical to good health. Since most writers readily acknowledged that brain and intestinal tract were linked, much printer's ink was spilled over the "intensity" of modern life. Scholars, as Celsus had already claimed in antiquity, seemed to be particularly prone to diseases of tension. American authors frequently attributed ailments to a lack of exercise, as we have noted above. The height of credulity seems to have been reached by Dr. L.P. Yandell of a well-known Kentucky medical family, who in an 1834 article on dyspepsia remarked on the problem of German scholars. "They remain so long inactive, we are informed, that they almost lose the use of their legs. . . ."[14] Yandell suggested that it was far healthier to engage in severe studies early in the day and to use the two or three hours before bedtime for light music or amusing conversation.

Much of the discussion of etiology of so-called nervous dyspepsia, or the variety that is not caused by organic diseases such as cancer or gastritis, concerned diet. Dr. James Robbins of Massachusetts, for instance, summed up the principal causes of American dyspepsia in 1882 as follows: 1.Rapidity in eating. The literature surrounding this supposedly peculiarly American trait, is voluminous. There was apparently an old adage among farmers to the effect that quick to eat meant quick to work. Unsuitable or improperly prepared food was, of course, equally to blame. 2.Over-eating. 3.The use of ice water. 4.The use of fine white flour. Actually as late as 1921, Dr. Simon Fraser wrote a letter to the *British Medical Journal* saying that he had in the previous few months seen twelve cases of severe dyspepsia caused by white bread. All, Fraser claimed, returned to normal within a week after wholemeal bread was substituted for the ordinary white bread in their diet. Dr. Robbins in 1882, however, made an astute epidemiological observation when he pointed out that ". . . we must acknowledge that the poorer classes who subsist most largely upon white flour, are not the greatest sufferers from stomach failure."[15]

One could spend much more time in discussing the supposed etiology of dyspepsia. By the last decade of the nineteenth century, there was some sentiment for discarding the term altogether as a pathological entity. Hypersecretion of acid and hypermotility of the gastro-intestinal tract were coming to be better understood.[16] By 1915 a study of 1,000 cases reported in the *Johns Hopkins Hospital Bulletin* was couched in diagnostic categories with which we still deal. In this series appendicitis and cholecystitis accounted for 35 percent of cases of indigestion; peptic ulcer and neuroses for 10 percent each; cancer accounted for 5 percent, chronic gastritis, adhesions and visceroptosis for 10 percent; and diseases of other organs with concomitant indigestion for 25 percent of all cases.[17]

As to frequency of dyspepsia, the historian has some trouble in evaluating the data. In the first place, the data are rarely expressed in numbers because the disorder was usually not fatal, not reportable, and was for so long mired in a maze of varying nomenclature. There is little doubt, however, that one should agree with George M. Beard's assessment that "dyspepsia is one of the most common, most fashionable, and most annoying nervous symptoms of our modern society."[18] Beard claimed that in the quarter of a century prior to 1879 it had increased in frequency with great rapidity. This was in contrast to Austin Flint's assessment at about the same time that dyspepsia was "undoubtedly less prevalent than it was a quarter of a century ago."[19]

Nevertheless, it is abundantly clear from the clinical literature that the perceptions of physicians in the late nineteenth century were expressed by Dr. J.H. Montgomery in the *JAMA* in 1898: "Probably there is no complaint more frequently encountered in practice than disordered digestion. It is seen at all seasons, at all ages, and in all ranks of life."[20] Or as an author of "Hints of Dyspeptics" in the *Eclectic Magazine of Foreign Literature, Science and Art* put it in 1881:

> Of all the ills that flesh is heir to, few are more insidious or distressing than dyspepsia, a disease unhappily so common that it seldom attracts sympathy. It is like a toothache in this respect. Because it does not kill exactly, we scarcely give it pity. Perhaps this is owing to the fact that the dyspeptic in nine cases out of ten is the author of his own miseries.[21]

A look through the medical literature reveals that in the 1830's there was a definite increase of interest in dyspepsia. One lay writer, himself a sufferer for many years, may well have been correct when he ventured in 1831: "The principal reason of their apparent increase [of digestive disorders], seems to be, that what are now enumerated as symptoms of one disease, were then considered and treated as distinct affections. Thus many affections, which were formerly known under different names and treated accordingly, as the Spleen, Vapours, Indigestion, Low Spirits, and Nervous Disease, are now generally comprehended under the sweeping term Dyspepsia."[22] In addition, he wrote, dyspepsia was becoming a fashionable complaint—the Gourmand and the Tippler would much prefer to be known as dyspeptics.

At the same time Edward Hitchcock, who later became president of Amherst college, lectured to the students at that school on diet, regimen, and employment. Published as a 451-page book in 1830 and again in 1831 as *Dyspepsy Forestalled and Resisted,* Hitchcock warned his young charges about the insidious nature of dyspeptic symptoms that could be caused by intemperance in diet, drink, or work. The mental symptoms as well as the physical, Hitchcock stressed, will take their toll. No nation becomes rich and prosperous without also becoming luxurious and debilitated. "They were eupeptics who carried the gospel over the earth in primitive times. They were eupeptics who in modern times have successfully engaged in the same work; and they must be eupeptics who are to bring on the millenium."[23]

There are many areas for future research. Obviously I have touched only upon some aspects of this fascinating and vexatious clinical phenomenon known as dyspepsia. For example, much further work needs to be done in elucidating the relationship of dyspepsia to George Beard's ideas about neurasthenia. Beard himself wrote on the subject, as have a number of subsequent medical writers and some historians.[24]

The descriptions of dyspepsia in the lay medical press and in the popular and family health guides are other obvious sources that need further exploration. O. Halsted's little book of 1831 on a *New Method of Curing Dyspepsia* was widely circulated and received a number of book reviews, most of them unflattering. One writer, probably a physician, in *The American Quarterly Review* warned readers about Mr. Halsted's four methods of treatment: tickling, pickling, ironing, and "throwing up the bowels." The ironing was done on towels laid on the abdomen on which a hot water bottle or a common flat iron was applied. This was to be as warm as the patient could stand it for fifteen to twenty minutes. But most of the reviewer's scorn was saved for throwing up the bowels:

> Fancy Mr. Halsted seated on the right side of his patient, and facing him; then placing his right hand upon the lower part of the abdomen, in such a manner, as to effect a lodgement as it were, under the bowels, suffering them to rest directly upon the edge of the extended palm, and then by a quick but not violent motion of the hand in an upward direction, the bowels are thrown up much in the same manner as in riding horseback, being communicated like that produced by a slight blow. (It is difficult to imagine who is entitled to the greatest admiration, the practitioner or the patient.)[25]

This is reminiscent, it might be noted, the so-called chiropractic thrust.

Much of the criticism of Mr. Halsted's apparently quite popular book pointed out that it was medical quackery. Dr. David M. Reese of New York in his *Humbugs of New York: Being a Remonstrance Against Popular Delusion* (1838), wrote that there was no better instance of the success of quackery than the "tribe of dyspeptic doctors, with which the city has been visited within a few years. The habits of high living, gluttony, intemperance, and sensual indulgence, in which all classes of the population have been growing worse and worse, have resulted in the almost universal prevalence of indigestion; to every variety of which the name dyspepsia has been stupidly and indiscriminantly applied; and to suffer from this disease has become so fashionable, that scarcely anyone has escaped its symptoms. . . ."[26] He then went on to deride the thumping cure. Obviously much remains to be done in order to further our understanding of dyspepsia and quackery.

The occurence of dyspepsia in biography also deserves further study. Winslow, in his study of Darwin's malady devoted a chapter to "Some Famous British Dyspeptics," as I have indicated. It may serve as a convenient starting place.[27] The theme of dyspepsia in literature has not been explored at all, so far as I know. Shakespeare, in *Coriolanus,* for instance described the stomach:

> It is the storehouse, and the shop
> Of the whole body. True it is,
> That it receives the general food at first;
> But all the cranks and offices of man,
> The strongest nerves, and small inferior veins,

From it receives that natural competence
Whereby they live.

Percival Wilde wrote a short, one act play entitled *The Dyspeptic Ogre,*
who was fond of eating little girls, suitably cooked.

The epidemiology of dyspepsia deserves much more study. I have
indicated some of the problems that such work will entail. An interesting by-product of following the evolution of our clinical knowledge of
dyspepsia in the nineteenth century, as it evolved into peptic ulcer
disease and other familiar modern medical entities, is the parallel
growth of our knowledge of the digestive function. Virtually all the
nineteenth-century writers on dyspepsia, for instance, incorporated
parts of William Beaumont's work into their own. In the early twentieth century, the physiologist Walter B. Cannon and the clinician
Walter C. Alvarez worked on intestinal motility and on the further
elucidation of the meanings of functional disease.[29]

Finally, then, returning to a point I made at the beginning, I
believe that a careful study of a disorder such as dyspepsia will lead us
to a much better understanding of nineteenth-century medical practice. Our medical colleagues frequently promulgate the false belief
that prior to mid-twentieth century antibiotic and hormone therapy,
coupled with great advances in surgery, medicine was mainly harmful
at worst or simply ineffective at best. Witness what two distinguished
professors of medicine had to say in the very first paragraph of their
recent book on two centuries of American medicine:

> Most of the advances have occurred during the second of these centuries.
> In the first century of American history, the role of the physician was that
> of the Good Samaritan. His success depended upon his sympathy, his
> humanity, and his art. Lacking a scientific base, his therapy for the more
> serious maladies was founded upon false hypotheses and fanciful systems
> and was for the most part ineffective.[30]

Now no one would deny that the physician's humanity has always
been a basis for his successful care of patients. There was a time, now
too often forgotten, when the mere presence of the doctor in the
patient's doorway led to a measurable sigh of relief and reassurance.
This was not owing only to the doctor's role as Good Samaritan. Many
physicians and historians have concentrated on effective therapy as the
yardstick for medical practice. The physician-patient encounter, however, cannot be so simply described. L.J. Henderson is usually credited
with the saying that it was not until about 1910 that the random patient

seeking help for a random illness from a randomly chosen physician had more than a 50–50 chance of benefitting from the encounter. Yet surely physicians have always provided help to the sick and suffering. As dyspepsia, with its intricate symptoms that interplay with general psychic, social, and cultural factors, so amply demonstrates, it was the doctor's management of the patient that led to relief. Whether it was the prescribed change, change in diet, change in mode of work, rest, exercise, or locale, or the mild acids or alkalis that the physician ordered, it was his prescription that was important. If dyspepsia was as common as it may well have been, then there was indeed much the doctor could do—at least much more than we are commonly led to believe.

Notes

1. George Rosen, "People, Disease, and Emotion: Some Newer Problems for Research in Medical History, *Bull. Hist. Med.*, 41 (1967), p. 9. A few months later Erwin H. Ackernecht made a similar point in his "A Plea for a 'Behaviorist' Approach in Writing the History of Medicine," *J. Hist. Med.*, 22 (1967), pp. 211–214. Very few have heeded their advice. A notable exception is Charles Rosenberg's "The Practice of Medicine in New York a Century Ago," *Bull. Hist. Med.*, 41 (1967), pp. 223–253.

2. Tinsley R. Harrison, *Principles of Internal Medicine*, 6th ed. (New York, 1970), p. 1462. This well-known textbook is now edited by seven eminent American clinicians.

3. Under the heading of "Unsettled Questions" *The Lancet* recently published a paper entitled "Is Duodenitis a Dyspeptic Myth?" June 4, 1977, pp. 1197–1198. See also editorial, "The Place of Dyspepsia in General Neurology," *Boston Med. and Surg. J.*, 126 (1892), pp. 667–68.

4. One paper with an intriguing title actually says little about the history of the disease: Thomas Hunt, "Doubt, Dogma and Dyspepsia," *Trans. Med. Soc. London*, 67 (1971), pp. 185–212.

5. George Pickering, *Creative Malady* (London, 1974, Delta reprint, 1976); Ralph Colp, Jr., *To Be An Invalid, The Illness of Charles Darwin* (Chicago, 1977); John H. Winslow, *Darwin's Victorian Malady, Evidence for its Medically Induced Origin* (Philadelphia: American Philosophical Soc., 1971). Despite Winslow's extensive discussion of dyspepsia, he attempted to prove that Darwin's gastro-intestinal symptoms were those of a chronic arsenic poisoning caused by the use of Fowler's solution.

6. Joseph E. Bogen, "Some Student Concepts of Functional Disease," *J. Med. Educ.*, 31 (1956) pp. 740–745.

7. "Dyspepsia," *Southern Rev.*, 4 (1892) p. 208.

8. *Ibid.*, p. 209.

9. *Ibid.*, p. 241.

10.   W.O. Huston, "The American Disease," *Columbus Med. J.,* 16 (1896), p. 1.

11.   John H. Kellogg, *The Stomach: Its Disorders and How to Cure Them,* (Battle Creek, 1896), p. 17.

12.   Austin Flint, *A Treatise on the Principles and Practice of Medicine,* (Philadelphia, 1866), p. 364. See also A.P. Dutcher, "Indigestion—Its Causes and Treatment," *Cincinnati Lancet and Observer,* 8 (1865), pp. 73–83; Arthur Leared, "The Causes of Dyspepsia," *Pop. Sci. Mo.,* 1 (1872), pp. 75–82; H. Illoway, "Nervous Dyspepsia," *Med. Record,* 47 (1895), pp. 7–15; Elbridge G. Cutler, "General Remarks on Gastric Dyspepsia," *Boston Med. and Surg. J.,* 137 (1897), pp. 249–55.

13.   A.K. Bond, *How Can I Cure My Indigestion* (1902).

14.   Lunsford P. Yandell, "Remarks on Dyspepsia," *Transylvania J. of Med. and Assoc. Sci.,* 7 (1834), 498.

15.   James H. Robbins, "American Dyspepsia," *Boston Med. and Surg. J.,* 107 (1882), pp. 132–134. Simon Fraser, Letter to the Editor, *British Med. J.,* 2 (1921), pp. 1011.

16.   See the general discussion of this trend in the chapter on "Functional Diagnosis," in Knud Faber, *Nosography in Modern Internal Medicine,* (New York, 1923), pp. 112–171.

17.   Douglas VanderHoof, "The Causes of Indigestion—A Study of 1000 Cases, *Johns Hopkins Hosp. Bull.,* 26 (1915), pp. 151–153.

18.   George M. Beard, *The New Cyclopedia of Family Medicine: Our Home Physician* (New York, 1879), p. 615. In the preface to the first edition of this massive book Beard wrote in 1869 that dyspepsia, along with hysteria, insanity, many skin and ear diseases, and rhinitis, all of which had been until recently ignored by the profession, were now treated with signal success.

19.   Flint, *Principles and Practice,* p. 365.

20.   J.H. Montgomery, "Some Disorders of Digestion of Frequent Occurence," *J.A.M.A., 30* (1898), p. 1494.

21.   *97* (1881) p. 762.

22.   O. Halsted, *A Full and Accurate Account of the New Method of Curing Dyspepsia, Discovered and Practised by O. Halsted,* 2nd. ed. (New York, 1831), p. 14. For a recent article on vapors see E.P. Scarlett, "The Vapors," *Arch. Int. Med., 116* (1965), pp. 142–146. I am indebted to Robert Hudson for this reference. See especially Hudson's recent article on chlorosis which poses many of the same problems for the historian as does a study of dyspepsia. Robert P. Hudson, "The Biography of a Disease: Lessons from Chlorosis," *Bull. Hist. Med., 51* (1977), pp. 448–463.

23.   2nd ed. (1831), pp. 332–333.

24.   The related literature is fairly extensive. For Beard see especially Charles E. Rosenberg, "The Place of George M. Beard in Nineteenth Century Psychiatry," *Bull. Hist. Med., 36* (1962), pp. 245–259. The first chapter, "The Nervous Century," in John S. and Robin M. Haller, *The Physician and Sexuality in Victorian America,* (Champaign Urbana, 1974, New York, Norton, 1977) is also a good summary.

25.   *American Quart. Rev., 9* (1831), p. 242. See also another anonymous review that appeared as a lead article in the *Boston Med. and Surg. J., 3* (1830), pp. 729–738, followed by an editorial pp. 740–42. The lay medical advice books, such as Beard's already cited

or R.V. Pierce's and many others, all carried articles on dyspepsia as did the eleventh edition of the *Encylopedia Britannica.* See especially the many references in the recent collection edited by Guenter B. Risse, Ronald L. Numbers, and Judith W. Leavitt, *Medicine Without Doctors, Home Health Care in American History* (New York, 1977). Dyspepsia does not, however, appear in the index.

26.   p. 121.

27.   But it is a mere beginning. Winslow discusses mainly the cases of Thomas Huxley and George Eliot, mentioning also the Carlyles, Herbert Spencer, and Thomas De-Quincy.

28.   The Dyspeptic Ogre may be found in Percival Wilde's, *Eight Comedies For Little Theatres* (Boston, 1922), pp. 37–68.

29.   Walter Alvarez also wrote books on the subject of dyspepsia: *Diseases of the Stomach,* (New York, 1924); *The Mechanics of the Digestive Tract* (New York, 1922, 2nd ed., 1928); *Nervous Indigestion* (New York, 1930); and *Nervousness, Indigestion, and Pain* (New York, 1943). The Cannon Papers at the Countway Library of Medicine in Boston contain a correspondence between Cannon and Alvarez describing some of their work. I wish to thank Saul Benison for calling these letters to my attention.

30.   James Bordley and A. McGehee Harvey, *Two Centuries of American Medicine* (Philadelphia, 1976), p. vii. For a different view, see Charles E. Rosenberg, "The Therapeutic Revolution: Medicine, Meaning and Social Change in Nineteenth Century America," *Perspectives in Biology and Medicine,* 20 (1977), pp. 485–506.

From Social Medicine
to Social Psychiatry:
The Achievement of
Sir Aubrey Lewis

MICHAEL SHEPHERD

Among George Rosen's most impressive gifts was his capacity to demonstrate how the historical perspective can illuminate and clarify contemporary issues. Nowhere is this exemplified more clearly than in his essay on the origins of social psychiatry[1], a term which has caused much discussion in recent years. The situation has been pungently described by Barbara Wootton:

> In the past decade or so, it has become increasingly fashionable to attach the adjective 'social' to 'psychiatry,' and to suggest that practically every field of human activity falls within the province of the social psychiatrist. Thus in the United States Dr. Alexander H. Leighton has written enthusiastically of the possible contribution of social psychiatry in the spheres of law, government, education, industry, and the armed forces; while at the Madrid Congress of the World Psychiatric Association it is reported that papers were presented dealing with subjects as diverse as drug addiction, criminology, mental disturbance and art, architecture and psychiatry, problems of sleep and dreaming, the biochemistry of the mind, the application of electronics to psychiatry, and the theory of sexual perversion. Some of this, one suspects, is simple empire building or an attempt to cash in on what has become a laudatory adjective—akin to the practice of euphemistic renaming which is to-day so popular in my own country, where unemployment has become 'redeployment,' deflation 'disinflation,' and a hobo a 'person without a settled way of living.' But in a more sober mood, the time is perhaps ripe for critical evaluation of the circumstances in which psychiatry, which can only be literally construed as the healing of the individual psyche, can justifiably call itself 'social.'[2]

George Rosen's paper shows that the concept of social psychiatry has been confusing long before modern times. In his own words: " . . . approaches to the elucidation of the problem have been coloured by various non-scientific views and considerations. In short the analy-

191

sis of this problem must be considered in terms of the sociology of knowledge as well as an aspect of the history of psychiatry." Much the same conclusion is drawn from his searching analysis of the development of social medicine.[3] Here, he not only traces striking parallels in the evolution of the two concepts, but suggests that the future of social medicine should be based on the "pattern of inquiry based on critical common sense" associated with the Swiss-American psychiatrist Adolf Meyer, whose guiding principles of psychobiology paid due regard to social factors. In the event, however, the task of demonstrating how such inquiries could be conducted, and thereby of establishing the scientific foundations of social psychiatry was not to be achieved by Meyer himself, but by the most eminent of his many pupils, Sir Aubrey Lewis (1900–1975). It is the purpose of this paper to indicate the genesis of a major achievement.

It is convenient to begin at the mid-point of Lewis' career, with a paper published during World War II entitled "Psychiatric Investigation in Britain."[4] Surprisingly, the bulk of the paper was an account of of officially sponsored surveys—surveys of mental ill-health in the industrial and ex-service populations; surveys of delinquency and maladjustment; surveys of the effects of wartime conditions on the mental health of the civilian population. A final section focuses on the measures being developed for the rehabilitation of psychiatrically disabled and handicapped persons. Hardly a word is devoted to the various clinical, therapeutic, or scientific advances which were being developed at the time. "Psychiatry," he concludes, "is not only a matter of mental hospitals and psychotherapeutic consulting rooms, but an integral part of medicine, especially of social medicine."

How had the author reached so far-sighted a conclusion? His educational development indicates the path he followed. Lewis' earliest interests had been in literature, history, and languages, so much so that the school teachers in his home town of Adelaide, Australia, predicted a distinguished career for him in the humanities.[5] He took up medicine with an eye at first on anthropology, and his first scientific paper was a report of a series of psychological observations on the aborigines of southern Australia.[6] Turning to psychiatry more or less *faute de mieux*, he was awarded a Rockefeller Fellowship and, at the Phipps Clinic of the Johns Hopkins Hospital, he imbibed the broad psychobiological concepts of medicine which had been developed by Adolf Meyer. During the following year in Heidelberg and Berlin, he was also to encounter the sophisticated approach to the *Grenzgebiete* of psychiatry associated with clinicians of the stature of Birnbaum, Kronfeld, Gruhle, and Jaspers. These men were all familiar with the work of such great European social theorists as Weber, Durkheim, and Simmel, and sought to apply their ideas to psychiatry. Aubrey Lewis was to absorb their teachings in a spirit of clear-sighted eclecticism and a full awareness of the historical continuity of their thinking. "The socially oriented psychiatry of today," he acknowledged 25 years later, "is the child of Adolf Meyer's teaching, but also of a rapidly developing social psychology which gets its stimulus and methods from many sources."[7]

In 1929 Lewis accepted a junior staff position at the Maudsley Hospital, the institution with which he was to remain associated for the rest of his working life. There, over the next decade, he built up a reputation as an outstanding clinician, research worker, and administrator. At the same time his interest in the history of medicine, which had been evident since his medical student days, was applied to the material that he collected for the historical section of his masterly study of melancholia.[8] The paper elicited a characteristic comment from Charles Singer: "The work appears to me to be both interesting and important. . . . The only criticism that I have to make is your treatment of Aretaeus of Cappadocia. Aretaeus wrote in Greek, and there is no case for quoting him in Latin."[9]

The various papers in the 1930's are permeated with an awareness of the social dimensions of clinical psychiatry, and the account of the facts and theory of eugenic legislation in National Socialist Germany illustrates his awareness of the wider implications of his discipline.[10] His formal entry into what would now be called social psychiatry, however, was signalised by a small-scale enquiry carried out in 1931: an examination, prompted by the then current concern with unemployment, of a group of men who had been without work for years because of neurotic disorders. His approach was characteristically direct and hard-headed:

> I found that there was no text or summarizing review of what was known about the psychiatry of unemployment, but that there was a very large amount of contingent information . . . and I recognised that the manifold problems revealed were not soluble by clinical study of individuals alone, but required that social data of an exact, well-organised sort should be ascertained and analysed, by methods which psychiatrists had not used in collecting the social information they needed in order to understand and treat individual patients.[11]

To obtain the necessary data, he supplemented the standard clinical information with a social history obtained from a relative by a psychiatric social worker and also by a further interview conducted in the patients' homes by a research social worker at a later date. His conclusions are worth noting:

> These men are as much social as medical problems. The majority of them are evidently unable to support themselves, the grounds for this are not to be found only in the economic circumstances which are responsible for unemployment in the country as a whole. Their previous history and present state are evidence of inherent deficiencies of adaptation to their environment. In their present circumstances may be seen a continuation of the external factors which for the greater part of their lives have interacted with inherited predispositions to make them in various ways unsatisfactory.[12]

Here, then, was the prototype of a novel form of investigation, but one which in its day was difficult to categorize. The term 'social psychiatry' had been introduced at about the same time in the United States by social scientists concerned with mental disorder and, even as late as 1948, H.W. Dunham was still able to claim it as ". . . a creation of sociologists to designate the interest of certain of their numbers who are doing research in the field of personality disorder."[13] The use of the concept in the context of psychiatry, with its public health and administrative overtones and its basis of empirical research, had more in common with the nascent discipline of social medicine which was emerging in Britain as a separate discipline from clinical medicine under the guidance of John Ryle.[14] With the coming of the Second World War, the potential significance of this viewpoint was rapidly acknowledged. One of the outstanding British figures in public health, Sir Wilson Jameson, devoted his Harveian Oration in 1942 to the seemingly paradoxical theme of 'War and the advancement of social medicine,' pointing out that armed conflict ". . . though a great destroyer of things worth preserving, may yet almost overnight open the door to progress and reform that in other times would have cost years of constant striving."[15] His was not an isolated voice. Nor was it as remote from the then current climate of opinion as might be imagined, for Jameson was a key member of Sir William Goodenough's Interdepartmental Committee on Medical Schools, which had been set up in 1942 to enquire into the organization of medical schools, with particular regard to clinical teaching and research in the government's post-war policy. In retrospect there is an almost visionary aspect to the notion of such concerns receiving official attention in the darkest days of the war. However, this was no routine report. Drafted simultaneously with the famous White Paper on "A National Health Service," its far-reaching proposals were based on a basic tenet: "Properly planned and carefully conducted medical education is *the* essential foundation of a comprehensive health service."[16]

Social medicine was, clearly, very much in the air, with a number of university departments already created for the development of the newly recognized discipline whose cognate bonds with psychiatry were explicitly acknowledged in the Goodenough report: "The relations between psychiatry and social medicine must . . . be close. Both branches have a strong interest in prevention, and a psychiatrist cannot fail to take account of social factors, any more than a worker in social medicine can avoid taking account of psychological factors."[16] This statement echoed the views of Aubrey Lewis who was one of only three psychiatrists invited to appear before the committee and whose opinions were already much the most influential. He had by then devoted much of his war-time research activities to the larger social problems of mental health in war-time conditions, and his commitment to social psychiatry had come into its own. The result was a stream of papers with largely self-explanatory titles, none of them concerned with the preoccupations of most clinical psychiatrists at the time: "Incidence of neurosis in England under war conditions,"[17] "Neurosis in soldiers: a follow-up study,"[18] "Social effects of neurosis,"[19] "Mental health in war-time,"[20] "Social causes of admission to a mental hospital for the aged,"[21] "Vocational aspects of neurosis in soldiers,"[22] "The industrial resettlement of the neurotic,"[23] "Psychiatric advice in industry."[24]

During this period Lewis became increasingly concerned to introduce some of these ideas to the psychiatric profession at large. Later, he was to reflect:

> . . . although I am not one of those who consider that we were in the Dark Ages in our approach to problems of neurosis and personality maladjustment until the war gave us enlightenment, it is still of course true that psychiatrists who had worked in the almost conventual isolation of some remote mental hospitals were brought face to face with social issues affecting mental health which might otherwise have remained as peripheral to their daily thinking and direct experience as trypanosomiasis or the structure and functions of the hypothalamus.

Following Lewis' appointment as honorary secretary to a Neurosis Sub-Committee of the Royal Medico-Psychological Association which was formed in 1942, a number of projects were initiated. The sub-committee, under his guidance, produced a series of memoranda on topics which were far removed from those which might have been anticipated. The first of these documents was concerned with the implications for social psychiatry of the famous Beveridge Report, which was to be one of the keystones of the post-war Welfare State in Britain.[25] The memorandum begins by examining the relevance to psychiatry of poverty, unemployment, old age, workers' compensation, social failure, and malingering. It then comments in some detail on various aspects of the Beveridge proposals—principles, benefit rates, contributory payments, and care of the injured—before going on to consider administrative measures and to advance no fewer than fifteen recommendations "to foster a healthy mental health outlook, as well as physical well-being, in our country."[26]

The sub-committee also considered the problems of neurosis in the merchant navy and prepared a memorandum on the residential treatment of chronic neurotics in colonies offering training, remunerative work, and rehabilitation. This concluded that "The conduct of a hostel or settlement should be primarily the concern of those who benefit from it—*viz.* the patients—and it should be self-supporting. Control would be vested in the health authority which provided the initial capital outlay; health insurance benefits would help towards maintenance costs. The occupational colony should be run by the health authority."[27] Finally, acting on the premise that much that is done by psychiatrists should be handled by the properly trained general practitioner, alive to the social and psychiatric aspects of his work, the committee prepared a forward-looking handbook for general practitioners to guide them in the psychiatric aspects of their work.

Within a few months, however, it was apparent that the concept of social psychiatry represented by these activities was being challenged by another group of claimants to the term. Their approach had also emerged from the experiences of the war but in an altogether different context, being based essentially on the extension of the group psycho-therapeutic principles which had been widely applied in the military setting. In the grandiose words of one of the best-known advocates of social psychiatry in this guise, the term was to be used as "an 'elastic' concept, to include all social, biological, educational and philosophical considerations which may come to empower psychiatry in its striving towards a society which functions with greater equilibrium and with fewer psychological casualties."[28] From this mode of thinking, emerged the nebulous but pervasive idea of the 'therapeutic community' which has been so widely linked to social aggregates of all varieties, varying from the family and institutions to the community at large. So superficially promising an outlook achieved rapid and uncritical acceptance. By 1959 a W.H.O. Expert Committee on Mental Health defined social psychiatry as "the preventive and curative measures which are directed towards the fitting of an individual for a satisfactory and useful life in terms of its own environment."[29]

The radical differences between these two contrasted notions of social psychiatry have been lucidly summarized by Hare:[30]

> The first school sees social psychiatry as a new discipline; the second sees it as an old one for which a new name has been found. The first school emphasizes treatment as the major activity of social psychiatry; the second emphasizes research. The first school sees the means of prevention as fundamentally the same as those of treatment; the second holds that prevention is in its infancy and that adequate measures will depend on a much greater knowledge of social causes than we have at present— hence its emphasis on research. Finally, the first school considers that social psychiatry has close links with psychotherapy and psychodynamics: the W.H.O. Expert Committee, for example, specifically notes the indebtedness of social psychiatry to these subjects and adds that 'the goals of psychotherapy and social psychiatry can be said to overlap'; the second school sees no such links and, indeed, Professor Lewis has written that 'the claims of psycho-analysis to explain all human behaviour diverted attention from the social causes, and effects, of mental abnormality.'

The incompatibility of these views was soon to become apparent in post-war Britain. In 1946 the Royal Medico-Psychological Association formed a Section of Social Psychiatry, with Aubrey Lewis as its chairman. Within a year, however, he resigned, and shortly thereafter the section was significantly renamed that of Social Psychiatry and Psychotherapy. Thenceforward, Lewis was to develop his own view of the subject in his own way, based squarely on the lessons drawn from the productive turmoil of wartime, as he made clear in his review of the post-war situation:

> The pressure of wartime demands in Britain has driven home, even to the minds of the abominators of statistics and the abhorers of planning, that it is better to build an Ark than to wait to be drowned; and that it is a good thing to study the weather and have good shipyard specifications pre-

pared well in advance of any major or minor deluge. . . . There is not such
a clear line between fundamental and applied science in the social field,
nor such a plentitude of fundamental work in social medicine, that we can
regard official investigations, and the more or less experimental action
taken on their findings, as anything but an indispensable part of research,
without which many lines of research would be closed. So far as psychiatry
is conceived as a branch of social medicine and public health, it must rely
for its advancement upon methods which require accurate statistics such
as it is the business of official intelligence to supply, as well as upon the
more individual and perhaps more original methods which are in keeping
with its main tradition.[31]

The moral which he drew from his experience was characteristically pragmatic: "It is in the interplay between the gross survey and
the refined experiment, each stimulating and reinforcing the other,
that research in social medicine finds its parallel to the marriage between bedside observation and laboratory studies that has been so
fruitful in clinical research. The social side of psychiatry, having lagged
behind here, is now hopefully labouring to make up for lost time."[32]
Lewis was soon to acquire the means to practice his ideas. Shortly after
his appointment to the vacant chair of psychiatry at the Maudsley
Hospital as a post-graduate school of the University of London in
1946, Lewis submitted a memorandum to the Medical Research Council outlining a programme of research in social psychiatry. In 1948 he
assumed the honorary directorship of an M.R.C. unit, the first time
that a psychiatrist had been entrusted with such a position. The unit
was multi-disciplinary from the outset, consisting of a psychiatrist, five
psychologists, and an economist. Its title was the Occupational Psychiatry Research Unit, and its modestly stated objectives were threefold:
to evaluate the conditions in which the mentally handicapped might
undertake useful work; to examine certain psychological characteristics of workers in industry; and to study the psychiatric interview as a
technique for the assessment of mental health.[33]

Three years later the unit was renamed the Unit for Research in
Occupational Adaptation in an attempt to define its expanded functions more precisely. During the 1950's the work came to include
several clinical and social problems associated with chronic psychosis
and field studies of attitudes towards mental illness. Throughout these
early years, Lewis continued to adopt a wary, step-by-step plan of
research. In the mid-1950's, he commented of his unit's programme:
"Though still in the stage at which methods have to be worked out,

and practical difficulties can sometimes be frustrating, it is essential that it should be diligently cultivated: otherwise our contemporary emphasis on social psychiatry will lack an assured foundation."[34] Not until 1958, and only after considerable hesitation, did Lewis agree to adopt the title of Social Psychiatry for his unit. He did so because its research activities had come to extend far beyond industrial psychiatry and because by then he felt he had laid down sufficiently firm foundations to justify its use of so slippery a term. What this was to mean in practical terms was amply demonstrated by the impressive body of research carried out under Lewis' direction which has been fully described elsewhere.[35] More relevant here is the approach to social psychiatry which he developed and the conclusions which he drew in the light of his mature experience.

The approach is best illustrated by the various investigations focused on the chronically ill psychiatric patient. Whether suffering from neurosis, psychosis, or mental subnormality, the point of entry was always the status of the patient as a disabled person, with down-to-earth rehabilitation rather than starry-eyed prevention or cure as the goal. The move in this direction was closely related to the climate of the times:

> A bold policy has led to the discharge from mental hospitals of many patients still plainly exhibiting symptoms of schizophrenia; this has been practised largely on a trial and error basis, without much regard to the reorientation within the hospital nor the conditions in the family or community outside hospital which might be supposed necessary. No one, of course, could be sure what conditions were called for inside and outside the hospital to promote sound development of this discharge policy, since insufficient research had been carried out. Hence the sense of urgency in getting on with it. It is arguable whether a sense of urgency is the best motive force for research and whether an atmosphere of reformist zeal is one in which research flourishes. But the research was obviously needed, and the changing conditions provided material for study and, in certain favourable areas, for planned experiment.[36]

It was this philosophy that inspired the series of studies into rehabilitation, where the social dimension is central. Rehabilitation is equated with 'treatment from the social point of view'; handicaps become 'symptoms relevant to social conduct' which call for measurement; 'attitudes,' as precursors to action, are called in and adapted from social psychology.[37]

The strategy of the research was clearly enunciated: "In the investigations which the Social Psychiatry Research Unit has been carrying out, we have found it necessary at each stage to pass backwards and forwards from laboratory to ward and from ward to laboratory, and to pass from both to the outer world where relatives live and conditions of work and daily life may make or mar the chronic schizophrenic's chance of staying outside hospital for good."[38] The tactics were explicitly interdisciplinary: "These social issues call for research untrammelled by customary professional divisions, untrammelled also by over-confident claims or over-ingenious word-play with the problem. . . . Boundaries between branches of knowledge are vicious if they hinder true research: it is therefore, I think, proper that one man, or several men together, should use at once social, psychological and clinical psychiatric methods and modes of thought to throw light on problems not obviously or traditionally included in psychiatry, but likely to be illumined by such study."[39] Testifying to the success of the program is the impressive list of workers who worked on the unit under Lewis' direction and then, following his retirement, continued the tradition either within the unit or elsewhere. They include J. Tizard, N. O'Connor, and P. Venables (psychology), G.M. Carstairs, K. Rawnsley, J.K. Wing, and M. Rutter (psychiatry), G.W. Brown (sociology), J.B. Loudon (social anthropology), R. Goldman-Eisler (linguistics).

Throughout his career Aubrey Lewis turned his attention afresh to some of the basic theoretical problems associated with social psychiatry, drawing constantly on the results obtained and problems posed by the work in hand. Adhering to Henry Sigerist's dictum that the development of medical science is determined by non-medical factors, he drew on a rich store of erudition and critical capacity to relate these factors to the development of the subject. Thus, in his survey of the content of social psychiatry,[40] he concentrated on the relevant methods of social investigation which had illuminated psychiatry. These included: epidemiology; studies of social class, marital status, exile and emigration; ecology; cultural and familial influences; and the social aspects of treatment. At all times, however, he insisted on separating the social from the biological basis of the morbid states under discussion, as he made explicit in a well-known paper on "Health as a Social Concept."[41] Further, the infiltration of Lewis' social thinking into the structure of clinical psychiatry led to an increasing emphasis on its place therein. In an interview after his retirement, he was asked whether he saw the development of social psychiatry as a way out of the dilemma of the organic and psycho-dynamic dichotomy. His reply was unequivocal:

> "I would not have it seen as a dilemma. I think that there is a proper place for the dynamic and the organic approaches very clearly, but the social side of psychiatry is so obtrusive at every point and has been in the history of psychiatry at all times, that I cannot see how it could have been so neglected if the methods of investigation had been better formed. In particular, the whole field of sociology is still embryonic. Otherwise, the crying need for better knowledge of the social aspects of psychiatry would surely have been fully recognized; they pervade, for example, legal issues, drug addiction, or the conditions within which certain forms of mental disorder appear to be generated or fermented.

In addition, Aubrey Lewis never forgot the historical roots of the empirical studies for which he was responsible. In his Adolf Meyer Lecture on "The Study of Defect," for example, the account of his unit's work on mental subnormality is accompanied by an exposition of the development of the concept of defect from the eighteenth century to the present day.[42] His Galton Lecture, devoted to "Fertility and Mental Illness," outlines Morel's 'degeneration' theory which carried so much weight in the nineteenth century.[43] The Hobhouse Lecture, "Agents of Cultural Advance," traces the evolution of the complex notions of culture and progress in relation to related ideas in psychology and psychiatry. In retrospect it is apparent that his basic theme was the grounding of social psychiatry in both social and medical history, an argument which he developed explicitly in his Bertram Robert's Lecture, 'Ebb and Flow in Social Psychiatry.'[44] Here, appropriately enough at Yale, he took over the baton from George Rosen to demonstrate the continuity and "strangely cyclical course" of thought among the early twentieth-century pioneers in the field, and his firsthand experience of the multiple facets of social psychiatry enabled him to do full justice to the contributions of early workers in the field: "The moral of this tale," he observed, "is that we do ill to think lightly of our predecessors in social psychiatry. The ablest among us need not be so humble as to say, with Bernard of Chartres, that we are dwarfs sitting on the shoulders of giants; but neither need it be supposed that we are giants sitting on the shoulders of dwarfs, or sitting on nobody's shoulders at all." And the paper itself pleads for "action research and laboratory experiments" rather than for reformist enthusiasm. In his own words: "The philosophers thought it proper to put not one but two mottoes on the temple at Delphi: one, the better remembered, was 'Know Thyself'; but the second, equally imperative, enjoined 'Nothing in Excess.' It might be worth inscribing that over the temple of psychiatry."

George Rosen's blueprint for the future of social psychiatry emphasized the need for research "on several levels" if progress is to be made. Aubrey Lewis demonstrated what this meant in practice and to what it must be related. His own careful, empirical work has given the subject a scientific basis, but he himself never lost sight of its derivations:

> The social influences to which the patient has been exposed within his family, at school, at work, during war, in marriage, through religion and politics and recreation, are all necessary to our understanding of how he has become what he is. We concern ourselves with his relatives, endeavouring to understand and perhaps to modify their feelings and attitudes so that it will be to his advantage, and often also to theirs. We use all the socialising influences we can while the patient is under our care in hospital, and we take pains to fit him for his return to society, perhaps by altering much of the social setting to which he will return. We take full advantages of the social provisions set up by the state. In all this, the psychiatrist is practising social medicine.[45]

Notes

1. Rosen, G. (1959): "Social Stress and Mental Disease from the Eighteenth Century to the Present: Some Origins of Social Psychiatry," *Milbank Memorial Fund Quarterly*, 37, pp. 5–32, p. 31.

2. Wootton, B. (1968): "Social Psychiatry and Psychopathology: A Layman's Comments on Contemporary Developments" in *Social Psychiatry,"* edited by Zubin, J. and Freyhan, F.A. (Grune & Stratton: New York) pp. 283–299; p. 283.

3. Rosen, G. (1947): "What is Social Medicine?" *Bulletin of the History of Medicine*, 21, pp. 674–733.

4. Lewis, A. (1945): "Psychiatric Investigation in Britain," *American Journal of Psychiatry*, 101, no. 4, pp. 486–493; p. 491.

5. Shepherd, M. (1977): *The Career and Contributions of Sir Aubrey Lewis*, Eyre & Spottiswoode for the Bethlem Royal and Maudsley Hospitals.

6. Lewis, A. and Campbell, T.D. (1926): "The Aborigines of South Australia: Anthropometric, Descriptive and Other Observations Recorded at Ooldea," *Trans. R. Soc.S. Aust.*, 50, pp. 183–197.

7. Lewis, A. (1951): "Social Aspects of Psychiatry," *Edinburgh Medical Journal*, LVIII, pp. 214–247; p. 245.

8. Lewis, A. (1934): "Melancholia: A Historical Review," *Journal of Mental Science*, 80. pp. 1–42.

9. Singer, C. (1932): Unpublished letter.

10. Lewis, A. (1934): "German Eugenic Legislation: An Examination of Fact and Theory," *Eugenics Review*, 26, pp. 183–191.

11. Lewis, A. (1959): "Changes in Social Psychiatry," Address to the Royal, Medico-Psychological Association (unpublished).

12. Lewis, A. (1935): "Neurosis and unemployment," *Lancet*, II, pp. 293–297; p. 297.

13. Dunham, H.W. (1948): "The Field of Social Psychiatry," *American Sociological Review*, 13, pp. 183–197; p. 183.

14. Ryle, J.A. (1948): *Changing Disciplines* (Oxford University Press: London).

15. Jameson, W.W. (1942): "War and the Advancement of Social Medicine," *Lancet*, II, pp. 475–479; p. 475.

16. Ministry of Health and Department of Health for Scotland (1944): *Report of the Inter-departmental Committee on Medical Schools* (H.M.S.O.: London).

17. Lewis, A. (1942): "Incidence of Neurosis in England under War Conditions," *Lancet*, II, pp. 175–183.

18. Lewis, A. and Slater, E. (1942): "Neurosis in Soldiers: A Follow-up Study," *Lancet*, I, pp. 496-498.

19. Lewis, A. (1943): "Social Effects of Neurosis," *Lancet*, I, pp. 167–170.

20. Lewis, A. (1943): "Mental Health in War-time," *Public Health*, 57, pp. 27–30.

21. Lewis, A. and Goldschmidt, H. (1943): "Social Causes of Admissions to a Mental Hospital for the Aged," *Sociological Review*, 35, pp. 86–98.

22. Lewis, A. and Goodyear, K. (1944): "Vocational Aspects of Neurosis in Soldiers," *Lancet*, II, pp. 105–109.

23. Lewis, A. (1945): "The industrial Resettlement of the Neurotic," *Labour Management*, 27, pp. 40–43.

24. Lewis, A. (1945): "Psychiatric Advice in Industry," *British Journal of Industrial Medicine*, 2, pp. 41–42.

25. Council of the Royal Medico-Psychological Association (1944): *Memorandum on Social Insurance and Allied Services in Their Bearing on Neurotic Disorder* (R.M.P.A.: London).

26. Special Article (1943): "Social Insurance and Neurotic Disorder," *Lancet*, II, pp. 775–776; p. 775.

27. Reconstruction (1944): "Colonies for Neurotics," *Lancet*, II, pp. 154–155.

28. Jones, M. (1968): *Social Psychiatry in Practice* (Penguin Books: London), p. 30.

29. World Health Organization (1959): *Social Psychiatry and Community Attitudes*, Technical Report Series, No. 177 (W.H.O.: Geneva).

30. Hare, E.H. (1969): "The Relation between Social Psychiatry and Psychotherapy," in *Psychiatry in a Changing Society*, edited by Foulkes, S.H. and Prince, G.S. (Tavistock: London), p. 10.

31. Lewis, A., *op. cit.* in fn. 4 above, p. 492.

32. *Ibid.*, p. 491.

33. O'Connor, N. (1968): "The Origins of the Medical Research Council Social Psychiatry Unit," in *Studies in Psychiatry*, edited by Shepherd, M. and Davies, D.L. (Oxford University Press: London), pp. 11–13.

34. Lewis, A. (1953): "Research in Occupational Psychiatry," *Folia Psychiatrica, Neurologica et Neurochirurgica Neerlandica*, 56, no. 5, pp. 779–786.

35. Shepherd, M. and Davies, D.L., editors (1968): *Studies in Psychiatry* (Oxford University Press: London).

36. Lewis, A. (1962): "Rehabilitation." Unpublished manuscript.

37. Lewis, A. (1956): "Rehabilitation Programs in England," in *The Elements of a Community Mental Health Program* (Milbank Memorial Fund: New York), pp. 196–206.

38. Lewis, A. (1958): "Between Guesswork and Certainty in Psychiatry," *Lancet*, I, pp. 227–230.

39. Lewis, A., *op. cit.* in fn. 7 above, p. 245.

40. Lewis, A. (1957): "Social Psychiatry," in *Lectures on the Scientific Basis of Medicine*, 6 (Athlone Press: University of London) pp. 116–142.

41. Lewis, A. (1953): "Health as a Social Concept," *British Journal of Sociology*, 4, pp. 109–124.

42. Lewis, A. (1960): "The study of defect," *The American Journal of Psychiatry*, 117, pp. 289–305.

43. Lewis, A. (1958): "Fertility and mental illness," *Eugenics Review*, 50, pp. 91–106.

44. Lewis, A. (1962): "Ebb and flow in social psychiatry," *Yale Journal of Biology and Medicine*, 35, pp. 62–83; p. 83.

45. Lewis, A., *op. cit.* in fn. 7 above, p. 217.

C.-E.A. Winslow: His Era and His Contribution to Medical Care

ARTHUR J. VISELTEAR

He who sees only ideals accomplishes little. He who sees only facts, even less. He who grasps both facts and ideals, who moulds the actual to the form of a vision, is the man who helps to build a better world.

> C.-E. A. Winslow, "Strategic position of the dispensary in the public health campaign," *The Nation's Health*, 1926, *8*, p. 4.

When C.-E. A. Winslow died in 1957, a month short of his eightieth birthday, he was universally regarded as the elder statesman of public health. His genius and versatility were evident in every branch of public health, including bacteriology, epidemiology, sanitary engineering, health education, occupational health, public health nursing, mental health, housing, and medical care. "He was a writer of distinction, a teacher of renown, a man whose counsel was prized, a favored speaker before his colleagues, a world citizen in the realm of health, a great statesman, a man who was always doing, never still—a simply extraordinary man"[1] He received his early training from William Sedgwick at M.I.T., taught biology and bacteriology at both the University of Chicago and the College of the City of New York, served in the New York State Department of Health under Biggs, and, in 1915, was called to Yale to occupy its first chair in public health, where he remained for 30 years as professor and chairman. He served as first editor of the *Journal of Bacteriology,* chairman of the New York State Commission on Ventilation, director of the John B. Pierce Laboratory of Hygiene, president of the American Public Health Association, vice-chairman and chairman of the Executive Board of the Committee on the Costs of Medical Care, and consultant to the World Health Organization. Toward the end of his career, when failing eyesight forced his retirement in 1954, he had served for a decade as editor of the *American Journal of Public Health,* writing a prodigious number of insightful editorials which revealed his catholicity of interests and progressive thinking, especially about medical care.

Winslow began his career as one of the new breed of public

health professionals who appeared at the turn of the century. Trained by Sedgwick at M.I.T., he became a prototype of the non-medical sanitary scientist, one with skills in biology, sanitary engineering, bacteriology, statistics, and health administration. He matured when public health was beginning to emerge from an aggregate of specialties to a profession whose principal objectives were the advancement of sanitary science, the promotion of organizations and measures for the practical application of public hygiene, and the control of communicable disease. Within these objectives great achievements had occurred. Water supplies, food, and drugs had been purified, milk pasteurized, houses ventilated, children immunized, laborers protected—and if our cities, towns, and work places had not become utopias, they had at least become more habitable and safer and we ourselves more healthy.

But despite the substantial progress, much more needed to be done, and during Winslow's lifetime public health underwent marked and fundamental changes. Community cleanliness, the application of the principles of the new science, and education in personal hygiene —the standard desiderata of the public health campaign—were deemed too narrow in focus, too limited in scope, and new definitions of public health were advanced to reflect new needs and missions.

Winslow's own definition of public health, prepared in 1920, indicates these new dimensions:

> Public health is the science and the art of preventing disease, prolonging life, and promoting physical health and efficiency through organized community efforts for the sanitation of the environment, the control of community infections, the education of the individual in principles of personal hygiene, the organization of medical and nursing service for the early diagnosis and preventive treatment of disease, and the development of the social machinery which will ensure to every individual in the community a standard of living adequate for the maintenance of health.[2]

Such expressions of social objectives—which gradually included the sensible coordination of private medical practice with public health, the recognition that social and environmental factors were threatening to health, and the solution of the problems attendant on the organization, financing, and delivery of health care—were examples of Winslow's view of the new public health, one which functioned in a society which accepted its fundamental responsibility for housing, economic security, and medical care—in fact, for the control of all factors that affected physical and mental well-being.[3]

Winslow's entry into the field of medical care was as subtle as it was deliberate, the product of an orderly progression in thinking as both events and new knowledge came his way. He had mastered the science of controlling the physical environment, experienced the period when the new science had been applied to control the acute communicable diseases, and had been part of the next phase of the public health movement which called for popular health education in the principles of personal hygiene. He had also witnessed the battles waged for social insurance,[4] read the studies describing the cyclical relationship between poverty and illness,[5] and studied the reports of various medical economic and social insurance commissions and surveys.[6] But it was not until his work with Hermann Biggs in New York and his membership on an American Red Cross mission to Russia that he began fully to appreciate the fourth phase of the modern public health campaign—the organization of medical services for the early diagnosis and prevention of disease.

In 1917, Winslow left for Russia and a year later reported on the Russian system of public health administration.[7] Much of what he observed impressed him, especially the Zemstvo system of free medical care for health protection for the rural population which they "regarded as the natural duty of society rather than as an act of charity."[8] Russia's major developments in public health had come along medical and bacteriological lines, in the control of the acute communicable diseases, and in the field of vital statistics. Certainly, much was yet to be done in Russia—their anti-tuberculosis campaign was still in its infancy as were their programs for venereal diseases and infant mortality—but Winslow believed that great progress had been made, based on the administrative structure and on the "remarkable development of social medicine along curative lines and the consequent close connection between curative and preventative work."[9] He wrote further that:

> Russia, on account of the peculiar acute needs of the rural population, has already developed the State care of the sick to a point of which we are only beginning to dream, and after the war the new republican government will no doubt pursue this social ideal to a much higher point of perfection. The opportunity for developing preventive educational work with such a system is practically unlimited. . . . We may therefore look in the future, as Zemstvo and municipal medicine develop and acquire the educational and preventive quality which is in accord with modern prog-

ress, for unprecedented successes in the control of preventable diseases in the great sister Republic.[10]

Russia did not live up to its potential as both war and internal political upheavals eroded the "unprecedented successes" that Winslow had reported. But the potential for establishing a truly preventive system of health care in the United States, organized along lines that were variations of themes that he had witnessed in Russia, was to color his thinking and excite his imagination for some time. The problem was how to excite his colleagues in the United States when many were concerned with what came to be called the "Red scare." Such arguments, which were already being heard when social reformers in New York, California, and other states attempted to enact programs for health insurance,[11] were exacerbated as the Bolsheviks gained control in Russia. Winslow referred to the Russian situation in a 1919 speech to the National Conference of Social Work.[12] What had happened in Russia, he said, was unfortunate. As bad as America's post-war problems were, however, "we must not dash upon the rocks and founder as Russia is foundering today." But we must also not be so frightened as to forget that "the health of the American people must be one of our ideals" and must be:

> ensured by the application of sanitary science and preventive medicine on a scale far greater than we have ever dared to dream. It must be ensured by a reorganization of medicine and nursing service on some social plan so that the rich and poor may receive the gifts of medical science and may receive them at a state when they can operate effectively and not, as today, when it is too late to do much more than ease the sufferer into his grave.[13]

But the battle was to be hard and up-hill. Winslow did not desist in his attempt to seek a rational solution to the question of how best to organize and finance services in the United States. He spoke of it in simple, but irresistably logical terms, in much the same way, for example, as did Biggs when advancing a program for health centers in New York State.[14] But Biggs had also run into the "Red scare" and had been defeated with such arguments as: "too much power to the laity and too little to the medical profession"; "a step toward centralization of government and paternalism"; "a measure which, to a great extent tends to or does deprive us of our liberties"; "the entering wedge toward state medicine."[15] Winslow, who had testified for the health center bill, was appalled by such attacks, which he later blamed on the "overactive hormonal secretions" of his opponents. But such irrationality, nevertheless, was a warning. Hereafter, he would continue to press on for reform—, but with caution.

In the 1920s, Winslow's speeches and writings touched on many different elements of health services reform. In a Yale address entitled "The Evolution and Significance of the Modern Public Health Campaign"[16] he spoke of the need to adopt "new machinery" to meet the challenges of the new concerns—tuberculosis, diseases of infancy, mental hygiene, venereal diseases, cancer, and heart disease. If such diseases were to be conquered, then the private practitioner would have to become a "real force in prevention." The arbitrary line separating private medicine from public health would have to be "obliterated," just as it had been for child health services, and were beginning to develop in connection with venereal diseases and tuberculosis.[17] But before medicine could become truly preventive, he said, something had to be done about payment.

> It is extremely unlikely that the average individual will ever resort to his physician until he experiences compelling symptoms of disease if incurring of an immediate financial obligation is specifically involved. The maintenance of physical health will surely call for the provision of some social machinery superior to the happy-go-lucky methods of the past. How the desired end can be attained is the major problem before the physicians and the public health profession of the present day.[18]

His address in 1923 was exploratory. He did not offer an answer as to how the "desired end" could be achieved. He said merely that solutions had already been proffered—compulsory health insurance, state medicine, health centers linked to dispensaries and hospitals under public or private auspices, or by regionalization (a "distinctly promising" step taken in England)—but whatever the ultimate recommendation it was clear to Winslow that solutions were to be:

> found only through patient and earnest and dispassionate adventure on the part of the medical profession. Preventive medicine must come, as a reality and not a pious phrase, through a fundamental change in the attitude of the physician and through a fundamental change in the attitude of the medical schools where he is trained.[19]

When Winslow became chairman of the newly established Department of Public Health at Yale in 1915, he addressed this issue of "attitude." Unlike Harvard or John Hopkins, which in the same period were to develop public health in separate and independent schools, cognate with the schools of medicine and law, Yale's program was constituted as one of the eight fundamental divisions of the medical school.[20] Winslow envisioned the integration as fundamental to the development of medical practice.

> For the past twenty years medical orators have revelled in the elaboration of the theme of preventive medicine; and it is indeed a fact that the progress of science and of social organization demands a fundamental realignment in the entire attitude of the physician toward his patient and toward the community. It is quite certain that the doctor of the future must be a family adviser on hygiene and sanitation quite as much as an ameliorative agent in respect to evils already largely consummated. It is very probable, too, that a large proportion of the doctors of the future will not only be doing a new kind of work but doing it in a new way, as parts of an organized community health service.[21]

It was Winslow's hope that his program, integrally related to the other departments of the medical school, would imbue the Yale Medical School graduate with a pervasive preventive spirit, "not as a form of words, but as a vital conception in the student's mind."[22]

But Winslow found that both physicians and medical students, even at Yale, were unwilling to embark on the adventure of social and professional coordination for which he had hoped.[23] If one could not effect the needed change in the medical schools, then perhaps the changes would come by structuring and rationalizing community health services. In a speech presented to the American Hospital Association in September, 1926, he considered the strategic position of the dispensary in the public health campaign.[24]

He began by noting that changes were already apparent. A hospital, for example, was no longer merely a shelter for the sick poor; a dispensary, similarly, was no longer a place for dispensing drugs to the same class of people; and a health department was no longer an office for the sanitary policing of the streets and yards of the city. A convergence or "interfusion" of roles had occurred. The hospital was becoming a "social agency" where anyone who needed services could receive care; the dispensary was also "reaching out"; and the health officer was moving from the field of sanitary law to the "broader realm of public health." What was needed was a "common meeting ground" to unite the best principles extant in the community. And for Winslow this point was the out-patient department of the hospital, which he envisioned as a "polyclinic" relating, on the one hand, to the specialized services of the hospital and, on the other hand, to a "generalized district service" comprised of major and minor health centers and a home nursing service.[25]

This hypothetical scheme did not consider personal jealousies, vested interests, or territorial imperatives, but:

> if we could once visualize an abstract ideal of organization as we would like to see it if we could, then we would have made the first step toward progress. The art of statesmanship in its essence consists of formulating an ideal and then so dealing with circumstances and with personalities that we approach that ideal instead of receding from it—even though our rate of progress may be infinitesimal.[26]

In this early period, while Winslow was refining his thinking about medical care, others had also begun to address the need for a broader, functional view of public health. In 1921, the Sheppard-Towner Act had been passed, providing federal grants to the states for infant health clinics.[27] APHA's Committee on Municipal Health Practice (which in 1925 changed its name to Committee on Administrative Practice to reflect a broader public health mandate than just the city) had begun to work cooperatively, through its Subcommittee on the Organized Care of the Sick, with the American Hospital Association in an endeavor to determine, for example, a community's need for hospital beds.[28] As a member and officer of APHA, Winslow had heard a few health officers call as early as 1921 for "state medicine." Articles in the *Survey,*[29] the *American Journal of Public Health,*[30] and the *New York State Journal of Medicine*[31] were similarly recommending a reorganization of health services or outlining the "next steps" which would bring to the people the benefits of modern medical science: a movement to chronic disease control, the teaching of preventive medicine in medical schools, adequate post-graduate medical instruction and periodic reexamination of physicians, annual physical exams, the reincarnation of the "old family physician" as hygienic adviser, an insurance mechanism to pool risks, and the extension of clinic and dispensary medical facilities on a pay basis for wider groups in the population.[32]

By the mid-1920s, however, the problems had grown worse. Medical care had become too expensive and costs were rising so rapidly that, except for the rich and the very poor, medical care was unavailable. Other reports revealed geographic and specialty maldistribution of health care providers; that there had been no cooperative efforts to rationalize the confusion; and that medical care was not preventive, but attempted alleviation after the event. In 1926, Winslow had refined his thinking sufficiently to join a small group of experts, a committee of five,[33] representing economics, medicine, and public health, who subsequently arranged an informal conference held in Washington, D.C. to consider the economic factors affecting the organization of medicine. Those in attendance considered a series of questions respecting medical costs: How rapidly had medical care costs risen? How much of a family's budget was being spent on medical care? From what source should a physician obtain his capital and operating budget? Could hospital policy be altered to provide care for patients of moderate means? Why were there no clinics for the average income earner? And according to what principles should the proposals to reduce or extend the functions of the state in the field of public health and medical care be judged?[34]

In October, 1926, Winslow employed many of the refinements and case examples he had heard discussed, or discussed himself, at these informal meetings in his presidential speech delivered to APHA.[35] The speech united many of the threads of principles and themes that he had expressed earlier and was a more comprehensive and ambitious attempt to emphasize a new direction for his parent organization and the health officers of the nation.

He began his address by noting the unprecedented successes that had been achieved by APHA in previous years and then turned his attention to future problems. APHA was standing at a "crossroads," he said, and how the new problems would be approached would determine not only the profile of the APHA of the future, but would have far-reaching consequences for "the welfare of the people of this continent."[36] His principal point was to summon public health officials to concern themselves with new challenges and responsibilities, to be aware of the "tendencies of the times," and to concern themselves with the organization of medical care:

> Future progress in the reduction of mortality and in the promotion of health and efficiency depends chiefly on the application of medical science to the early diagnosis and preventive treatment of disease. . . . In the last analysis, it will be the duty of the health officer of the future to see that the people under his charge, in city or country, in palace or tenement, have the opportunity of receiving such service and on terms which make it economically and psychologically easy of attainment.[37]

Without mentioning the group with which he had aligned himself, he said that there were hopeful signs that some attempts were being made to resolve the problems attendant to medical care costs. There were also some interesting programs in operation in both Europe and the United States, for example, which needed careful evaluation. Some of these programs were sound and significant, others frivolous and superficial, but "the habit of condemning any attempt at intelligent community action by labeling it 'socialistic' or 'bureaucratic' is an example unworthy of serious-minded men." Some things were better done by the individual, some better by the state; but the "catchwords would not help us to determine to which class a given activity belonged,"[38] he concluded.

Winslow said that he favored no single solution. He was not for group practice, state medicine, health insurance, "or any other panacea," as each system could be legitimately criticized. There were "very serious dangers" in almost any plan for the better organization of medical service, and only the "maximum broad-minded statesmanship" on the part of both health officials and the medical profession would assure a satisfactory solution.[39] A programmatic solution might not be forthcoming for "twenty years," he said; but if his speech served the purpose he had intended, the health officer of the future, and his parent organization, would lose no time in embarking upon a program of research and demonstration in cooperation with the medical profession to resolve the issues as he had outlined them.

A few months later, the committee of five, now comprised of Winifred Smith, Lewellys Barker, Michael M. Davis, Walton H. Hamilton, and Winslow, with Harry H. Moore, acting as secretary, submitted their report to their parent body, the Conference on the Economic Factors Affecting the Organization of Medicine. The report recommended that an organization be established with the title "The Temporary Committee on Medical Economics" the principal functions of which would be to analyze the problem of medical organization, particularly of its economic factors, and to interest professional groups and the public in the facts about medical service.[40] In a subsequent meeting, an executive committee was appointed, with Davis, Haven Emerson, and J. Shelton Horsley as members and Winslow as chairman.[41] Winslow was also vice-chairman of the "Temporary Committee," which in 1927 had taken the title "Committee on the Cost [*sic*] of Medical Care."[42]

CCMC, founded in 1927, went into high gear a year later. Funded by eight foundations and chaired by Ray Lyman Wilbur, it at first had 48 members, from the healing arts, public health, health institutions, economics, and the general public, over half of whom held the medical degree. Its principal objective was mainly a fact-finding one, and between 1929 and 1932, CCMC issued 27 volumes, a veritable library on medical circumstances and the problems of the time.

The year-by-year progress of CCMC and an analysis of CCMC's internal affairs, staff and field work, analytic studies, and accomplishments and frustrations—a bittersweet episode in the annals of medical care—is another story.[43] But what can be divined from the minutes of CCMC and from Winslow's correspondence and his published writings are his efforts to guide CCMC through a rather tortuous path marked at every turn by conflicting ideologies and ambiguity. This was where Winslow brought his special administrative genius to play. His style of leadership is best illustrated in a speech[44] he gave in 1930 at the Henry Street Visiting Nurse Service.

There was a new leadership abroad in the land, he said, a leadership which was no longer "mastership," but which recognized that every human being has his own contribution to make to the common task. This new leadership was "centripedal and not centrifugal"; the leader did not "radiate force to receptive subordinates," but formed "a coordinating center and a channel of expression for a group of vitally functioning sources of independent power." The wise leader "comes not to get or to give but to share in a creative process." There was no conflict between minds, he said, but there was "a common conflict of all against the common enemy, which is old chaos." He quoted from Heraclitus—"Nature desires eagerly opposites and out of them it completes its harmony, not out of similars"—and concluded that out of such a meeting would come "not compromise but integration."[45] It was the integration of ideas, data, and concepts, based on "expert technical knowledge," that he attempted to win from the members of CCMC. In the end he only partially achieved his goal and began to realize that even the elegance of compromise had limitations.

The task to which CCMC committed itself reflected the confidence of its leadership that "concerted study, analysis, and reflection on the part of knowledgeable and concerned people could result in a program useful for dealing with problems calling for societal resolution."[46] As Winslow wrote to John A. Kingsbury, secretary of the Milbank Memorial Fund, one of CCMC's sponsors:

> I feel quite sure from my knowledge of the general field of public health that there is nothing within the entire field which is of such vital moment

as a fundamental analysis of the relationship between the medical profession and the public. This must be our major task for the next twenty years. In order to approach it with success it is necessary first of all to secure a fundamental body of exact data. . . . The Committee on the Cost of Medical Care will be a fact finding body. It will accumulate the data and draw conclusions as to existing conditions but will not formulate policies.[47]

The man most closely identified with physician interests in CCMC was Olin West, then executive secretary of the American Medical Association. In another letter to Kingsbury, Winslow wrote that CCMC was happy to have such a high ranking physician on board:

There are most encouraging indications of new influences at work in the AMA. Not only have they consented that Olin West shall be a member of the Committee on the Cost of Medical Care but they have also approved the appointment of a joint committee to discuss with the APHA points of friction and possibilities of cooperation between health departments and the medical profession. This is a great step forward and I think we owe it very largely to the influence of President Wilbur.[48]

Kingsbury was not as sanguine as Winslow: "I am glad to know that indications of new influences at work in the AMA are encouraging but beware of Greeks bearing gifts!"[49] Nevertheless, Winslow believed it vital to have the physicians' support and not to alienate them or to make them feel that they were in hostile territory. Much time was spent, for example, in trying to "educate" physicians about CCMC's origins, plans, and aims and in reassuring them that neither the staff nor the membership of CCMC held preconceived notions or were responsible to any previously established organization.[50]

On one side were physicians, Winslow felt, and on the other insistent reformers—both had to be held in line. To Kingsbury, Winslow offered the following reassurance:

I realize very fully that on this committee I am attempting the most delicate and dangerous thing that I have ever done. With the persons who are providing the funds [you are] animated by a very natural and logical resentment against the medical profession, and with Wilbur earnestly anxious to bring the medical profession into line and desirous of not antagonizing them. I know, however, that you will trust me not to sacrifice any essential interests and I think we can afford to step carefully relying on the logic of the situation and the underlying facts to keep us straight.[51]

In 1929, Winslow spent a summer in Europe as a member of an international commission appointed by the Health Organization of the League of Nations and the International Labor Bureau to study the relationship between health insurance and public health work. In a memorandum, he reflected on the European scene and considered lessons for the United States. "I have come to the fairly definite conclusion," he wrote, "that sickness insurance of the continental pattern would not fit into the social and economic conditions of America and is not likely to do so for some time to come." This was primarily owing to the "wide differences in political structure, in social conditions, and in national psychology." Both for the patient and physician, he had found as many dangers as he had advantages. The "right personal relationship between physician and patient," he wrote, formed "as essential a therapeutic agent as an x-ray machine." And, in considering reform in the United States, the "technical need for organization and the human need for individualization" would have to be balanced, one against the other.[52] "The principle of insurance against illness," he concluded, "seems an essentially sound one and appears capable of improving medical care on the one hand and increasing the aggregate income of the medical profession on the other. It seems to the writer, however, that the possibilities of voluntary insurance should be thoroughly explored before resorting to compulsion in the United States."[53]

In the memorandum, which was published in the *New England Journal of Medicine,* Winslow appeared to be reassuring physicians by limiting CCMC's recommendations.[54] In fact, he stated categorically that the United States was not yet ready for compulsory health insurance, despite the more radical arguments of Kingsbury and others. Organization in the provision of medical service, Winslow believed, was inevitable and desirable, but was not necessarily related to the insurance principle. Whatever would be done in this direction, he concluded, would have to be done "with the view to a minimum sacrifice of the personal relation between physician and patient and to the maintenance of the morale of the general practitioner."[55]

By defending the medical profession whenever possible and by effecting compromise and "integration" of conflicting views, Winslow and Wilbur sought a consensus for their ultimate objective. They even accepted the possibility of minority reports—"entirely sound procedures" in studies of this magnitude, as Wilbur wrote to Winslow.[56] But their collective hope that, if possible, the minority reports would be constructive and "point the way to the provision of more adequate medical care for all the people, rich and poor, at a cost within their means"[57] was not to be realized. Winslow soon recognized what they were up against. The physicians—"Follansbee, West, et al"—wrote Winslow to Lewellys Barker, "are, I am sorry to say, very much off the reservation, and there will certainly be a more or less vehement minority report on the conservative side." There will not be too much objection to a minority report, he continued, "if the minority is not too large," but it would be "a very serious matter if this minority report were signed by a large number of medical men for it would mean setting the stage for a war between the professionals and the public which is precisely the thing we have wanted to avoid."[58]

In the end, CCMC's majority report[59] was better than Winslow had feared. It included five recommendations, of which three were concerned with strengthening public health services, coordinating all health services, and with health manpower and training. The major recommendations were that: comprehensive medical care should be provided by organized groups of practitioners; that medical care costs should be placed on a group payment basis, whether through insurance, taxation, or both; and that payment through individual fee-for-service should continue to be available for those who preferred it. The principal minority report took issue with the call for group practice and group payment, recommending instead solo practice and business as usual; but, no matter, wrote Winslow, "I feel more and more sure that we are right and that the truth will ultimately prevail."[60]

Winslow was among those who discussed and defended the recommendations of CCMC immediately following the publication of its final report. He was responsible for presenting its conclusions and recommendations to a session held at the New York Academy of Medicine in November, 1932[61] and also prepared an analysis for *Science,* which appeared in January, 1933.[62] In both presentations he placed CCMC's activities in historical perspective by first discussing the changing role of the physician, from "priestly mission" to "half priest, half businessman, a servant of society in a world which has ceased to recognize service except as measured by financial return, a businessman in a field where the fundamental requirements of basic human need preclude the application of ordinary principles of economic individualism."[63] In the *Science* article he not only reviewed the principal findings and recommendations but also addressed the arguments of CCMC's critics.

The final report had been vigorously criticized,[64] which Winslow believed was "highly encouraging, since only platitudes receive easy and general acceptation,"[65] but some of the criticism was excessive and unfounded. CCMC, for example, had been charged with advocating socialism and communism—"inciting to revolution." Winslow dismissed this as spurious because CCMC's entire program had been based primarily on group practice in voluntary hospitals and on group purchase by privately organized bodies of citizens. General revenue taxes, he said, would be used only for rural areas where there were no other sources of funding and for the support of the indigent, which was already an accepted form of service provided in the United States.[66]

A second criticism was that CCMC advocated contract medicine, a practice considered unethical and which critics believed would lead to unfair competition among physicians. Winslow wrote that CCMC had found that group practice was viable and that physicians practicing in such groups were satisfactorily compensated; moreover, they furnished equivalent care to patients at costs lower than those of their colleagues practicing individually in the community. The advantages which accrued directly from the organized nature of group practice, he argued, were clearly in the interest of both the profession and the public and, "therefore, no condemnation of unfair competition which is based only on such advantages can ultimately be maintained."[67]

Critics also charged that laymen would "control" medical practice. CCMC, however, had stated unequivocally that lay groups "organized for profits" had no legitimate place in the provision of "vital public service." Yet such service also meant that there were also "vital public interests at stake." Medicine needed large capital outlays and the public had a right to participate in such matters. He concluded that the combination of a "lay board representing the public interests involved and a professional staff in full control of professional policies" was a rational solution to the problem.[68]

Another criticism was that group practice and prepayment would wipe out "the essential personal relationship between physician and patient." Winslow replied that this had not happened in the university or industrial services that had been studied by CCMC. In a properly organized medical center, moreover, the relationship between patient and family physician could be restored to a new importance and dignity "and freed from the constant inhibitions on both sides which are due to the intrusion of the element of pecuniary responsibility at every stage in what should be a free personal relationship."[69] Winslow concluded in characteristically lapidary style: "Experimental social planning along sound theoretical lines, but based on existing American institutions—this is the objective set before us for the solution of the economic problem of medical care."[70] Throughout the Depression, Winslow and others continued to search for an "American solution."

As the economic situation worsened and medical care and other social needs far exceeded the capacities of state and local governments and voluntary agencies, the federal government finally accepted its responsibility for the public's health. At the National Health Conference held during the summer of 1938 in Washington, D.C., the discussion centered on the national health program advanced by the Technical Committee on Medical Care of the Federal Interdepartmental Committee to Coordinate Health and Welfare Activities.[71] The Technical Committee, chaired by Dr. Martha Eliot, then assistant chief of the Children's Bureau, brought out new studies on the social needs of the nation. Their survey of more than 800,000 families revealed unemployment, starvation wages, shameful housing, inadequate nutrition, and the stark connection of poverty to sickness. The cost to the nation of sickness alone was estimated at $10 billion! The Technical Committee recommended a program which covered the areas of public health, maternal and child welfare, care of the indigent, hospitalization, and health and disability insurance.[72]

Winslow was one of many participants who spoke at the Conference. He favored a national program which included project and grant moneys for states wishing to develop a health program and which would also permit them to enact voluntary or compulsory health insurance programs. He again attempted to achieve consensus and avoid the acrimonious schisms of the past, but despite his appeals and those of such public health advocates as Paul Kellogg, Josephine Roche, John P. Peters, Martha Eliot, Alice Hamilton, and others, the AMA and its spokesman remained adamantly opposed to change. And in debating the advocates of the status quo, Winslow argued that national governmental action and compulsory health insurance were the only remedies for America's health problems.[73]

A year later, at a special APHA session on the public health aspects of medical care, Winslow discussed the Conference in the most exuberant terms. He believed that those whose reputations had been tarnished by association with CCMC had been vindicated. The Technical Committee's surveys had substantiated everything CCMC had found and had adopted the principal recommendations of CCMC's majority. "To many of us, it seems that at last our dreams of twenty years ago are coming true," he said.[74]

Between 1939 and his last active years in the 1950s, Winslow supported those government leaders advocating a national health program which included national health insurance. He continued to write and speak on behalf of national health causes throughout the war. In 1940, at a Town Meeting he discussed with Henry E. Sigerist and Terry M. Townsend the question: "Does America Need Compulsory Health Insurance?"[75] Winslow, representing "the consumer," was troubled by inaction. So much had been said and written about the subject that he was surprised to find himself again on a platform debating pros and cons of a matter that should be obvious to everyone. "We stand still and quarrel about details and about hypothetical damage to vested interests while men, women, and children suffer and die for the lack of the resources of modern medical science,"[76] he said.

> Let us forget slogans and avoid vague terminologies which arouse the secretions of the endocrine glands instead of stimulating the higher nerve centers. Let us recognize that the situation is serious and calls for action. Let us remember that there is no single easy solution of the problem, but that what we need is a national program so constructed as to enable the people of the United States to obtain and pay for the medical care that they need, whether they pay for it as individuals, as groups, or as taxpayers.[77]

In this address and in others delivered during the 1940s, he offered his solutions with renewed force and clarity:

> Medical care is not a luxury to be purchased at will by the wealthy. It is a fundamental necessity for normal human living. It can only be made really attainable on a systematic prepayment basis, by voluntary insurance for the group which can readily pay the average but not the emergency costs of illness; by compulsory health insurance, with supplement by subsidy when necessary, for the next lower economic group; and by tax support for the group which cannot pay even a part of its medical bills, or which cannot be readily organized under an insurance plan. Furthermore, in any of these categories a reasonable quality of service and reasonable economy of service must be ensured by group practice under competent medical supervision.[78]

Winslow supported the legislative proposals developed in 1939 and helped to draft a part of President Truman's National Health Program Message of November, 1945;[79] in the 1940s and early 1950s he served as consultant to the World Health Organization.[80] In 1944, when he was 67, he became editor of the *American Journal of Public Health*. Despite the years of stalemate and frustration, World War II, the new barbarism, and political reaction, Winslow was the "sweet voice of reason"—a philosopher, clarifier, interpreter, and visionary.

Although there were many themes to Winslow's editorials, the titles are deceptive, for although they concern standard public health subjects, the articles themselves include much more. Each subject was presented in a social context, revealing a technical knowledge not only of the field but also of its political, economic, and cultural underpinnings. In a Winslow editorial on medical care, for example, the reader could learn about democratic principles, social systems, and social justice;[81] in a discussion of slums, about exploitation, greed, and unheralded courage;[82] and in an article on the validity of data, about arrogance, humility, and the public health spirit.[83]

Winslow's editorials were masterfully written essays. There were references to the Bible, to Arnold, Carlyle, and Shakespeare, as well as to Pasteur, Panum, Simon, Biggs, Sedgwick, and Chapin. There were discussions of pending health legislation,[84] children,[85] the elderly,[86] and the tubercular.[87] There were summaries of annual APHA meetings,[88] and obituaries that were written with a grace and insight that captured the essence of his former colleagues-in-arms, their era, and their contributions.[89] There was a brilliance here, and an unbridled optimism; but there were also some editorials—those which dealt with man's ignorance, stupidity, and fear, for example—which revealed a sadness that man had not progressed far enough from the primitive state.[90]

His essay "Who Killed Cock Robin?", widely quoted in the literature, satirized the claim by the "National Committee for the Extension of Medical Service" that past achievements had been accomplished only by "American Doctors" operating under "the American system" —meaning, obviously, the private practice by individual physicians on a fee-for-service basis. "Let's look at the record," he wrote. Data revealed that "organized health forces representing the public interest" had been responsible for most of the reduction in mortality and morbidity and not the private practitioners, who had often strenuously opposed many of the public health initiatives when originally introduced.[91]

In an editorial summarizing APHA's 1944 annual meeting, he described the special session devoted to medical care. He was enthusi-

astic that a report, "Medical Care in a National Health Program," had
been adopted by APHA, at long last putting "APHA squarely on the
record in favor of a national program."

> This is a bold pronouncement [he wrote], which required real courage
> to adopt. The policy outlined is sound and will, we believe, receive the
> very serious consideration of legislators concerned with this challenging
> problem. It is fitting and proper that the first clear and constructive
> statement of a national program of medical care to be made by any
> national body of experts should come from the A.P.H.A.—since the
> health officer represents professional knowledge on the one side and
> community responsibility on the other. The physician is bound by a
> Hippocratic oath which calls for the highest standard of service to those
> individual patients who call upon his skill. The health officer is the one
> person whose oath of office lays upon him the responsibility of planning
> for the health of the community as a whole. That responsibility has been
> assumed—with modesty, but with a compelling sense of public duty—in
> the adoption of [this resolution.][92]

In an editorial devoted to APHA's medical care policy statement,
in which he also considered a report on "Principles of a New Health
Program" prepared by a Health Program Conference chaired by Michael M. Davis and one about a conference sponsored by the Physician's Forum for the Study of Medical Care, Winslow concluded that,
although the three differed in their emphasis in detail, they were iden-
tical in their essential trends. "It seems clear that the question before
the American people is not 'Whether' but 'How.' "[93]

And, in an editorial entitled "Galileo Was Right," which was
prompted by a Brookings Institution report on medical care which had
concluded that the experience of the United States since 1932 had
"demonstrated the wisdom" of CCMC's majority recommendations,
he reviewed the majority recommendations of CCMC, the American
Medical Association's criticism of CCMC's final report, and the
changed environment of 1948. Even the AMA, he wrote, had "moved
on to almost the exact position taken by CCMC." What was "socialism
and communism—inciting to revolution"—was now "accepted doctrine" in the minds of "such highly conservative groups" as the Brookings Institution and AMA, he wrote. "Public opinion necessarily moves
slowly; but the ground gained by cooperative thinking is most encouraging. . . . Galileo was right. The world does *move.* "[94]

It was his faith, too, that appears in the editorials, just as it had
in all that he had written throughout his life. One of his favorite books

was H.G. Well's fantasy *The Food of the Gods* in which a godlike youth, a giant, who had been raised by jealous and fearful men as a prisoner in a quarry and had been kept in ignorance of the world about him, escaped to London where he stood towering above the hurrying frightened crowds. Amazed at their numbers and activities, the youth cried out in wonder, "What are all you people doing with yourselves? What is it all for and where do I come in?"[95] In his valedictory address delivered in 1945 to the Yale Medical School, Winslow again asked: "What are you all for anyway?"[96] His answer—and his valedictory message—was a quote from Arnold's essay "Culture and Anarchy."

> . . . there is of culture another view, in which not solely the scientific passion, the sheer desire to see things as they are, natural and proper in an intelligent being, appears as the ground of it. There is a view in which all the love of our neighbour, the impulses toward action, help, and beneficence, the desire for removing human error, clearing human confusion, and diminishing human misery, the noble aspiration to leave the world better and happier than we found it—motives eminently such as are called social—come in as part of the grounds of culture, and the main and preeminent part. Culture is then properly described not as having its origin in curiosity, but as having its origin in the love of perfection; it is *a study of perfection.*[97]

It was man's duty to strive, to "leave the world better and happier" than he had found it, to be useful, to advance always with hope and courage—this was the motive for a life of service in the cause of humanity.[98]

Notes

1. R.W. McCollum, "Introduction," in A.J. Viseltear (ed.), "C.-E.A. Winslow Day: Proceedings of the June 3, 1977 Centenary Celebration," *Yale Journal of Biology and Medicine*, 1977, *50*, 603–630. The C.-E.A. Winslow Papers, extending for more than 150 linear feet, have been deposited in the "Contemporary Medical Care and Health Policy Collection" of Manuscripts and Archives, Yale University Library. Articles about Winslow have been mostly memorials. See I.V. Hiscock, "Charles-Edward Amory Winslow, February 4, 1877—January 8, 1957," *Journal of Bacteriology*, 1957, *73*, 295–296; "Charles-Edward Amory Winslow, 1877–1957," *American Journal of Public Health*, 1957, *47*, 153–167; John F. Fulton, "C.-E.A. Winslow, Leader in Public Health," *Science*, 1957, *125*, 1236. See also R.M. Acheson, "The Epidemiology of Charles-Edward Amory Winslow," *Journal of Epidemiology*, 1970, *91*, 1–18.

2. C.-E.A. Winslow, "The Untilled Fields of Public Health," *Modern Medicine*, 1920, *2*, 6–7.

3.   See Edgar Sydenstricker, "The Changing Concept of Public Health," *Milbank Memorial Fund Quarterly*, 1935, *13*, 301–310.

4.   See O.W. Anderson, *The Uneasy Equilibrium* (New Haven, 1968), pp. 57–88.

5.   In the Library of the Department of Epidemiology and Public Health, Yale University School of Medicine, where Winslow's Library was deposited, there is a collection of reprints from the *Public Health Reports*, bound and reissued by the U.S. Public Health Service dating from 1916 to 1917. See, for example, L.K. Frankel and L.I. Dublin, *Community Sickness Survey, Rochester, N.Y., September, 1915* (Washington, 1916).

6.   Also in Winslow's book collection is a copy of J.R. Commons and A.J. Altmeyer, "Special Report XVI. The Health Insurance Movement in the United States," in *Report of the Health Insurance Commission of the State of Illinois* (Springfield, 1919). See especially pp. 625–647.

7.   C.-E.A. Winslow, *Public Health Administration in Russia in 1917* (Washington, 1918), (Reprint No. 445 from the *Public Health Reports*, December 28, 1917, pp. 2191–2219.)

8.   *Ibid.*, p. 5.

9.   *Ibid.*, p. 30.

10.   *Ibid.*

11.   See, for example, Anderson, *op.cit.* (n.4), R.L. Numbers, *Almost Persuaded* (Baltimore, 1978), and A.J. Viseltear, "Compulsory Health Insurance in California, 1915–1918," *Journal of the History of Medicine and Allied Sciences*, 1969, *24*, 151–182.

12.   C.-E.A. Winslow, "Poverty as a Factor in Disease," *Proceedings of the National Conference of Social Work* (Chicago, 1919), pp. 153–156.

13.   *Ibid.*, p. 154.

14.   See Hermann M. Biggs, "The New York State Health Centers Bill," *New York State Journal of Medicine*, 1921, *21*, 6–9 and Milton Terris, "Hermann Biggs' Contribution to the Modern Concept of the Health Center," *Bulletin of the History of Medicine*, 1946, *20*, 387–412.

15.   See C.-E.A. Winslow, *The Life of Hermann M. Biggs* (Philadelphia, 1929), pp. 354–355.

16.   C.-E.A. Winslow, *The Evolution and Significance of the Modern Public Health Campaign* (New Haven, 1925). Originally delivered as an address under the auspices of the Gamma Alpha Fraternity of Yale University, 1923.

17.   *Ibid.*, pp. 50–57.

18.   *Ibid.*, pp. 61–62.

19.   *Ibid.*, pp. 63–64.

20.   These were anatomy, physiology and physiological chemistry, bacteriology and pathology, pharmacology, medicine, surgery, pediatrics, and obstetrics and gynecology.

21.   C.-E.A. Winslow, "The Place of Public Health in a University," *Scinece*, 1925, *62*, p. 337.

22.   *Ibid.*

23. *Ibid.*

24. C.-E.A. Winslow, "Strategic Position of the Dispensary in the Public Health Campaign," *The Nation's Health,* 1926, 8, 1–4.

25. *Ibid.,* pp. 3–4.

26. *Ibid.,* p. 4.

27. See Grace Abbott, "Federal Aid for the Protection of Maternity and Infancy," *American Journal of Public Health,* 1922, *12,* 737–742.

28. See A.J. Viseltear, *Emergence of the Medical Care Section of the American Public Health Association, 1926–1948* (Washington, 1972), pp. 4–5.

29. See D.B. and E.B. Armstrong, "What the Doctors Must Do," *Survey,* 1920, *44,* 707–710.

30. See, for example, W.S. Rankin, "The Next Step for State Health Departments," *American Journal of Public Health,* 1922, *12,* 1000–1002 and D.B. Armstrong, "Social Uses of Medicine," *ibid.,* 1920, *10,* 921–931.

31. L.F. Barker, "The Future of Medicine in America," *New York State Journal of Medicine,* 1921, *21,* 193–195.

32. Armstrong, *op. cit.* (n. 29), p. 707.

33. See, "Minutes of a Meeting of the Committee of Five of the Informal Conference to Consider the Economic Factors Affecting the Organization of Medicine, April 1, 1926 and April 15, 1926." Winslow Papers, Box 11.

34. *Ibid.,* April 15, 1926.

35. C.-E.A. Winslow, "Public Health at the Crossroads," *American Journal of Public Health,* 1926, *16,* 1075–1085.

36. *Ibid.,* p. 1077.

37. *Ibid.,* p. 1084.

38. *Ibid.,* p. 1082.

39. *Ibid.,* pp. 1082–1083.

40. Minutes of the Committee of Five, May 31, 1926. Winslow Papers, Box 11.

41. Reported by H.H. Moore, in "Report of a Conference on the Economic Factors Affecting the Organization of Medicine with Recommendations for a Committee to Conduct a Five Years' Study in this Field, March 27, 1927." Winslow Papers, Box 11.

42. On May 2, 1930, debate centered on changing the name of the Committee on the Cost of Medical Care "to avoid misunderstanding of its field of interest." During the same meeting, Haven Emerson suggested "The Committee on Medical Care." Later in the day, the name of the organization was approved as "The Committee on Costs of Medical Care," and on May 3, 1930, officially ratified as "The Committee on the Costs of Medical Care." Winslow Papers, Box 11.

43. See, D.S. Hirshfield, *The Lost Reform* (Cambridge, 1970) and Anderson, *op. cit.* (n. 4).

44. C.-E.A. Winslow, "The New Leadership," *Public Health Nurse,* 1931, *23,* 108–113.

45. *Ibid.*, p. 111.

46. I.S. Falk, "Medical Care in the U.S.A., 1932–1974," *Milbank Memorial Fund Quarterly*, 1973, *51*, p. 3. Professor Falk was the associate director of the Research Staff of CCMC, serving under H.H. Moore.

47. Winslow to Kingsbury, May 19, 1927. Winslow Papers, 19/40.

48. *Ibid.*, December 23, 1927.

49. Kingsbury to Winslow, December 23, 1927. Winslow Papers, 19/40.

50. Ray Lyman Wilbur to Dr. Morris Fishbein, May 29, 1928. Winslow Papers, Box 11.

51. Winslow to Kingsbury, January 5, 1928. Winslow Papers 19/40.

52. C.-E.A. Winslow, "Some Reflections on Sickness Insurance in Germany and Austria," *New England Journal of Medicine*, 1929, *200*, 1161–1163. See also Winslow's "Sickness Insurance in Central Europe and Its Lessons for Us in the United States," *Yale Journal of Biology and Medicine*, 1929, *1*, 391–402.

53. *Ibid.*, *Yale Journal*, p. 401–402.

54. Kingsbury, for example, wanted CCMC to take testimony from George F. McCleary of Great Britain. Harry H. Moore declined the offer. Kingsbury, however, had his way and McCleary subsequently met with a number of CCMC members. See Kingsbury to H.H. Moore. Winslow Papers, Box 11. See also G.F. McCleary, "English Health Insurance and the Standard of Medical Service," *Milbank Memorial Fund Quarterly*, 1933, *11*, 83–87.

55. Winslow, *Yale Journal, op. cit.* (n. 52), p. 402.

56. Wilbur to Winslow, September 12, 1932. Winslow Papers, Box 11.

57. *Ibid.*

58. Winslow to L.F. Barker, October 15, 1932. Winslow Papers, Box 11.

59. See *Medical Care for the American People, The Final Report of the Committee on the Costs of Medical Care.* Reprinted by the U.S. Department of Health, Education, and Welfare, Public Health Service (Washington, 1970).

60. Winslow to Moore, February 25, 1933. Winslow Papers, Box 11.

61. C.-E.A. Winslow, "The Recommendations of the Committee on the Costs of Medical Care," *New England Journal of Medicine*, 1932, *207*, 1138–1142.

62. Winslow, "A Program of Medical Care for the United States," *Science*, 1933, *77*, 102–107.

63. *Ibid.*, p. 102. See, also, Winslow, "The Physician—Priest or Businessman," *Bulletin of the Medical Library Association*, 1946, *34*, 310–319.

64. Despite the furor, Wilbur, Winslow and others accepted the criticism calmly, for they believed that in the long run they would succeed. Winslow sent the following message to Wilbur:

> "I am personally not at all disturbed about the controversy or about the immediate popular reaction [to the final report]. I suspect that the public as well as the medical profession will in general regard our recommendations as altogether too radical and that the report will appear during the next six months to have failed of its objectives. This is of no consequence, however. What we are looking for is the effect

of our analysis during the next ten years upon the thousand or two leaders in the various communities in America. While the tumult and the shouting is going on these men will be thinking, and if our conclusions are sound, as I think they are, they will work themselves out. I suggest that in 1942 we have a reunion dinner to consider progress, and I think we shall find it notable." Winslow to Wilbur, December 1, 1932. Winslow Papers, Box 11.

Wilbur concurred:

". . . all things considered, it seems to me that we are making progress at about the rate that could be expected. We will have to go through this preliminary period of personal attack etc., before the medical profession as a group actually settles down to face the issue. It is a new and trying experience for them and I can quite understand their reluctance to accept practical solutions." Wilbur to Winslow, February 20, 1933. Winslow Papers, Box 11.

65. Winslow, *op. cit.* (n. 62), p. 106.

66. *Ibid.*

67. *Ibid.*, pp. 106–107.

68. *Ibid.*, p. 107.

69. *Ibid.*

70. *Ibid.*

71. See, Viseltear (n. 28), pp. 7–8.

72. C.-E.A. Winslow, "The Public Health Aspects of Medical Care," *American Journal of Public Health*, 1939, *29*, 16–22

73. *Ibid.*, pp. 20–22.

74. *Ibid.*, p. 22.

75. "Does America Need Compulsory Health Insurance?," *Town Meeting*, 1940, *5*, 1–28. (January 22, 1940). Dr. Henry E. Sigerist was introduced as "Professor of the History of Medicine in Johns Hopkins University, leading exponent of socialized medicine in America; Dr. Terry M. Townsend, President of the Medical Society of the State of New York; and Dr. C.-E.A. Winslow, Professor of Public Health in Yale University."

76. *Ibid.*, p. 16.

77. *Ibid.*, pp. 16–17.

78. C.-E.A. Winslow, "The Future—Problems and Trends," in *The University and Public Health Statesmanship* (Philadelphia, 1941), pp. 21–33.

79. Winslow Papers, Box 12 (Addition, 1975).

80. See Winslow's, *The Cost of Sickness and the Price of Health* (Geneva, 1951).

81. See, for example, "Constructive Thinking about Medical Care," *American Journal of Public Health*, 1945, *35*, 159–162; "A Health Department Medical Care Program," *ibid.*, 1948, *38*, 555–557; "The National Health Assembly of 1948," *ibid.*, 851–852; and "The Morning After," *ibid.*, 1694–1696.

82. For example, "Friends of the Slum," *ibid.*, 1944, *34*, 387–388 and "The Key to Slum Elimination," *ibid.*, 1949, *39*, 1581–1582.

83. "Who Killed Cock Robin?," *ibid.*, 1944, *34*, 658–659.

84. For example, "The Wagner Bill of 1945," *ibid.*, 1945, *35*, 824–825; "Public Health in the Eightieth Congress," *ibid.*, 1948, *38*, 90–93 and "The Hospital Survey and Construction Program," *ibid.*, 1949, *39*, 1468–1469.

85. See "The Challenge of Child Care," *ibid.*, 1949, *39*, 1176–1177.

86. See "Health Problems of an Aging Population," *ibid.*, 1949, *38*, 1698–1699.

87. See "Administrative Judgment in the Control of Tuberculosis," *ibid.*, 1948, *38*, 557–559.

88. "The Atlantic City Meeting," *ibid.*, 1947, *37*, 1590–1592.

89. See, for example, "Milton Joseph Rosenau," *ibid.*, 1946, *36*, 530–531 and "Hugh S. Cumming," *ibid.*, 1949, *39*, 225.

90. See especially, "Who Is Un-American Now?," *ibid.*, 1947, *37*, 1592–1595.

91. *Op. cit.* (n. 83).

92. See "The Second Wartime Public Health Conference," *ibid.*, 1944, *34*, 1183–1185.

93. "Constructive Thinking," *op. cit.* (n. 81).

94. "Galileo Was Right," *ibid.*, 1948, *38*, 1275–1276.

95. *Op. cit.* (n. 24), p. 1.

96. C.-E.A. Winslow, "Yale Valedictory, 1945," *Yale Journal of Biology and Medicine,* 1945, *18*, 1–5.

97. *Ibid.*, p. 5

98. See "Sedgwick Memorial Medal Awarded to Dr. C.-E.A. Winslow," *American Journal of Public Health,* 1942, *32*, 1416–1417.

The American Journal
of Public Health
1957–1973

ALFRED YANKAUER*

In 1957, the *American Journal of Public Health,* official organ of the American Public Health Association, was just one year younger than its new editor, Dr. George Rosen. Rosen, a member of the *Journal's* Editorial Board for the preceding ten years, succeeded Abel Wolman, a distinguished sanitary engineer, as editor. Of the eight editors who preceded Rosen, only one, Dr. Mazÿck P. Ravenel, held the position for a comparable length of time. Both Ravenel and Rosen edited the *Journal* for sixteen years—Ravenel from 1924 to 1940 and Rosen from 1957 to 1973. These two sixteen-year spans, in contrast to the intervening and preceding periods, were times of great change for the public health infrastructure and the health care system of the United States.

The antecedents and early days of the *Journal* which Ravenel and Rosen edited were described by Rosen himself in 1972 in a broad summary that also comments briefly on the years of his own tenure.[1] Although preceded by other publications, the *Journal,* as the official organ of the American Public Health Association, first appeared in 1911, acquired its present name in 1912, expanded the name in 1927 to absorb another publication, *The Nation's Health,* and dropped the expanded name in 1971 when its parent organization initiated a monthly newspaper called *The Nation's Health.*[2] During Ravenel's tenure the *Journal* grew from a small organ—initially (in 1911) little more than a report of the annual meeting and a topically oriented newsletter to serve the 700-member Association—to a nationally recognized periodical speaking for what was then a cohesive American public health movement close to the summit of its influence and power.

Ravenel's tenure spanned the boom of the late 1920s, and the bust and slow recovery which followed. In the middle of his tenure at the zenith of the New Deal, the Social Security Act of 1935 was passed. This legislation was the most important federal action affecting the health field in the history of the United States up to that time. During

229

these sixteen years the growth of a public health organization rooted in local government prior tó the Social Security Act is illustrated by the increase in county health departments from 278 with a total budget of $3.5 million in 1924 to 610 with a budget of $9.2 million in 1931.[3] The Social Security Act strengthened this infrastructure and accelerated this growth by providing grants-in-aid to state health departments to initiate and expand public health programs.

For the American public health movement, the years of Ravenel's editorship were a time of consolidation and strengthening along traditional lines that were clearly defined and understood and which were further solidified by the Social Security Act of 1935. This tradition reached its peak and began to decline with the publication in 1945 of *Local Health Units for the Nation* by Haven Emerson and Martha Luginbuhl.[4] The undifferentiated nature of the growth of the public health movement during Ravenel's years is reflected by the fact that although active membership of the American Public Health Association doubled, rising from 3,049 in 1924 to 6,334 in 1940, only one new section, the Epidemiology section was formed within the organization during this decade and a half. In 1940, the *Journal* reached 2,000 subscribers in addition to the 6,334 APHA members and fellows. This addition did no more than round out, as sections within the Association, what Dr. Emerson and his contemporaries regarded as the basic public health activities: Statistics, sanitation, health education, nutrition, maternal and child health, and laboratory services already had their Association sections; with the epidemiology section, communicable disease control was now added to them. Rosen's tenure spanned a turbulent era that extended from the Cold War to Watergate, with the War on Poverty, the Vietnam War, the civil rights movement, and the youth revolt sandwiched between. The greatest changes in public health occurred under President Johnson when several major health care amendments (e.g., Medicare and Medicaid) were added to the Social Security Act. Simultaneously, other far-reaching health legislation was also enacted. These actions constituted the most important federal actions affecting the health field in 30 years.

Their net effect undermined the responsibilities and importance of the state and local health departments. Administration of the Medicare and Medicaid programs, which are essentially bill-paying mechanisms, became the responsibility of the Social Security Administration and the Social and Rehabilitation Service at the federal level, with little involvement by the Public Health Service; and, with rare exceptions, welfare departments became the designated state agencies for administration of Medicaid. Other categorical health programs aimed primarily at the needs of the poor (e.g., neighborhood health centers, model cities, maternity, infancy, and children's programs, and community mental health centers) were administered by a variety of local agencies or groups receiving federal grants or contracts. Only a minority of these projects were the responsibility of local health departments.

There were other important federal health initiatives (e.g., the Regional Medical Programs and comprehensive health planning) only peripherally related to the existing public health departments in the states and communities. Concurrently, the U. S. Public Health Service, which had provided professional leadership in public health since 1798, was virtually dismantled. In short, during the midyears of Dr. Rosen's term as editor, there was a virtual revolution in how the public's health business was conducted.

This essay does not seek to interpret the meaning of significance of these changes in U. S. health policy, but to describe how a journal sponsored by an association of public health professionals endured these troublesome times. The term public health is presently defined and understood differently by different people, including those who consider themselves public health practitioners, teachers, administrators, or researchers. On the one hand, it may be considered as any activity requiring the combination of professional skills which are needed to promote and protect the health of the people through social action at an organizational level. On the other, it may be viewed as a police function combined with a pot-pourri of health-related activities which have no other home. In any case, it is clear that its span is broad, its membership interdisciplinary, and its definition amorphous.

Both the *Journal's* circulation and its sponsoring organization's membership also doubled during Rosen's editorship. In 1957 the American Public Health Association had 12,736 active members and fellows; in 1973 there were 25,167. In 1973, the *Journal* reached 5,431 subscribers in addition to the 25,167 APHA members. However, the character of the growth in these latter years was very different from that in the Ravenel years. During the seventeen-year interim between Ravenel and Rosen, four new sections were formed within the Association (School Health, 1942; Dental Health, 1943; Medical Care, 1948; Mental Health, 1955.) In 1957, when Rosen became editor, the theme of the Association's Annual Meeting was: "Is Public Health in Tune with the Times?" 1957 also saw the passing of two giants of the public health movement, Haven Emerson and C.-E.A. Winslow, and of Reginald Atwater, executive secretary of the APHA for 22 of its halcyon years. During the 16 years of Rosen's editorship the Association created seven new sections, one-third of its 21 sections existing in 1973,[5] when more than half its active members were affiliated with sections that had been created since Ravenel's day. The bulk of its membership were no longer from official health agencies. The significance of these developments was clearly perceived and interpreted by Rosen himself in a *Journal* editorial of 1972 entitled "Specialization in Public Health."[6]

After pointing out that H.W. Hill, chairman of the first section (Laboratory) formed within the APHA, had discussed specialization in 1907, the editorial continues:

> Hill's description of specialization in public health and his analysis of its implications related to a relatively early stage in this process. But as he foresaw, specialization would increase and exert a growing influence on the organization of public health. Today, sixty-five years later, it is clear that the continuing specialization of public health is one of the important factors underlying the malaise and disarray which marks it. The centrifugal tendencies inherent in specialization could be effectively controlled as long as the goals of public health were clearly envisaged within an accepted program, and an institutional form was available to encompass the diversity of knowledge and professional identity which emerged with the expansion of public health in the earlier decades of this century. Essentially, this involved the control of bacterial pollution in the environment, the prevention of communicable diseases and conditions produced by defective nutrition, and the achievement of these aims through an official health agency, a local or a state health department, complemented in various ways by voluntary health agencies.
>
> The achievement of these aims to a considerable extent, the emergence of newer health problems, and the consequent change in the scope and focus of public health disrupted the previously existing situation, and left the various groups of public health workers without a generally accepted integrated program or an institutional structure through which it might be put into practice. In this situation centrifugal tendencies of special groups have led to a multiplication of agencies concerned with health problems. Fragmentation which appeared earlier in clinical medicine as a consequence of specialization is now fully apparent in public health. Recognition of this problem has not been lacking, but so far efforts to deal with it have not achieved much success.

Health services administration has emerged as a concept, but more than a concept is needed.

During the *Journal's* early years and extending through Ravenel's editorship, its content was an editorial distillate or selection of what the fellows and members of the American Public Health Association discussed with each other at their annual meetings. In 1940 three-quarters of the articles published by the *Journal* were annual meeting papers, while another fifteen percent were papers presented at the meetings of affiliated societies (regional and state public health associations). Indeed, the Association had ruled that all papers presented at all such meetings belonged to it and could not be submitted or published elsewhere without their express permission.

Thus, it is not surprising to find that in 1940 well over one-half of the principal authors of the papers published by the *Journal* were designated as fellows of APHA. Basically, although the *Journal's* reputation was enhanced, it was primarily an organ for members of the Association (predominately senior members or fellows) to communicate their opinions and experiences to each other. Junior members and outsiders might be allowed to listen and learn, but those who were already members of this privileged group had the advantage. In 1940 most of the authors were employed either by the U.S. Public Health Service or by state and local health departments. The others were likely to work for a voluntary health agency or a school of public health. Eighty-eight percent of the principal authors were men, and 70 percent were sole authors. Besides the laboratory oriented studies, relatively few articles contributed original research findings, and research grants were almost unknown. Most papers described programs and recounted lessons learned from experience in much the same way as had the clinical journals of the previous century.

By 1957 this situation had not changed greatly as the data in Table 1 demonstrate. The research grants program of the Public Health Service had been initiated in 1946, and its impact was beginning to become apparent. More graduate school faculty were contributing papers. Although not shown in the table, most articles continued to be derived from annual meeting papers which were still the property of the Association and screened for possible publication by the officers of each section (specialty) which sponsored the session at which they were presented. Only about ten percent of the content of the Journal was derived from contributed papers. This situation was analagous to that of contemporary state and local medical society journals. Most of the national journals published by medical specialty associations had already divorced the publication of their journal from papers presented at their annual meetings. For the *American Journal of Public Health* this divorce did not occur until 1963 when the Association relinquished its exclusive rights to annual meeting papers. By 1972 half of the published papers were contributed directly to the *Journal* rather than via annual meeting presentation. In 1976 78 percent of the published papers were contributed directly rather than after annual meeting presentation.[7]

Table 1, based on analyses of two three-year periods at the beginning and end of George Rosen's tenure, illustrates the alteration in the character of contributors to the *Journal*. The emergence of the *Journal* as a professional organ open to all contributors is reflected by the drop in fellows from more than half the principal authors to less than a third. In 1972 the Association, in line with the egalitarian trend of the times, abolished the category of fellowship, so that data for comparison are drawn from 1971 only.[8] More women authors, more joint authorship of articles, and more papers emanating from research grants reflect the changing times. Only one out of five principal authors was employed by an official health agency, while graduate school faculty formed the majority of contributors. This change in the distribution of authors' employers may express the publish-or-perish atmosphere of the university, or the harried plight of busy public health practitioners. In any case, the trend was not unique to public health. The shift in authors from practitioner to academician reflects the institutionalization of the research establishment, and the increasing distance between writers and doers throughout the biomedical and social sciences. For epidemiology, often called the basic science of public health, this gap was portrayed by Dr. Milton Terris, a former president of the APHA, in a 1972 *Journal* editorial in the following words:

> Many of the individuals who have been trained in epidemiology in schools of public health during the past decade—and some of their teachers— have never worked in a health department and have no appreciation of the problems involved in community disease control programs. Their attitude to the health officer and the community health organizer is too often like that of the academic physician to the lowly "LMD"; it tends to be arrogant and elitist, and hardly designed to assist in maintaining close ties between epidemiology and public health practice.[9]

Terris went on to describe other aspects of the practitioner-academician schism as it had affected the broad field of public health in recent years:

> Just as this revolution in epidemiology meant an expansion in scope from infectious disease to all disease, so the revolution in public health has created a parallel expansion from health services for infectious disease to health services for all disease. The movement to include medical care organization within the scope of public health was led by individuals with training and experience in public health. But, like the younger group of epidemiologists, the new generation in medical care organization has no such background; it comes directly from the universities or from medical care programs with an almost completely therapeutic orientation. Unfortunately many of these students—and some of their teachers—conceive of public health as part of medical care instead of understanding that medical care is only part of public health.

Terris' reference to the lowly "LMD" was highly apropos. His observations, as well as Rosen's analyses quoted earlier, had their parallel in the concerns of many medical and nursing leaders about the paths which their own professions had followed during the preceding decade or two: specialization and neglect of primary care with the disappearance of family physicians and the enhancement of research and the ivory tower mentality.

Accompanying this technological explosion, a plethora of new medical publications had appeared on the scene. Sir Theodore Fox remarked in 1963 on the occasion of his retirement as Editor of *The Lancet,* "When there were only a few journals the system was relatively efficient, because new information published in any one of them probably reached everyone interested in its subject. But today so much is printed in so many places that mere publication of a fact or an idea does not by any means ensure that it will reach all the people who need it for their practice or research."[10] In the biomedical field there were 712 journals of substance published in the United States in 1957 and still alive in 1973. By 1973, they had been joined by 1,079 more making a total of 1,791.[11]

Between 1957 and 1973 components of the American Public Health Association itself helped launch two new journals, *Medical Care* (1963) and *Health Laboratory Science* (1964), and the Association began publishing its own newspaper, *The Nation's Health* (1971). Numerous new journals touching public health interests appeared in specialty fields such as nutrition, family planning, mental health, etc. Examples of new American journals with broader interests that overlap with public health and which were first published during Rosen's tenure include: *J. Occ. Med.* (1959), *Inquiry* (1963), *Int. J. Health Ed.* (1963), *Health Serv. Research* (1966), *J. Pub. Health Dentistry* (1966), *Social Science & Med.* (1967), *Health Education* (1970), *Int. J. Health Serv.* (1971), *Int. J. Epid.* (1972), *Preventive Med.* (1972).

This explosion of new publications caused Sir Theodore Fox to predict that medical journals would disappear as recorders of research ("recorder" journals) and become what he called "clinical companions" and "newspapers for the profession—journals that inform, interpret, stimulate, criticize, integrate, reform, and even amuse."[12] Sir Theodore's predictions show no signs of materializing, however, either for medicine or for public health. As Franz Inglefinger pointed out in 1977 on the occasion of his retirement as editor of the *New England Journal of Medicine,* "the results of modern research are jet-diffused. It is a rare American investigator who does not know what is going on in his deep but narrow burrow of research long before descriptions . . . have appeared in print. Fox's recorder journal is in fact not obligatory for the brush-fire spread of medical research; rather periodicals of that type serve archival purposes. . . ."[13]

Neither have the well established medical journals become "newspapers" and "clinical companions" during this time. Instead, these roles have been played by frequent new editions of standard text books, by a variety of "give-away" periodicals colorfully produced, and by the marketing of self-supporting subscription journals, medical newsletters, and tape-recorded digests. Many of the "give-aways" and low-cost journals are supported by the pharmaceutical industry and heavily larded with advertising. Other new journals maintain themselves, in part, by charging authors a page fee for the articles published. Some of these new organs are (or attempt to be) newspapers in the true sense, including their format. Others resemble Fox's concept of a "clinical companion," although their contents may sometimes be biased and uncritical. There has been a comparable growth of "clinical companions" for nurses.

Although the APHA launched its own newspaper, *The Nation's Health,* no publications comparable to these "clinical companion" periodicals and tape-recorded casettes have appeared to serve the wide variety of specialists who cluster under the public health umbrella. Perhaps their very mixture and diversity discourages the advertising funds which subsidize so many of the "clinical companions" of the practicing physician and nurse.

In an attempt to discover how the *American Journal of Public Health* fared during the years when journals proliferated and technological advances ran rampant, I classified and counted *Journal* contents (exclusive of editorials, book reviews, regular columns and Association news) at the beginning and end of the Rosen era. The contents of a journal are less easy to categorize and count than the authors of its articles. Nevertheless, in Table 2 they are arranged according to their theme and their character. The arrangement is arbitrary and personal, and the count during the two periods has not been subject to reliability testing. The comparison between 1957–1959 and 1971–1973 shows relatively little change in the distribution of themes. There are somewhat more articles about the health care system in the later period, despite the mushrooming growth of other journals exclusively for medical care. The decline in articles about communicable disease (which may reflect the influence of *Health Laboratory Science* and the conquest of many epidemic diseases) is balanced by a rise in articles on family planning.

There was also relatively little change in the character of the published articles (Table 2), except that the proportion of original research papers rose somewhat to become almost half of the output in 1973. The remainder of the Journal's content might be described as an appropriate "clinical companion" to a public health practitioner, but one cannot be certain. The relative distribution of research and non-research pieces, astonishingly enough, is similar to that estimated by its editor for the *New England Journal of Medicine*.[14]

The quality of published material is even more difficult, if not impossible, to assess. However, it is probable that scholarly overviews of high quality, an important aspect of the "clinical companion", became more and more difficult to secure. As another editor has stated: "It is hard indeed in these days to persuade talented people to take time off from research and administration and writing of grant applications in order to present coherent accounts of the status of important problems. All these conflicting pressures have increased in recent years. . . . A generation ago, contributors delivered their reviews to us more or less on time; there were some delinquents but they were a minority. Today, a writer who is on time is the shining exception."[15]

Professional journals such as the *AJPH* are nourished entirely by the voluntary contribution of material whose publication repays its author only by the prestige it affords. Those most capable of preparing critical overviews of a field already possess such prestige, primarily through their original research or through writing books which return a royalty fee.

A voluntary communal enterprise such as the *American Journal of Public Health,* tends to limit the influence of its editor to the selection and editing process—to choosing and refining from among the offerings presented. As solicitation becomes more frustrating, the limitation becomes more stringent. On the other hand, to balance this limitation, as the choice becomes more discriminating and the published product more readable, so the offerings increase and improve, and the choice becomes less limiting. The process feeds on itself, since published articles and the prestige they accord are the signposts which entice future contributors to submit their manuscripts to a journal.

During the years of Dr. George Rosen's editorship, the source of offerings to the *Journal* expanded far beyond the lists of Association members and the papers presented at public health meetings. The number of submissions increased and the quality of published pieces improved. On his retirement, the years of his editorship were well summarized by his last editorial board chairman, M. Allen Pond:[16]

> When Dr. Rosen became Editor in 1957, he followed a tough act that had been playing for decades. He inherited a show that had been staged at one time or another by such public health stars as Livingston Farrand, Selskar Gunn, Henry Vaughan, Mazÿk Ravenel, Harry Mustard, C.-E.A. Winslow, and Abel Wolman. He also had to contend with the fact that the public health movement was in one of its periods of great and unusual ferment (as it is today). Additionally the Association itself was seriously re-examining its own mission. It was in this difficult context that Dr. Rosen took office. During the ensuing years he has acted with extreme sensitivity, keen historical perspective, and statesmanlike understanding of the aspirations and needs of his wide-ranging audience.

Notes

*Dr. Yankauer is Professor of Community Medicine, U. Mass. Medical School, Worcester, and Editor of the *American Journal of Public Health.*

1.   G. Rosen, "The American Journal of Public Health: Antecedents, Origin and Evaluation," *Am. J. Pub. Health,* 62 (1972), pp. 724–733.

2.   Editorial, "The Nation's Health," *Am. J. Pub. Health,* 61(1971), p. 1.

3. J.A. Ferrell and P.A. Mead, *A History of County Health Organization in the United States, 1908–1933* (Washington, D.C.: G.P.O., 1936 [Public Health Bulletin No. 222]).

4. H. Emerson and M. Luginbuhl, *Local Health Units for the Nation* (New York: Commonwealth Fund, 1945); H. Emerson and M. Luginbuhl, "Twelve Hundred Local Health Departments for the United States," *Am. J. Pub Health*, 35(1945), p. 898.

5. These new sections were Radiological Health (1964), Community Health Planning (1969), Veterinary Public Health (1970), Social Work (1970), New Professionals (1971), Injury Control and Emergency Health (1972), Podiatric Health (1972).

6. G. Rosen, "Specialization in Public Health," *Am. J. Pub. Health*, 62 (1972), pp. 624–625.

7. "The Nation's Health," *Am. J. Pub. Health*, 61 (1971), p. 1.

8. Between 1957 and 1973 an unknown proportion of principal authors were "members" rather than "fellows" of the Association, but the membership category of authors cannot be estimated from available data. In 1976, half of the principal authors were members of the Association and half were non-members.

9. M. Terris, "The Epidemiologic Revolution," *Am. J. Pub. Health*, 62 (1972), pp. 1439–1441.

10. T. Fox, *Crisis in Communication: The Functions and Future of Medical Journals* (London: Athlone Press, 1965).

11. Data made available through the National Library of Medicine computer-based, on-line system SERLINE. M.E. Corning and M.M. Cummings, *Advances in American Medicine: Essays at the Bicentennial*, vol. 2, J.Z. Bowers and E.F. Purcell, eds., (New York: Josiah Macy Foundation, 1976).

12. Fox, *Op. cit.*

13. F.J. Inglefinger, "Shattuck Lecture—The General Medical Journal: for Readers or Repositories?," *New Engl. J. Med.*, 296 (1977), pp. 1258–1264.

14. *Ibid.*

15. J.T. Edsall, "Acceptance Speech" (CBE Meritorious Award, 1977), *Council of Biology Editors Newsletter*, June, 1977.

16. M.A. Pond, "Retirment of our Editor," *Am. J. Pub. Health*, 63 (1973), pp. 1019–1020.

Table 1

Selected Characteristics of Principal Authors and Articles
Published by *The American Journal of Public Health*

	1957–1959 (N: 400)	1971–1973 (N: 580)
Characteristics of Principal Author	%	%
Male	84.9	73.1
Sole Author	61.7	51.1
APHA Fellow	54.5	31.3*
Acknowledged Funding	14.2	36.8
HEW	(5.0)	(23.2)
Other Govt.	(5.4)	(9.1)
Pvt. Foundation	(3.8)	(4.5)
Principal Author's Employer		
HEW	22.1	9.4
State Health Dept.	11.8	4.4
Local Health Dept.	11.0	6.9
Medical School	10.8	19.5
Public Health School	13.8	17.3
Other University	4.4	15.9
Remainder	26.1	26.6

*1971 only (N: 214)

Table 2

Percentage Distribution of Themes and Character of
Articles Published by *The American Journal of Public Health*

	1957–1959 (N: 400)	1971–1973 (N: 580)
Theme		
Health Care[1]	18.1	26.0
Comm. Disease	20.0	6.3
Environment	7.7	7.0
Child Health	8.7	7.2
Mental Health	9.7	10.0
Dental Health	4.3	3.7
Health Education[2]	5.6	6.0
Food & Nutrition	5.6	3.3
Maternal Health[3]	1.5	14.0
Chronic Disease	4.1	5.8
Radiological Health	3.1	3.3
All Other	12.6	7.4
Total	100.0	100.0
Character		
Research	39.2	47.6
Review	22.8	13.5
Progammatic[4]	28.0	24.8
Methodologic	1.8	4.6
Commentary[5]	8.2	9.5
Total	100.0	100.0

[1] Administration, management, planning, evaluating and delivering organized health services.

[2] Health behavior and education to change behavior.

[3] Includes family planning.

[4] Description of program, evaluation, policy analysis.

[5] Not editorials but editorial-like (opinion) pieces.

Dr. George Rosen:
An Appreciation

SAUL BENISON

When George Rosen died on July 27, 1977, in Oxford, England, he left a singular legacy to both history and medicine. While these disciplines on their face are different, they were in his mind inextricably linked. I would like to examine briefly, how this legacy came into being, and to sketch some of its subsequent development and substance.

George Rosen was born to Jewish immigrant parents in Brooklyn, New York, on June 23, 1910. Although his father worked in the shirt waist industry, the family was not poor. Their moderate circumstances were perhaps best attested to by the fact, they had accumulated sufficient substance by 1912 to leave the teeming slums of the lower East Side of Manhatten, for a home amidst the relative comforts of Brooklyn, then widely regarded as a bedroom of New York. The first generation of the sons and daughters of immigrants to the United States, Jew and gentile alike (especially those who later became intellectuals), were endowed with a special vision. They not only acquired the ability to see the particular limitations of their parents' heritage in the New World; they could also see the shortcomings of the society they were born into, and whose life, language, and dreams they came to share. In sum, their vision prepared them to become critics of both the old and new. As critics, many embraced history as a tool and guide to understanding and action. It offered the solace of continuity between past, present, and future, and in their hands it became the sybil who could answer the mysteries of life, the messiah who had the power and understanding to design and build a new society.

New York City, for all of its shortcomings, did, in the early twentieth century, provide an incomparable education for the children of its inhabitants. Dr. Rosen was educated in the primary and secondary schools of the city. Upon graduation from Peter Stuyvesant High School (a school for the specially gifted) in 1926, he entered the College of the City of New York. The College, one of the earliest urban institutions of higher learning in the United States, was a singular school. It exacted no fees, and since each class had but a lim-

242

ited number of places, it chose its students solely on the basis of merit. To be considered, a student needed at least a grade average of 80 percent. However, such was the competition for place, that the real average for entrance, in any one year, was well above 90 percent. The student body, therefore, was selectively bright and competitive. Combined with a distinguished faculty, they created a contentious, probing atmosphere. In this environment Dr. Rosen came of age intellectually.

It is difficult to say when he decided to become a doctor, but when he graduated from college in 1930, however, he had great difficulty in getting into medical school. This difficulty had little to do with his ability—for he was a bright and talented student—rather it lay with the medical schools, many of which at the time embraced a policy of *numerus clausus,* specially designed to restrict the entrance of Jews into the medical profession. Silent, polite, and always proper, this policy of segregation, ended the dreams of a career in medicine for scores of students whose major defect was being Jewish and bright.[1] The ultimate social cost of such a policy has never been estimated. Many of those who were rejected sought their education abroad. In 1930, Dr. Rosen and two companions entered the medical faculties of the University of Berlin.

History has its special ironies. Prejudice ultimately served George Rosen well. First: As a medical student in Berlin, he gained an early understanding of the danger to the human spirit and to life itself, in the then rising tide of Nazism. Second: as a foreigner at the medical school, he was required to learn German, in which he became very proficient and which opened the important literature of scientific and social medicine to him. Third: he fell in love with a fellow student, Beata Caspari, who later married him and became his helpmate. And fourth: he was introduced to the history of medicine.

At that time, the medical faculties of the University of Berlin required that all candidates for the M.D. degree write a thesis. Dr. Paul Diepgen, the German historian of medicine, with whom Dr. Rosen studied suggested that he write to Dr. Henry Sigerist, then the Director of the Institute for the History of Medicine at The Johns Hopkins Medical School, for a thesis topic. Dr. Sigerist urged him to investigate the reception given in Europe to the researches of William Beaumont, the nineteenth-century American physician-physiologist. The thesis, published in German in 1935[2] and in English translation in 1942,[3] not only studied the reception of Beaumont's unique physiological research in Germany, England, and France, it also traced in detail the influence of that work on the subsequent development of gastric physiology and pathology. It is of interest that Dr. Rosen's findings that German, English, and French physicians and scientists reacted differently to the same research data, developed by Beaumont, remained unchanged until 1957 when Dr. F.N.L. Poynter, the distinguished British historian of medicine discovered new data on the reception of Beaumont among English physiologists.[4]

Upon his return to America, Dr. Rosen took an internship at the Beth-El Hospital in Brooklyn and later began medical practice with a specialty in ophthalmology and otolaryngology. Unfortunately, he was not successful as a medical practitioner, in part because he alienated that large group of patients who often come to doctor's offices with nebulous complaints and no real illness. Aware that his practice would not support his growing family, he took a civil service examination for a post in the New York City Department of Health. His grades were the highest achieved in the examination, and in 1941 he joined the Department of Health as a clinic physician in the Bureau of Tuberculosis. Later he became a District Health Officer and ultimately Director of the Bureau of Health Education. His work in public health is important as one of the keys necessary for an understanding of his later historical and sociological investigations. There are other keys as well.

In 1936, following a symposium on the history of industrial and occupational disease, held at the New York Academy of Medicine, Dr. Rosen met Dr. Henry Sigerist in person for the first time. From his arrival in the United States in 1932, Dr. Sigerist became one of the dominant forces in the development of the history of medicine in this country. Although there had been historians of medicine in the United States long before Henry Sigerist, few, however, had shared his singular vision of the tasks of that discipline. His philosophy of the history of medicine was perhaps best expressed in his valedictory address at Johns Hopkins in 1947:

> The history of medicine is both history and medicine. It is one aspect of the history of civilization and a part of the theory of medicine. The historical analysis is a method that can be applied profitably in medicine as in other fields, to clarify concepts, to make trends and developments conscious, so that we may face them openly and may act more intelligently. When you pursue your historical studies into the present, you imperceptibly enter the field of sociology, and begin to see that an infinite number of non-scientific factors, social, economic, political, philo-

sophical, religious, may well determine success or failure of medicine, factors which must be investigated.[5]

Dr. Sigerist's enthusiasm for the history of medicine was infectious, and he found a willing follower in Dr. Rosen. The meeting in 1936 was the beginning not only of a long and fruitful relationship between Sigerist and Rosen, but also between Rosen and the young and happy company of the Institute, including among others, Owsei Temkin, Erwin Ackerknecht, Genevieve Miller, and Ludwig Edelstein. The new relationship bore a rich and immediate fruit. Dr. Rosen's linguistic ability led to translations of Jacob Henle's *On Miasmata and Contagia*[6] and Paracelsus' *On the Miners' Sickness and Other Miners' Diseases,*[7] both of which were published by The Johns Hopkins Press. The introductions which Dr. Rosen provided for these translations, not only placed the works in historical perspective, they also displayed his perception and definition of historical problems as well. Typical was one of his remarks on Henle's seminal essay: "In translating this paper I have attempted to retain the author's style as far as possible. I have done this not only for the purpose of permitting the logical cogency of Henle's reasoning to speak for itself, but also in order that one of the factors which in my opinion militated against the rapid acceptance of the theory might become more apparent." Dr. Rosen found this factor to be terminology and conceptual structure. "The lack of a satisfactory terminology or of concepts with which the investigator can operate," he continued, "can have the effect of retarding or even of bringing to a standstill the most promising advances."[8]

In 1943, Henry Schuman published Dr. Rosen's first major study *A History of Miner's Diseases.*[9] The study undertaken at Dr. Sigerist's suggestion, not only meticulously traced the development of clinical and pathological knowledge of various diseases that afflicted miners, it also correlated the growth of such knowledge with the varying social and economic conditions that contributed to such diseases.

Dr. Rosen did other work worthy of comment during the late 1930's and early 1940's. To supplement his income during this period he often undertook to translate German studies into English. These works were not exclusively medical in content. Many for example, were historical and philosophical studies, among others: Arthur Rosenberg's *Democracy and Socialism,*[10] Fritz Kahn's *Man in Structure and Function,*[11] and Philipp Frank's *Einstein His Life and Times.*[12] Late in 1937, the Ciba Corporation asked Dr. Rosen to edit The *Ciba Symposia,* small booklets in the history of medicine which were distributed free to physicians as a promotional device. Originally Ciba thought that Dr. Rosen would simply translate into English the German version of The *Symposia* published in Switzerland. And the earliest numbers of The *Symposia* published in America were in fact translations. Very quickly, however, Dr. Rosen put his own imprimatur on the American *Symposia.* Between 1938 and 1944 with the assistance of his wife Beata, who served as co-editor, a spate of booklets were turned out monthly covering topics ranging from Salernitan medicine and Arabian pharmacology, to medical education in the United States, and the history of metabolic disease. Some of the numbers were written by Dr. Rosen or by his wife, others by members of the Institute for the History of Medicine, or by physician enthusiasts in the field. Not only were The *Symposia* beautifully written and researched, they were superbly illustrated as well, reflecting Dr. Rosen's deep conviction of the importance of paintings and photographs as historical documents in their own right. The issues edited by Dr. and Mrs. Rosen are prized to this day, and a single year's run will bring from $30 to $50 in the scholarly book market.

Soon after joining the New York City Department of Health, Dr. Rosen, convinced that he needed more formal training in the social sciences, became a graduate student in the sociology department in the Graduate Faculty of Political Science, History, and Philosophy at Columbia University. Here, under the tutelage of Robert Lynd, Robert Merton, and Robert MacIver, he immersed himself in the study of medical sociology. In 1944 he was awarded a doctorate in sociology. His dissertation *The Specialization of Medicine: with particular reference to ophthalmology*[13] was an examination of the social genesis of specialized occupational groups within the medical profession. It was a complex study involving an analysis of the scientific and technological basis of modern medical specialization, of the social forces that either opposed or encouraged the physician to limit his work to a special field, and of the various medical institutions through which the physician carried on his activities. The dissertation proved to be the first of several studies dealing with the professionalization of medicine. In 1946 he published *Fee and Fee Bills,*[14] an examination of the economic aspects of medical practice in nineteenth-century America. Two years later with the aid of his wife, he published *Four Hundred Years of A Doctor's Life,*[15] an anthology largely based on physician autobiographies, which was designed to illuminate various aspects and activities of physician's lives ranging from family history, education, and practice, to marriage, scholarship, scientific investigation, and politics.

The substance and volume of Dr. Rosen's early historical and sociological work is all the more remarkable when one realizes that it was accomplished while he was in practice, working full time in the New York City Department of Health, engaged in graduate studies, and, above all, served in the war as a medical intelligence officer in The Division of Preventive Medicine, Surgeon General's Office, in The European Theatre. This last service was especially satisfying at the war's end, when he served as an interpreter during the interrogation of Nazi generals in London.

In 1946, Dr. Rosen returned to the New York City Health Department and once more immersed himself in public health work, initially as a Health Officer in charge of preparing a Manual of District Health Administration. At the same time he continued formal studies in public health at The School of Public Health at Columbia University. In 1947 he was granted a masters degree in public health and three years later became a Diplomate of The American Board of Preventive Medicine. His growing skill and expertise in public health administration and education was recognized in 1950, when he was appointed Director of The Division of Health Education and Preventive Services, of The Health Insurance Plan of Greater New York. A year later, he joined The School of Public Health and Administrative Medicine at Columbia University as Professor of Public Health Education—a post he held until he went to Yale in 1969.

One of the keys to the success of Dr. Rosen's work in public health was his continuous research in the history and sociology of medicine. History became his tool for dealing with problems in preventive medicine. Indeed, he used it much as the clinician uses the stethoscope or x-ray to examine patients, or the microbiologist uses the microscope in his research. The meaning of history for him was perhaps best expressed in the first editorial he wrote for *The Journal of The History of Medicine and Allied Sciences,* which John Fulton and Henry Schuman helped him to found in 1946, and which he served continuously either as editor or on the editorial board until his death. "History," he wrote,

> is one of the most powerful driving forces in human development. Every situation that man has faced and every problem that he has had to solve have been the product of historical developments and processes. Further-

more, the way in which we act is in large measure determined by the mental image of the past we have created to understand our own society. To be capable of playing a role in our own civilization we must have knowledge of the actions of the past . . . and of the mental struggles, the ideological and philosophical conflicts that preceded that action.[16]

It has often been said that Dr. Rosen was not a teacher until he came to Yale in 1969 as Professor of the History of Medicine. That statement is only true if one defines teacher by institutional affiliation. As editor of *The Journal of the History of Medicine and Allied Sciences* and as editor and member of the editorial board of the *American Journal of Public Health* (from 1948 to 1973), he literally instructed a postwar generation of medical historians and sociologists and thousands of public health workers and physicians in the history and sociology of medicine. He was midwife to the papers of hundreds of aspirants in these disciplines. Between 1946 and his death in 1977, he himself wrote more than 173 papers, some of which later provided the substance of his *History of Public Health*[17] and his *History of Preventive Medicine,*[18] while others were published as anthologies in such volumes as *From Medical Police to Social Medicine*[19] and *Madness in Society.*[20] His work covered myriad phases of medical thought, practice, and care, and he used a variety of devices in his writing to deal with them.

Biographical studies of physicians, for example, were used to inform and analyze a larger number of subjects and problems than their titles might initially suggest. A sketch of Christian Fenger[21] became the vehicle for an exploration of the transmission of European pathological thought and practice to the United States in the last quarter of the nineteenth century. A note on Nicholas Senn[22] became an investigation of the contributions of surgeons to early cancer research. A portrait of Billroth[23] became an analysis of the organization of Prussian Military Medical Service and wound surgery in the mid-nineteenth century. One of the questions that absorbed him during the 1950's and early 1960's was how social and cultural factors determined and defined the mentally ill in various societies during different historical periods. His investigations of this species of human alienation demonstrated the extraordinary unity and continuity between such phenomena as the melancholia of the late middle ages, the witchcraft mania of the sixteenth and seventeenth centuries, the messianic movements of Jews in eighteenth-century Poland, the Ghost Dance Religion of American Plains Indians in the late nineteenth century, and the

Cargo Cults of the South Seas in our own time.[24]

His learning in the history and sociology of medicine was profound. It was also often the bane of younger historians and sociologists who cherished what they believed to be original findings, only to learn that Dr. Rosen had written a paper on the very same subject 20 or 25 years before. Above all he was always concerned with the utility of his research. The past was queried and prodded to inform the present and the future. This concern is nowhere better demonstrated than in his later work in urban history[25] and in particular the questions he posed at the conclusion of his study of the rise and fall of the neighborhood health center movement:

> Analysis of the earlier health center movement raises certain questions about current neighborhood health centers. These too have come into being to provide for the needs of the urban poor, of people who have migrated to the city and who live under circumstances highly adverse to health. These centers clearly fill an immediate need, and no doubt fulfill their purpose better than did the earlier centers. Today they are located in impoverished areas. But what should happen if and when the economic status of the population changes? One aim of the centers is job training, which implies a change in economic conditions. Is it not possible that improved economic circumstances may lead to a change in population, and thus to a loss of health center clientele? Or is there an unexpressed assumption that the poor will always be with us and a separate system is needed for them. Furthermore, should neighborhood centers remain purely local, or should they become part of a larger system of health care toward which we appear to be moving? Should they become a part of a national health insurance system and of a larger health care delivery system? Obviously such questions have no immediate answers, but they do arise from a consideration of the earlier health center movement.[26]

George Rosen has left us a living legacy, one that will grow and develop in the years to come, as young minds use his analyses and findings to address the varied problems facing contemporary medical thought, practice, and care. With the poet Rilke we can say. "Golden thread you are part of the weaving now."

Notes

1. Dr. Julius Axelrod, denied entrance to medical school when he graduated from The College of the City of New York in 1933, became a biochemist. In 1970 he won a Nobel Prize for his work on the role of certain chemicals in the transmission of nerve impulses. Zuckerman, Harriet, *Scientific Elite: Nobel Laureates in the United States* (New York: Free Press, 1977), p. 73.

2. Rosen, George, *Die Aufnahme der Entdeckung William Beaumont's durch die europaische Medizin: Ein Beitrag zur Geschichte der Physiologie im 19. Jahrhundert (Abhandlung zur Geschichte der Medizin und der Naturwissenschaften, Heft 8)* (Berlin: E. Ebering, 1935).

3. Rosen, George, *The Reception of William Beaumont's Discovery in Europe* (New York: Schuman's, 1942).

4. Poynter, F.N.L., "The Reception of William Beaumont's Discovery in England Two Additional Early References," *Journal of the History of Medicine,* 12 (1957), pp. 511–512. *Cf.* Rosen, George. "The Reception of William Beaumont's Discovery. Some Comments on Dr. Poynter's Note," *Journal of the History of Medicine,* 13 (1958), pp. 404–406.

5. Sigerist, Henry, E, "Medical History in the United States: Past-Present-Future: A Valedictory Address," in Felix Marti-Ibanez (editor), *Henry E. Sigerist on the History of Medicine* (New York: MD Publications, 1960), p. 245.

6. Rosen, George (translator), Jacob Henle: *On Miasmata and Contagia* (Baltimore: The Johns Hopkins Press, 1938).

7. Rosen, George, "Paracelsus: On the Miner's Sickness and Other Miner's Diseases," translated from the German with an introduction in: *Four Treatises of Theophrastus von Hohenheim, called Paracelsus,* edited by Henry E. Sigerist (Baltimore: The Johns Hopkins Press, 1941).

8. Rosen, George (translator), Jacob Henle, *op. cit.,* p. 3.

9. Rosen, George, *The History of Miner's Diseases, A Medical and Social Interpretation* (New York: Schuman's, 1943).

10. Rosenberg, Arthur, *Democracy and Socialism, A Contribution to the Political History of the Past 150 Years,* (New York: Alfred A. Knopf, 1939).

11. Kahn, Fritz. *Man in Structure and Function,* 2 vols. (New York: Alfred A. Knopf, 1943).

12. Frank, Philipp, *Einstein, His Life and Times* (New York: Alfred A. Knopf, 1947).

13. Rosen, George, *The Specialization of Medicine* (New York: Froben Press, 1944, reprinted Arno Press, 1972).

14. Rosen, George, *Fee and Fee Bills: Some Economic Aspects of Medical Practice in 19th Century America* (Baltimore: The Johns Hopkins Press, 1946).

15. Rosen, George, with Beata Caspari-Rosen, *400 Years of a Doctor's Life* (New York: Henry Schuman, 1947).

16. Rosen, George, "What is Past is Prologue," *Journal of the History of Medicine,* 1 (1946), p. 3.

17. Rosen, George, *A History of Public Health* (New York: MD Publications, 1958).

18. Rosen, George, *Preventive Medicine in the United States, 1900–1975. Trends and Interpretations* (New York: Science History Publications, 1975).

19. Rosen, George, *From Medical Police to Social Medicine. Essays on the History of Health Care* (New York: Science History Publications, 1974).

20. Rosen, George, *Madness in Society. Chapters in the Historical Sociology of Mental Illness* (Chicago: University of Chicago Press, 1968).

21. Rosen, George, "Christian Fenger, Medical Immigrant," *Bulletin of the History of Medicine,* 48 (1974), pp. 129–145.

22. Rosen, George, "Nicholas Senn's Experimental Work on Cancer Transmissibility," *The American Journal of Surgical Pathology* (1977), pp. 85–87.

23. Rosen, George, "Billroth in 1870," *Surgery,* 72 (1972), pp. 337–344.

24. Rosen, George, "Psychopathology in the Social Process: 1. A Study of the Persecution of Witches in Europe as a Contribution to the Understanding of Mass Delusions and Psychic Epidemics," *Journal of Health and Human Behavior,* 1 (1960), pp. 200–211;

Discussion of Alexander H. Leighton: "Cultures as Causative of Mental Disorders, Causes of Mental Disorders: A Review of Epidemiological Knowledge," 1959, *Milbank Memorial Fund Quarterly* (July, 1961), pp. 471–485;

"Psychopathology in the Social Process. II. Dance Frenzies, Demonic Possession, Revival Movements and Similar so-called Psychic Epidemics. An Interpretation," *Bulletin of the History of Medicine,* 36 (1962) pp. 13–44 (Garrison Lecture);

"Emotion and Sensibility in Ages of Anxiety: A Comparative Historical Review," *American Journal of Psychiatry,* 124 (1967), pp. 79–92 (Benjamin Rush Lecture).

25. "Disease, Debility and Death," in *The Victorian City, Images and Realities,* edited by H. J. Dyos and Michael Wolff, 2 vols. (Routledge and Kegan Paul, London, 1973), vol. II. "Social Variables and Health in an Urban Environment: The Case of the Victorian City," *Clio Medica,* vol. 8: no. 1, (1973), pp. 1–17.

26. Rosen, George, "The First Neighborhood Health Center Movement: Its Rise and Fall," *American Journal of Public Health,* 61 (1971), p. 1637.

George Rosen
Bibliography

Books

Die Aufnahme der Entdeckung William Beaumont's durch die europäische Medizin: Ein Beitrag zur Geschichte der Physiologie im 19. Jahrhundert (Abhandlungen zur Geschichte der Medizin und der Naturwissenschaften, Heft 8). Berlin: E. Ebering, 1935.

The Reception of William Beaumont's Discovery in Europe. New York: Schuman's, 1942.

The History of Miners' Diseases. A Medical and Social Interpretation. New York: Schuman's, 1943.

The Specialization of Medicine. New York: Froben Press, 1944 (Reprinted Arno Press, 1972).

Fees and Fee Bills: Some Economic Aspects of Medical Practice in 19th-Century America. Baltimore: Johns Hopkins Press, 1946.

(With Beate Caspari Rosen) *400 Years of a Doctor's Life.* New York: Henry Schuman, 1947 (German translation: *Ich der Doktor. 400 Jahre aus dem Leben des Arztes.* München, 1956).

A History of Public Health. New York: MD Publications, 1958 (Japanese translation, Tokyo, 1974).

Madness in Society. Chapters in the Historical Sociology of Mental Illness. London: Routledge and Kegan Paul; Chicago: University of Chicago Press, 1968. Also appeared as Harper Torchbook, Harper & Row, 1968. (Spanish translation, 1974).

From Medical Police to Social Medicine. Essays on the History of Health Care. New York: Science History Publications, 1974.

Preventive Medicine in the United States, 1900–1975. Trends and Interpretations. New York: Science History Publications, 1975.

Translations

Jacob Henle. *On Miasmata and Contagia.* Baltimore: The Johns Hopkins Press, 1938.

Fritz Kahn. *Our Sex Life, A Guide and Counselor for Everyone.* New York: Alfred A. Knopf, 1939.

Arthur Rosenberg. *Democracy and Socialism, A Contribution to the Political History of the Past 150 Years.* New York: Alfred A. Knopf, 1939.

Paracelsus. *On the Miners' Sickness and other Miners' Diseases.* In: *Four Treatises of Theophrastus von Hohenheim, called Paracelsus.* Edited by Henry E. Sigerist. Baltimore: The Johns Hopkins Press, 1941.

Fritz Kahn. *Man in Structure and Function* 2 vols. New York: Alfred Knopf, 1943.

Philipp Frank. *Einstein, His Life and Times.* New York: Alfred A. Knopf, 1947.

Articles*

John Elliotson—Physician and Hypnotist," *Bull. Inst. Hist. Med.,* 4:600–603, 1936.

"Carl Ludwig and His American Students," *Bull. Inst. Hist. Med.,* 4:609–650, 1936.

"Social Aspects of Jacob Henle's Medical Thought," *Bull. Inst. Hist. Med.,* 5:509–537, 1937.

"On the Historical Investigation of Occupational Diseases: An Apercu," *Bull. Inst. Hist. Med.,* 5:941–946, 1937.

"Negative Factors in Medical History. A Preliminary Inquiry Into Their Significance for the Dynamics of Medical Progress," *Bull. Inst. Hist. Med.,* 6:1015–1019, 1938.

"A Note on the Reception of the Stethoscope in England," *Bull. Inst. Hist. Med.,* 7:93–94, 1939.

"Claude Bernard's Work on Experimental Pneumoconiosis," *Bull. Hist. Med.,* 7:412–416, 1939.

"Occupational Diseases of English Seamen during the Seventeenth and Eighteenth Centuries," *Bull. Hist. Med.,* 7:751–758, 1939.

"Early Observations on Indian Baths," *Ciba Symposia,* 1:163, 1939.

"Dr. Barter's Cattle Bath," *Ciba Symposia,* 1:164, 1939.

"Trepanation in Cornish Miners," *Ciba Symposia,* 1:197, 1939.

"Remarks on the Doctor's Office in America," *Ciba Symposia,* 1:288–290, 1939.

"A Theory of Medical Historiography," *Bull. Hist. Med.,* 8:655, 1940.

"The Miner's Elbow," *Bull. Hist. Med.,* 8:1249–1251, 1940.

"Some Ancient References to Sexual Abnormalities," *Ciba Symposia,* 2:492, 1940.

"Homosexuality in Primitive Societies," *Ciba Symposia,* 2:495, 1940.

"The Production of the Homunculus," *Ciba Symposia,* 2:495–496, 1940.

"Jacques Gautier D'Agoty (?–1785)," *Ciba Symposia,* 2:496, 1940.

"Sarah Toft and Her Remarkable Confinement," *Ciba Symposia,* 2:496, 1940.

"The Roman Nurse," *Ciba Symposia,* 2:558–559, 1940.

"Taoism," *Ciba Symposia,* 2:622, 1940.

"Chinese Materia Medica," *Ciba Symposia,* 2:622, 1940.

"Alcoholic Beverages in China," *Ciba Symposia,* 2:622, 1940.

"Leeches and Cupping," *Ciba Symposia,* 2:622–623, 1940.

"Jacob Henle and William Farr," *Bull. Hist. Med.,* 9:585–589, 1941.

"Disease and Social Criticism: A Contribution to a Theory of Medical History," *Bull. Hist. Med.,* 10:5–15, 1941.

"Experimental Intersexuality," *Ciba Symposia,* 2:721–722, 1941.

*Book reviews and editorials contributed to various journals have been omitted from this bibliography.

"John Ferriar's 'Advice to the Poor'," *Bull. Hist. Med.,* 11:222–227, 1942.

"Changing Attitudes of the Medical Profession to Specialization," *Bull. Hist. Med.,* 12:-343–354, 1942.

"New York City in the History of American Ophthalmology," *N.Y. State Jour. Med.,* 43:754–758, 1943.

"The Worker's Hand," *Ciba Symposia,* 4:1307–1318, 1942.

"Early Medical Photography," *Ciba Symposia,* 4:1344–1355, 1942.

"Notes on the Reception and Influence of William Beaumont's Discovery," *Bull. Hist. Med.,* 13:631–642, 1943.

"The Medical Aspects of the Controversy Over Factory Conditions in New England, 1840–1850," *Bull. Hist. Med.,* 15:483–497, 1944.

"Left-Wing Puritanism and Science," *Bull. Hist. Med.,* 15:375–380, 1944.

"An Eighteenth Century Plan for a National Health Service," *Bull. Hist. Med.,* 16:-429–436, 1944.

"Medicine in Utopia from the 18th Century to the Present," *Ciba Symposia,* 7:188–200, 1945.

"What is Past, Is Prologue," *Jour. Hist. Med.,* 1:3–5, 1946.

"(With Beate Caspari-Rosen) "Autobiography in Medicine," *Jour. Hist. Med.,* 1:290–299, 1946.

"The Philosophy of Ideology and the Emergence of Modern Medicine in France," *Bull. Hist. Med.,* 20:328–339, 1946.

"Mesmerism and Surgery: A Strange Chapter in the History of Anesthesia," *Jour. Hist. Med.,* 1:527–550, 1946.

L.L. Finke: "On the Different Kinds of Geographies, But Chiefly on Medical Topographies, and How to Compose Them," translated from the German, with an introduction by George Rosen, *Bull. Hist. Med.,* 20:527–538, 1946.

"Janus, 1846–1946," *Jour. Hist. Med.,* 2:5–9, 1947.

"Victor Robinson (1866–1947)," *Jour. Hist. Med.,* 2:117–120, 1947.

"Tribute to a Pioneer," *Physicians Forum Bulletin,* 8:14, 1947.

"Some Recent European Publications Dealing with Paracelsus," *Jour. Hist. Med.,* 2:-537–548, 1947.

"What is Social Medicine? A Genetic Analysis of the Concept," *Bull. Hist. Med.,* 21:-674–733, 1947.

"Dream and Nightmare in Reginald Scot's Discovery of Witchcraft," *Ciba Symposia,* 10:956, 1948.

"Special Medical Societies in the United States after 1860," *Ciba Symposia,* 9:787–790, 1947–1948.

"Approaches to a Concept of Social Medicine. A Historical Survey," *Milbank Memorial Fund Quarterly,* 26:7–21, 1948.

"From Mesmerism to Hypnotism," *Ciba Symposia,* 9:838–844, 1947–1948.

"Two Nineteenth Century Medical Examination Papers," *Victor Robinson Memorial Volume.* New York: Froben Press, 1948. Pp. 343–352.

"Biography of Dr. Johann Peter Frank . . . Written by Himself," translated from the German . . . by George Rosen, *Jour. Hist. Med.,* 3:11–46, 279–314, 1948.

"The Place of History in Medical Education," *Bull. Hist. Med.,* 22:594–627, 1948.

"Society and Medical Care. An Historical Analysis," *McGill Medical Journal,* 17:410–425, 1948.

"Changing Concepts of the Relation of Medicine to Society in the Age of Enlightenment," in *Social Medicine. Its Derivations and Objectives.* New York: Commonwealth Fund, 1949. Pp. 13–29.

"Origins of Medical Specialization," *Ciba Symposia,* 11:1126–1156, 1949.

"Medicine under Hitler," *Bull. N.Y. Acad. Med.,* February, 1949, pp. 125–129.

"The Health Educator's Bookshelf," *A. J. P. H.,* 39:433–442, 1949.

"Five Years in the Practice of a 19th Century New York Physician—Dr. William H. Van Buren," *N. Y. State Jour. Med.,* April 15, 1949, pp. 932–935.

"Osler and Public Health," *N. C. Med. Jour.,* 10:277–279, 1949.

"Osler and Miner's Phthisis," *Jour. Hist. Med.,* 4:259–266, 1949.

"The Idea of Social Medicine in America," *Can. Med. Assoc. Jour.,* 61:316–323, 1949.

"Puritanism and the Orientation of Thomas Sydenham's Medical Thought," *Festschrift zum 80. Geburstag Max Neuburgers.* Vienna: Verlag Wilhelm Maudrich, 1948. Pp. 401–403.

"Levels of Integration in Medical Historiography: A Review," *Jour. Hist. Med.,* 4:460–467, 1949.

"Public Health Problems in New York City During the Nineteenth Century," *N. Y. State Jour. Med.,* January 1, 1950, pp. 73–78.

"The Diaries and Letters of Peter Solomon Townsend, M.D.," *The Academy Bookman,* 3:3–7, 1950.

"William Henry Welch, 1850–1934," *Jour. Hist. Med.,* 5:233–235, 1950.

"Politics and Public Health in New York City (1838–1842)," *Bull. Hist. Med.,* 24:444–461, 1950.

"Facts Do Not Speak for Themselves, or the Importance of Meaning in Medical History" (mimeographed paper prepared for distribution to a society of surgeons), 1950.

"Polydore Vergil—Renaissance Historian of Medicine," *Ciba Symposia,* 11:1377, 1951.

"The Library of the New York Academy of Medicine," *Special Libraries,* 42:86–89, 1951.

"Romantic Medicine: A Problem in Historical Periodization," *Bull. Hist. Med.,* 25:149–158, 1951.

"An American Doctor in Paris in 1828. Selections from the Diary of Peter Solomon Townsend, M.D.," *Jour. Hist. Med.,* 6:64–115, 209–252.

"Multiphasic Screening," *A. J. P. H.,* 41:94–95, 1951.

"The Application of Science to Medicine," *Am. Jour. Pharm. Ed.,* 15:290–307, 1951.

"The New History of Medicine, A Review," *Jour. Hist. Med.,* 6:516–522, 1951.

"The Writing of Medical History," *Ciba Symposia*, 11:1350–1357, 1951.

"History of Medical Education," *Ciba Symposia*, 11:1358–1366, 1951.

"Clear Thinking on Multiple Screening," *A. J. P. H.*, 42:304–305, 1952.

"Political Order and Human Health in Jeffersonian Thought," *Bull. Hist. Med.*, 26: 32–44, 1952.

"A Medical Painting by Toulouse-Lautrec," *Jour. Hist. Med.*, 2:388–389, 1947.

Letter to the Editor (Criticism of the article "Anthropology and its Contribution to Public Health," by G.P. Murdock, *Am. Jour. Pub. Health*, January, 1952), *A. J. P. H.*, 42:443–445, 1952.

"Health Education and Preventive Medicine—'New Horizons in Medical Care'," *A. J. P. H.*, 42:687–693, 1952.

"Operations Research and Public Health," *A. J. P. H.*, 42:1306–1307, 1952.

"Cameralism and the Concept of Medical Police," *Bull. Hist. Med.*, 27:21–42, 1953.

"History of Medical Hypnosis," in *Hypnosis in Modern Medicine*, edited by Jerome C. Schneck. Springfield, Illinois: Charles C. Thomas, 1953. Pp. 3–27.

"Medical Care and Social Policy in Seventeenth Century England," *Bull. N. Y. Acad. Med.*, 29 (2nd ser.): 420–437 (May, 1953).

"Economic and Social Policy in the Development of Public Health. An Essay in Interpretation," *Jour. Hist. Med.*, 8:406–430, 1953.

"Occupational Health Problems of English Painters and Varnishers in 1825," *Br. J. Ind. Med.*, 10:195–199, 1953.

"Charles Turner Thackrah in the Agitation for Factory Reform," *Br. J. Ind. Med.*, 10:-285–287, 1953.

"Leonhard Ludwig Finke and the First Medical Geography," *Science, Medicine and History. Essays on the Evolution of Scientific Thought and Medical Practice Written in Honour of Charles Singer.* Oxford University Press, 1953. Pp. 186–193.

"The Historical Significance of Some Medical References in the *Defensor Pacis* of Marsilius of Padua," *Sudhoffs Archiv für Geschichte der Medizin und der Naturwissenschaften*, 37: 350–356, 1953.

"The Community and the Health Officer—A Working Team," *A. J. P. H.*, 44:14–17, 1954.

"A Conceptual Framework and a Code for the Analysis and Evaluation of Preventive Services in Medical Care," in C.G. Sheps and E.H. Taylor: *Needed Research in Health and Medical Care, A Bio-social Approach.* Chapel Hill: University of North Carolina Press, 1954. Pp. 199–211.

"Acute Communicable Diseases," in *The History and Conquest of Common Diseases* edited by Walter R. Bett. Norman: University of Oklahoma Press, 1954. Pp. 3–70.

"Problems in the Application of Statistical Analysis to Questions of Health: 1700–1880," *Bull. Hist. Med.*, 29:27–45, 1955.

"Metabolism: The Evolution of a Concept," *Jour. Am. Dietetic Assoc.*, 31:861–867, 1955.

"Hospitals, Medical Care and Social Policy in the French Revolution," *Bull. Hist. Med.*, 30:124–149, 1956.

"An Orientation Course in the History of Medicine," *Jour. Med. Ed.* 31:680–683, 1956.

"The Biological Element in Human History," *Medical History,* 1:150–159, 1957.

"The Fate of the Concept of Medical Police, 1780–1890," *Centaurus,* 5:97–113, 1957.

"H.E. Sigerist, Social Historian of Medicine," *Science,* 126:551, 1957.

"Community Health—Yesterday, Today and Tomorrow, A Symposium. Medical Care," *Bull. Med. Lib. Assoc.,* 46:17–32, 1957.

"Purposes and Values of Medical History," in Iago Galdston (editor): *On the Utility of Medical History.* New York: International Universities Press, 1957. Pp. 11–19.

"Haven Emerson, October 19, 1874—May 21, 1957," *A. J. P. H.,* 47:1009–1011, 1957.

"The American Public Health Association (1872–1957)," *Hospital Management,* 85:30–32, 1958.

"The Physician in Health Education," *Health Ed. Jour.,* 16:70–75, 1958.

"Critical Levels in Historical Process, *Jour. Hist. Med.,* 13:179–185, 1958.

"Henry E. Sigerist (1891–1957)," *Isis,* 49:170–171, 1958.

"Trends in American Public Health, from the Colonial Period to the Present," *International Record of Medicine,* 171:507–515, 1958.

"The Reception of William Beaumont's Discovery. Some Comments on Dr. Poynter's Note," *Jour. Hist. Med.,* 13:404–406, 1958.

"Hospital," *Encyclopedia Americana,* Vol. XIV, 1958, pp. 427–433.

"William Hallock Park," *Dictionary of American Biography,* Supplement II, June, 1958, pp. 513–514.

"Health Education for the Later Years," *Gerontological Newsletter,* Vol. V, No. 3, September, 1958.

"Toward a Historical Sociology of Medicine. The Endeavor of Henry E. Sigerist," *Bull. Hist. Med.,* 32:500–516, 1958.

"Provision of Medical Care History, Sociology and Innovation," *Pub. Health Reports,* March, 1959, pp. 199–209.

"Victor Robinson, A Romantic Medical Historian." (First Annual Victor Robinson Lecture in History of Medicine, Temple University School of Medicine). The *Pharos* of Alpha Omega Alpha; separate printing and distribution by Wyeth Laboratories, 1959.

"Social Stress and Mental Disease from the 18th to the Present. Some Origins of Social Psychiatry," *Milbank Memorial Fund Quarterly,* January, 1959, pp. 5–32.

"The Conservation of Energy and the Study of Metabolism," in the *Historical Development of Physiological Thought,* edited by C. McC. Brooks and P.F. Cranefield. New York: Hafner, 1959. Pp. 243–263.

(With Edward Wellin) "A Bookshelf on the Social Sciences and Public Health," *A. J. P. H.,* 49:441–454, 1959.

"Mercantilism and Health Policy in Eighteenth Century French Thought," *Medical History,* 3:259–275, 1959.

"A Healthier World," in *The Nation's Children* (3 vols.). New York: Columbia University Press, 1960. Vol. 1.

"Reflections on Education for Prevention," *Can. Jour. Pub. Health*, January, 1960, pp. 8–13.

(With Odin Anderson) *An Examination of the Concept of Preventive Medicine*, Health Information Research Series 12, New York, 1960.

(With John J. Hanlon and Fred B. Rogers) "A Bookshelf on the History and Philosophy of Public Health," *A. J. P. H.*, 50:445–458, 1960.

"Patterns of Discovery and Control of Mental Illness," *A. J. P. H.*, 50:855–866, 1960.

"Psychopathology in the Social Process: I. A Study of the Persecution of Witches in Europe as a Contribution to the Understanding of Mass Delusions and Psychic Epidemics," *Jour. Health and Human Behavior*, 1:200–211, 1967.

"Health Programs for an Aging Population," in *Handbook of Social Gerontology*, edited by Clark Tibbitts. Chicago: University of Chicago Press, 1960. Pp. 521–548.

"Editorial Viewpoints," *Internat. Record Med.*, 173:437–440, 1960.

"Cross-Cultural and Historical Approaches," *Psychopathology of Aging*, edited by P.H. Hoch and J. Zubin. 1961. Pp. 1–20.

"Discussion of Alexander H. Leighton: Cultures as Causative of Mental Disorders, *Causes of Mental Disorders: A Review of Epidemiological Knowledge*. 1959," *Milbank Memorial Fund Quarterly*, July, 1961, pp. 471–485.

"Man and His Changing Environment. Historical Perspective," *A. J. P. H.*, 51:1013–1017, 1961.

"Some Substantive Limiting Conditions in Communication between Health Officers and Medical Practitioners," *A. J. P. H.*, 51:1805–1816, 1961.

"Evolving Trends in Health Education," *Can. Jour. Pub. Health*, 52:499–506, 1961.

"Psychopathology in the Social Process II. Dance Frenzies, Demonic Possession, Revival Movements and Similar So-called Psychic Epidemics. An Interpretation," *Bull. Hist. Med.*, 36:13–44, 1962 (Garrison Lecture).

"The Why and the How of Sociology in Medical Training," *Arch. Environmental Health*, 4:638–642, 1962.

"Thoughts on Social Science and Public Health." Presented to Health Officers Section, 90th Annual Meeting American Public Health Association, October 18, 1962. Published in *Newsletter* of Health Officers Section, A.P.H.A.

"Purposes and Values of Medical History," *Jour. Albert Einstein Med. Ctr.*, 10:92–97, 1962.

"The Evolution of Social Medicine," in *Handbook of Medical Sociology*, edited by H.E. Freeman, S. Levine, and L.G. Reeder. Englewood Cliffs, N.J.: Prentice Hall, 1963. Pp. 17–61.

"The Hospital: Historical Sociology of a Community Institution," in *The Hospital in Modern Society*, edited by Eliot Freidson. 1963. Pp. 1–36.

"Public Health and Mental Health: Converging Trends and Emerging Issues. Historical Background," in *Mental Health Teaching in Schools of Public Health*. New York: Columbia University School of Public Health & Administrative Medicine, 1961. Pp. 1–75.

"Social Attitudes to Irrationality and Madness in 17th and 18th Century Europe," *Jour. Hist. Med.*, 18:220–240, 1963 (Beaumont Lecture).

"Community Orientation and the Next Stage in Medical Evolution," *Arch. Environmental Health,* December, 1963.

"Medical Care: Health Needs and Resources in the United States," *N. E. Jour. Med.,* 270:81–88, 1964.

"Human Health, Community Life, and the Rediscovery of the Environment," in *Man— His Environment and Health.* Supplement to *A. J. P. H.,* January, 1964, Part II, pp. 1–6.

"The Impact of the Hospital on the Physician, the Patient and the Community," *Hospital Administration,* 9:15–33, 1964.

"The Mentally Ill and the Community in Western and Central Europe during the Late Middle Ages and the Renaissance," *Jour. Hist. Med.,* 19:377–388, 1964.

"The Bacteriological, Immunologic and Chemotherapeutic Period, 1875–1950," *Bull. N.Y. Acad. Med.,* 40:483–494, 1964.

"Plague," *Encyclopedia Americana,* 22:143–146, 1964.

"Patterns of Health Research in the United States 1900–1960," *Bull. Hist. Med.,* 39:-201–219, 1965.

"Noah Webster: Historical Epidemiologist," *Jour. Hist. Med.,* 20:97–114, 1965 (Beaumont Lecture).

"Public Health," *Encyclopedia Americana,* 1965.

"Modes of Feeling and Intellectual Attitudes Toward Medical Problems from the Late Fifteenth to the Seventeenth Centuries, Current Problems in the History of Medicine," *Proceedings XIX International Congress of the History of Medicine.* Basel: 1964; S. Karger, 1966. Pp. 142–154.

"Is Saul also Among the Prophets?" *Gesnerus,* 23:132–146, 1966.

"Harry Friedenwald, M.D., Physician, Bibliophile, Historian," in *The Jews and Medicine,* edited by Harry Friedenwald. KTAV Publishing House, 1967. Pp. IX–XVIII.

"Health is a Community Affair," *A.J.P.H.,* 57:572–583, 1967.

"People, Disease and Emotion: Some Newer Problems for Research in Medical History," *Bull. Hist. Med.,* 41:5–23, 1967.

"Emotion and Sensibility in Ages of Anxiety: A Comparative Historical Review," *Am. Jour. Psychiatry,* 124:79–92, 1967, (Benjamin Rush Lecture).

"Some Notes on Greek and Roman Attitudes Toward the Mentally Ill," in *Medicine, Science and Culture, Historical Essays in Honor of Owsei Temkin,* L. G. Stevenson and R. P. Multhauf (eds.). Baltimore: Johns Hopkins Press, 1968.

"Enthusiasm: A Dark Lanthorn of the Spirit," *Bull. Hist. Med.,* 42, 1968, (Noguchi Lecture).

"Pierre Louis," *International Encyclopedia of the Social Sciences,* Vol. 9, pp. 478–479, 1968.

"Public Health," *International Encyclopedia of the Social Sciences,* Vol. 13, pp. 164–170, 1968.

"Benjamin Rush," *International Encyclopedia of the Social Sciences,* Vol. 13, pp. 588–589, 1968.

"What Medical History Should Be Taught to Medical Students," *Education in the History of Medicine,* edited by John B. Blake. New York: Hafner, 1968. Pp. 19–34.

"The Revolt of Youth. Some Historical Comparisons," *Yale J. Biol. Med.,* 1969, 42,

86–98. Also published in *The Psychopathology of Adolescence*, J. Zubin and A.M. Freedman (eds.). New York: 1970. Pp. 1–14.

"Mental Disorder, Social Deviance and Culture Pattern: Some Methodological Issues," in G. Mora and J. L. Brand (eds;), *Psychiatry and its History. Methodological Problems in Research.* Springfield, Illinois: Charles C. Thomas, 1970. Pp. 172–194.

"William Beaumont," in *Dictionary of Scientific Biography*, Vol.1, Charles C. Gillispie, ed. New York: Charles Scribner's Sons, 1970. Pp. 542–545.

"Sir William Temple and the Therapeutic Use of Moxa for Gout in England," *Bull. Hist. Med.*, 44:31–39, 1970.

"The Medical Library. A Laboratory for Research," *Yale Univ. Lib. Gaz.*, 44:210–213, 1970.

"Medicine as a Function of Society," in *Mainstreams of Medicine*, ed. Lester S. King. Austin, Texas and London: University of Texas Press, 1971. Pp. 26–38.

"Auenbrugger on Suicide," in *Medizingeschichte in unserer Zeit*, ed. Hans-Heinz Eulner, *et al.* Stuttgart: Enke, 1971. Pp. 294–299.

"History in the Study of Suicide," *Psychological Medicine*, 1971.

"The First Neighborhood Health Center Movement: Its Rise and Fall," *A. J. P. H.*, 61:1620–1637, 1971.

"Historical Trends and Future Prospects in Public Health," in *Medical History and Medical Care*, eds. G. Maclachlan and T. McKeown. London: Oxford University Press, 1971. Pp. 59–84.

"Social and Health Problems Are Inseparable," *A. J. P. H.*, 61:2311–2312, 1971.

"The Sociological Section of the American Public Health Association, 1910–1922," *A. J. P. H.*, 61:2515–2517, 1971.

"Changing Attitudes of the Medical Profession to Specialization," *Medical Men and their Work*, eds. Eliot Freidson and Judith Lorber. Chicago and New York: Aldine-Atherton, 1972. Pp. 103–112 (orig. in *Bull. Hist. Med.*, 1942).

"The Committee of One Hundred on National Health and the Campaign for a National Health Department, 1906–1912," *A. J. P. H.*, 62:261–263, 1972.

"Michael M. Davis (November 19, 1879-August 19, 1971): Pioneer in Medical Care," *A. J. P. H.*, 62:321–323, 1972.

"Some Recollections of Wilson G. Smillie. Selected and edited by G. Rosen," *A. J. P. H.*, 62:431–434, 1972.

"Tenements and Typhus in New York City (1840–1875)," *A. J. P. H.*, 62:590–593, 1972.

"The American Journal of Public Health, Origin, Antecedents and Evolution," *A. J. P. H.*, 62:724–733, 1972.

"The Richmond Meeting of the American Public Health Association in 1878," *A. J. P. H.*, 62:880–882, 1972.

"Billroth in 1870," *Surgery*, 72:337–344, 1972.

"Forms of Irrationality in the Eighteenth Century," *Studies in Eighteenth Century Culture*, vol. 2. In *Irrationalism in the Eighteenth Century*, edited by H. Pagliaro. Cleveland: Press of Case Western Reserve University, 1972. Pp. 255–288.

"Psyche and History," *Psychological Medicine,* 2:205–207, 1972.

"Percussion and Nostalgia," *Jour. Hist. Med.,* 27:48–450, 1972.

"Freud and Medicine in Vienna," *Psychological Medicine,* 2:332–344, 1972.

"Social Change and Psychopathology in the Emotional Climate of Millennial Movements," *American Behavioral Scientist,* 16:153–167, 1972.

"Disease, Debility, and Death," in *The Victorian City. Images and Realities,* edited by H.J. Dyos and Michael Wolff, 2 volumes. London: Routledge and Kegan Paul, 1973.

"Health, History and the Social Sciences," *Social Science and Medicine,* Vol. 7, 1973, pp. 233–248.

"Social Variables and Health in an Urban Environment: The Case of the Victorian City," *Clio Medica,* Vol. 8, No. 1, pp. 1–17, 1973.

"A Backward Glance at Noise Pollution," *A.J.P.H.,* 64:514–517, 1974.

"Ellen H. Richards (1842–1911), Sanitary Chemist and Pioneer of Professional Equality for Women in Health Science," *A.J.P.H.,* 64:816–819, 1974.

"Carl Friedrich Wilhelm Ludwig," *Dictionary of Scientific Biography,* Vol. 8, New York: Charles Scribners, 1973. Pp. 540–542.

"Christian Fenger, Medical Immigrant, The Seventeenth Annual Samuel Clark Harvey Lecture in the History of Surgery, February 28, 1972," *Bull. Hist. Med.,* 1974, pp. 129–145.

"Historical Evolution of Primary Prevention," *Bull. N.Y. Acad. Med.,* 51: No. 1, p. 9–26, 1975.

"History [of suicide]," in *A Handbook for the Study of Suicide,* edited by Seymour Perlin. New York: Oxford University Press, 1975. Pp. 3–29 (originally published in *Psychological Medicine,* 1971).

"Medical Care for Urban Workers and the Poor: Two 19th century Programs," *A. J. P. H.,* 65: 299–303, 1975.

"From Frontier Surgeon to Industrial Hygienist: The Strange Career of George M. Kober," *A. J. P. H.,* 65:638–643, 1975.

"The Case of the Consumptive Conductor, or Public Health on a Streetcar: A Centennial Tribute to Alfred F. Hess, M.D.," *A. J. P. H.,* 65:977–978, 1975.

"Nostalgia. A 'Forgotten' Psychological Disorder," *Clio Medica,* 10:28–51, 1975. Also in *Psychological Medicine,* 5:340–354, 1975.

"Health in the City: A Comparative Approach," *Ethics in Science and Medicine,* 2:89–95, 1975.

"Lorenz Heister on Acupuncture: An Eighteenth Century View," *Jour. Hist. Med.,* 30:-386–388, 1975.

"The Efficiency Criterion in Medical Care, 1900–1920: An Early Approach to an Evaluation of Health Service," *Bull. Hist. Med.,* 50:340–354, 1975.

"A Slaughter of Innocents: Aspects of Child Health in the 18th Century City," *Studies in 18th Century Culture,* vol. 5, Madison, Wisconsin: University of Wisconsin Press, 1976. Pp. 293–316.

"Medicine in the American Revolution," *Yale Medicine,* 11:2–7, 1976.

"Benjamin Rush on Health and the American Revolution," *A. J. P. H.,* 66:397–398, 1976.

"John Shaw Billings and The Plan for a Sanitary Survey of the U.S.," *A. J. P. H.,* 66:492–495, 1976.

Library of Congress Cataloging in Publication Data

Main entry under title:

Healing and history.

   Bibliography: p.
   1. Medicine--History--Addresses, essays,
lectures. 2. Social medicine--History--Addresses,
essays, lectures. 3. Rosen, George, 1910-1977
--Addresses, essays, lectures. I. Rosen, George,
1910- 1977 II. Rosenberg, Charles E.
R131.H35   362.1'09   78-12089
ISBN 0-88202-180-X